The Difficult Hair Loss Patient

Ralph M. Trüeb

The Difficult Hair Loss Patient

Guide to Successful Management of Alopecia and Related Conditions

Springer

Ralph M. Trüeb
Dermatologische Praxis & Haarcenter
Wallisellen (Zürich)
Switzerland

ISBN 978-3-319-19700-5 ISBN 978-3-319-19701-2 (eBook)
DOI 10.1007/978-3-319-19701-2

Library of Congress Control Number: 2015946863

Springer Cham Heidelberg New York Dordrecht London

Printed on acid-free paper

Springer International Publishing AG Switzerland is part of Springer Science+Business Media (www.springer.com)

Preface

A physician is not angry at the intemperance of a mad patient,
nor does he take it ill to be railed at by a man in fever.
Just so should a wise man treat all mankind,
as a physician does his patient,
and look upon them only as sick and extravagant.

Lucius Annaeus Seneca (4BC–AD65)

Every physician comes into the situation of having to care for patients who are perceived as difficult because of behavioral or emotional aspects that affect their interrelationship. From experience, few dermatologic complaints carry as much emotional overtones as those related to hair loss.

Difficulties may be traced to the patient, to the physician, or to the underlying dermatologic condition itself. Patient factors include psychiatric disorders, personality disorders, and behavioral traits. Physician factors include overwork, poor communication skills, low level of experience, and discomfort with uncertainty. Finally, some dermatologic conditions may be challenging both in terms of differential diagnosis and effective treatment.

Usually, a detailed patient history, systematic physical examination, pertinent screening blood tests, and a biopsy will establish a specific diagnosis, and once the diagnosis is certain, treatment appropriate for that diagnosis is likely to control the problem. Nevertheless treatment options remain limited, both in terms of indications and efficacy.

Success depends both on comprehension of the underlying pathology and on unpatronizing sympathy from the part of the physician. Ultimately, patients need to be educated about the basics of the hair cycle and the nature of their condition and why considerable patience is required for effective cosmetic recovery. Communication is an important component of patient care. For a successful encounter at an office visit, one needs to be sure that the patient's key concerns have been addressed. Physicians should recognize that alopecia goes well beyond the simple physical aspects of hair loss. Patients' psychological reactions to hair loss are less related to physicians' ratings than to patients' own perceptions. Some patients have difficulties adjusting to hair loss. The best way to alleviate the emotional distress is to eliminate the hair problem that is causing it.

Finally, patients with hypochondriacal, body dysmorphic, somatoform, or personality disorders remain difficult to manage. Therefore, patients should also be assessed carefully for untreated psychopathology, and as indicated, physicians should seek professional care or support from peers. The physician should be careful not to be judgmental or scolding because this may rapidly close down communication.

Treatment success ultimately relies on patient compliance. Rather than being the patient's failure, patient noncompliance results from failure of the physician to ensure confidence and motivation. The influence of the prescribing physician should be kept in mind, since inspiring confidence versus skepticism and fear clearly impacts the outcome of treatment. Sometimes the patient gains therapeutic benefit just from venting concerns in a safe environment with a caring physician.

You could read every textbook available on hair growth and disorders and still not be able to treat hair loss effectively. This book is a thorough guide going beyond the technical aspects of trichology and evidence-based medicine, providing specialists and primary care physicians experienced in the basic management of hair loss with the extra know-how to master the ultimate challenge of the difficult hair loss patient.

Wallisellen, Switzerland Ralph M. Trüeb

Author

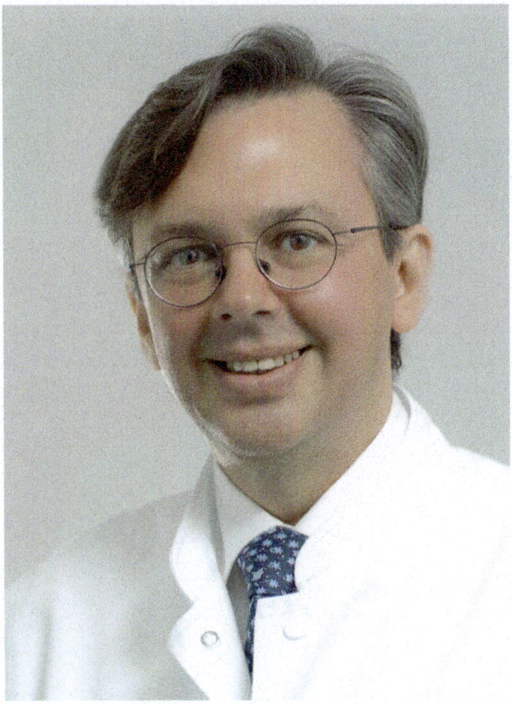

Posteriores enim cogitationes, ut aiunt, sapientiores solent esse
(Second thoughts are best as the proverb says)

Marcus Tullius Cicero, Philippicae (XII, 2)

Ralph M. Trüeb is a Professor of Dermatology. He received his MD and Swiss Board Certification for Dermatology and Venereology as well as for Allergology and Clinical Immunology from the University of Zurich, Switzerland. In 1994-5 he spent a year at the University of Texas Southwestern Medical Center at Dallas with Rick Sontheimer and at the Howard Hughes Medical Institute in Dallas with Bruce Beutler (Nobel Prize Laureate for Medicine, 2011) to complete his Fellowship in Immunodermatology. After 20 years[1] tenure at the Department of Dermatology, University Hospital of Zurich, where he established and was head of the Hair Consultation Clinic, in 2010 he set up a private Center for Dermatology and Hair Diseases in Zurich-Wallisellen. He is past

President of the European Hair Research Society (2008-11) and founding President of the Swiss Skin and Hair Foundation (2011). His clinical research interests focus on hair loss in women, inflammatory phenomena, hair aging and anti-aging, and patient expectation management. He is the author of more than 170 peer-reviewed scientific publications and author or editor of a number of textbooks on hair, including the Springer books Male Alopecia:Guide to Successful Management (2014), Aging Hair (2010), and Hair Growth and Disorders (2008).

Acknowledgment

> *There is something good in all seeming failures. You are not to see that now. Time will reveal it. Be patient.*
>
> Swami Sivananda (1887–1963)

I would like to acknowledge all my difficult hair loss patients, who have challenged me and herewith taught me the most.

Contents

1 Introduction: Defining the Difficult Hair Loss Patient

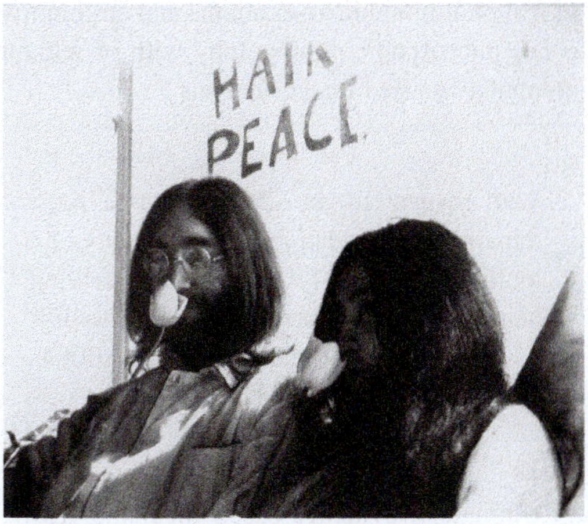

Hair Peace, John Lennon and Yoko Ono, Amsterdam, 1969, B/W photo (by Nico Koster, Center for Dermatology and Hair Diseases Professor Trüeb)

There are three secrets to managing.
The first secret is have patience.
The second is be patient.
And the third most important secret is patience.

Chuck Tanner (1928–2011)

The difficult patient can be defined as one who impedes the clinician's ability to establish a therapeutic relationship. Data from physician surveys suggest that nearly one out of six outpatient visits are considered difficult.

The recent past has seen an increase in study of the difficult patient, with the literature warning against viewing the patient as the only cause of the problem. It suggests, rather, that the clinician–patient relationship constitutes the proper focus for understanding and managing difficult patient encounters. Therefore, communication between clinicians and patients is a key factor in understanding and caring for patients who are perceived to be difficult.

> Probably the most frequent cause for difficult patient encounters are prior negative patient experiences with physicians; others are specific psychopathological disorders related to the somatic complaint that again have to be identified as such.

R.M. Trüeb, *The Difficult Hair Loss Patient: Guide to Successful Management of Alopecia and Related Conditions*, DOI 10.1007/978-3-319-19701-2_1

Prerequisites for a successful management of hair loss are twofold: on the technical and on the psychological level.

On the *technical level*, prerequisites for success are a specific diagnosis, a profound understanding of the underlying pathophysiology, the best available evidence gained from the scientific method for clinical decision making, and regular follow-up of the patient combining standardized global photographic assessments and epiluminiscence microscopic photography with or without computer-assisted image analysis.

With respect to the diagnosis, one must remain open minded for the possibility of a multitude of cause relationships underlying hair loss and therefore also for the possibility of combined treatments and multitargeted approaches to hair loss.

Ultimately, evidence-based medicine (EBM) guidelines do not remove the problem of extrapolation to different populations or longer time frames. Even if several top-quality studies are available, questions always remain about how far, and to which populations, their results may be generalized. Certain groups have been historically under-researched, such as special age groups, ethnic minorities, and people with comorbid conditions, and thus the literature is sparse in areas that do not allow for generalizing. EBM applies to groups of people, but this does not preclude clinicians from using their personal experience in deciding how to treat each patient.

Therefore, good medical practice (GMP) means integrating individual clinical expertise with the best available external evidence from EBM.

On the *psychological level*, for a successful encounter at an office visit, one must be sure that the patient's key concerns have been directly and specifically solicited and addressed: acknowledge the patient's perspective on the hair loss problem, explore the patient's expectations from treatment, and educate the patient into the basics of the hair cycle and why patience is required for effective cosmetic recovery. One must recognize the psychological impact of hair loss.

Physicians should recognize that alopecia goes well beyond the simple physical aspects of hair loss. Patients' psychological reactions to hair loss are less related to physicians' ratings than to patients' own perceptions.

Some patients have difficulties adjusting to hair loss. The best way to alleviate the emotional distress is to eliminate the hair disorder that is causing it. Only a minority of patients suffer from true imaginary hair loss. These have varied underlying mental disorders ranging from overvalued ideas to delusional disorder. In these cases, one must aim at making a specific psychopathological diagnosis.

Communication is an important part of patient care and has a significant impact on the patient's well-being. Successful communication is the main reason for patient satisfaction and treatment success, while failed communication is the main reason for patient dissatisfaction, irrespective of treatment success.

Communication skills require a genuine interest in the problem of hair loss on the technical level and a genuine interest in the patient on the psychological level.

In almost any subject, your passion for the subject will save you. To succeed, you need the qualities that are essential in any endeavor: desire amounting to enthusiasm, persistence to overcome all obstacles, and the self-assurance to believe you will succeed. At the same time, try your best to develop the ability to let your patients feel into your head and heart.

2 Prerequisites for Successful Management of Hair Loss

Try not to become a man of success, but rather try to become a man of value.

Albert Einstein (1879–1955)

As with any medical problem, the patient complaining of hair loss requires a comprehensive medical and drug history, physical examination of the hair and scalp, and appropriate laboratory evaluation to identify the cause. The clinician also has a host of diagnostic techniques that enable classification of the patient's disorder as a shedding disorder or a decreased density disease and documentation of true pathology or only perceived pathology.

> Prerequisite for delivering appropriate patient care is an understanding of the underlying pathologic dynamics of hair loss and a potential multitude of cause relationships. By approaching the hair loss patient in a methodical way, commencing with the simplest and easiest to recognize objects, and ascending step by step to the knowledge of the more complex, an individualized treatment plan can be designed.

It must be borne in mind that hair loss often does not result from a single cause effect, but from a combination of factors that all need to be addressed simultaneously for success. Therefore, it is wise to divide each of the difficulties under examination into as many parts as possible, and as might be necessary for its adequate solution, and finally to make enumerations so complete and reviews so general, so that nothing is omitted that might compromise success. For this purpose it is advisable to design a hair database sheet that enables a complete record of collected data.

2.1 Patient History

History taking is of paramount importance in assessing hair loss. By careful and systematic questioning, it is possible to assess the factors pertinent to differential diagnosis and particular lines of further investigation.

> In the course of history taking, it is advisable never to accept anything for true, neither from the patient nor from the referring physician, which is not clearly recognizable as such, that is to say, carefully to avoid precipitancy and prejudice and to comprise nothing more in one's judgment than what is presented to the mind so clearly and distinctly as to exclude all grounds of doubt.

R.M. Trüeb, *The Difficult Hair Loss Patient: Guide to Successful Management of Alopecia and Related Conditions*, DOI 10.1007/978-3-319-19701-2_2

HAIR DATA BASE SHEET

Patient History

Family History negative ☐ androgenetic alopecia ☐ other: ____________

Personal History

Drug History ____

Hair Cosmetic Procedures negative ☐ positive: ______________________________

Clinical Examination

Hair Loss Pattern androgenetic ☐ diffuse ☐ localized ☐

Scalp Examination ____

Felt Examination ____

Part Width Assessment ____

Hair Pull frontal ____/50 occipital ____/50 lesional ____/50

Hair Feathering normal ☐ pathologic ☐

Trichoscopy

Follicular Patterns peripilar sign ☐ yellow dots ☐ loss of follicular ostia ☐
empty follicles ☐ black dots ☐ follicular keratosis ☐

Vascular/Pigment Patterns vascular ☐ __________ pigment ☐ __________

Hair Shaft Patterns anisotrichosis ☐ other: ____________________

Exogeneous Materials ____

Trichogramm	Frontal	Occipital	Contralateral
Anagen with outer root sheath	____%	____%	____%
Anagen without outer root sheath	____%	____%	____%
Catagen	____%	____%	____%
Telogen	____%	____%	____%
Dystrophic	____%	____%	____%
Broken-off	____%	____%	____%
Miniaturized	____%		

Laboratory Evaluation

Biochemical Investigations ____

Microbiological Studies ____

Scalp Biopsy Specimen ____

Hair Counts

Daily ____

Hair Wash/Modified Wash ____

Final Diagnosis: ____

A detailed family history relating to hair loss is pertinent to the diagnosis of genetic disorders.

While monogenic disorders are usually determined by one gene that has a strong influence on the phenotype, polygenic traits are likely to be determined by a large number of genes that confer variable levels of risk. Moreover, complex polygenic traits usually are not binary in nature, that is, the trait does not exist as one state or the other, such as affected or not affected. More so, the trait presents as a continuous variable that shows a normal distribution across a population. Ultimately, genetic sequence variation is not the only contributing factor that determines the trait. Environmental influences also play a role. It is this synergistic interplay between genes and environment that determines a complex phenotype.

In everyday clinical practice, we are usually dealing with androgenetic alopecia that represents a complex polygenic trait. The genetic involvement is pronounced, and the importance of genes concurs with marked sex-dependent and racial differences in prevalence of androgenetic alopecia. The high frequency of androgenetic alopecia has complicated attempts to establish a mode of inheritance.

As a rule, the risk of premature hair loss usually rises with the frequency and extent of the balding trait within first-degree relatives, while a negative family history does not exclude the diagnosis in a particular individual.

The personal history encompasses on:

- Date of onset of the hair loss problem
- Periodicity of hair loss
- Rate of progression
- Previous investigations and treatments

- Present and past medical history
- Medications, including hormone active treatments (anabolics, oral contraceptives, hormone replacement therapy)

- Associated symptoms relating to the general health status
- Associated symptoms relating to the condition of the scalp

Associated symptoms relating to the condition of the scalp may be:

- Greasiness (seborrhea)
- Dryness (sebostasis)
- Itchiness (pruritus)
- Dandruff
- Burning sensations or hair pain (trichodynia)
- Scratching habit (15 min of scratching will lead to breakage of hair)

Women often blame hair cosmetics for their hair loss, while some men suspect wearing hats or helmets as the culprit.

The fact is that neither washing nor blow drying affects the condition of the hair follicle and therefore has no impact on hair growth. Nevertheless, overaggressive shampooing, toweling, and excessive heat from blow dryers may cause physical damage to the hair shaft resulting in brittle hair.

Unless a headdress is worn tight enough to cause long-standing pressure to the scalp or traction to the hair, wearing a hat does not cause hair to fall. The perception of hair loss in association with the wearing of hats or helmets derives from the fact that male pattern baldness typically starts at an age in which young men become active in the military or in professions with headgears. It represents nothing more than a temporal coincidence.

Frequently, patients claim of hair loss in association with the use of a particular shampoo, typically an anti-dandruff shampoo. This observation is easily explained either through the more intense scrubbing of the head with a special care shampoo causing more telogen hairs to be shed, or the shedding of telogen hairs trapped in scales, once these are effectively removed from the scalp.

Diffuse hair loss due to an inhibition of mitosis associated with long-term use of shampoos containing keratostatic anti-dandruff agents, such as selenium sulfide, has been discussed in the older literature, but remains controversial. However, absence of effects of dimethicone- and non-dimethicone-containing shampoos on hair loss rates has systematically been demonstrated.

With respect to hairstyling, it is rather the particular hairstyle than the styling product, such as gels, pomades, hair sprays, perm solutions, or coloring, that may result in hair loss. Anything causing long-standing traction to the hair, such as tight ponytails, cornrows, or chignons, will lead to focal hair loss, particularly in association with androgenetic alopecia. Ultimately, the use of chemicals and heat as well as braiding is relevant to central centrifugal cicatricial alopecia in black women.

Finally, acute telogen effluvium may be induced by allergic contact dermatitis to hair dyes, particularly to paraphenylenediamine. In these cases, patch testing will reveal the culprit.

For a proper appreciation of the condition of the hair shaft and hair breakage as it relates to hair care and grooming habits, inquiries should be made on:

- Frequency and type of shampooing
- Use of hair care products
- Hairstyling products
- Hair coloring agents
- Hair curling or hair straightening
- Hair grooming habits

The medical history should focus on most frequent causes of hair loss:

- Iron deficiency
- Thyroid disorder
- Lupus erythematosus
- Intake of drugs

Drug-induced hair loss is usually a diffuse non-scarring alopecia that is reversible upon withdrawal of the drug. Only a few drugs, mainly antimitotic agents, regularly cause hair loss, whereas many drugs may be the cause of isolated cases of alopecia. There is a long list of drugs that on occasion have been cited as causing hair loss: all anticoagulant and antithyroid drugs can produce hair loss; some psychotropic drugs are likely to induce a drug-related alopecia; it has been reported that some patients taking lithium developed hair thinning; case reports with tricyclic antidepressants rarely appear in the literature; hair loss is reported secondary to some anticonvulsant agents, mainly valproic acid; among antihypertensive drugs, ACE inhibitors and systemic or topic beta-adrenoceptor antagonists (for treatment of glaucoma) should be considered as possible causes of hair loss; hair loss from nonsteroidal analgesics occurs in a very small percentage of patients; and a few isolated cases have been reported with some hypocholesterolemic or anti-infectious agents.

Regularly, contraceptive pills or hormone replacement therapies with progestogens that possess net androgenic activity, such as norethisterone, levonorgestrel, and tibolone, induce hair loss in genetically predisposed women. It has been proposed that in the presence of a genetic susceptibility, it is the estrogen to androgen ratio that might be responsible for triggering hair loss in women. In the same line is the observation of hair loss induced in the susceptible women by treatment with aromatase inhibitors for breast cancer.

Diagnosis of drug-induced alopecia remains a challenge. The clinical identification of adverse drug reactions has been based largely on subjective criteria.

However, the possible culprit of an adverse drug reaction can systematically be assessed based on the following six variables: previous experience with the drug in the general population, alternative etiological causes (usually androgenetic alopecia or may be caused by the disease that is treated with the drug in question), timing of events, drug levels or evidence of overdose, patient reaction to removal of the suspected drug, and patient reaction to rechallenge.

Finally, a history should be taken of:

- Dietary behavior and alcohol abuse
- UV exposure
- Cigarette smoking
- Sexual risk behavior and drug abuse (syphilis, HIV infection)
- Stressful life events

The quantity and quality of hair are closely related the nutritional state of an individual. Normal supply, uptake, and transport of proteins, calories, trace elements, and vitamins are of fundamental importance in tissues with a high biosynthetic activity such as the hair follicle. Because hair shaft is composed almost entirely of protein, protein component of diet is critical for production of normal healthy hair. The rate of mitosis is sensitive to the calorific value of diet, provided mainly by carbohydrates stored as glycogen in the outer hair root sheath of the follicle. Finally, a sufficient supply of vitamins and trace metals is essential for the biosynthetic and energetic metabolism of the follicle.

In instances of protein and calorie malnutrition, deficiency of essential amino acids, of trace elements, and of vitamins, hair growth and pigmentation may be impaired. In general, malnutrition is due to one or more of following factors: inadequate food intake, food choices that lead to dietary deficiencies, and illness that causes increased nutrient requirements, increased nutrient loss, poor nutrient absorption, or a combination of these factors.

It appears that on a typical Western diet, the hair follicle should have no problem in producing an appropriate hair shaft.

Nevertheless, vitamin and nutritional deficiencies are not uncommonly observed in adolescents feeding on "junk food," people on fad diets, alcoholics, and the chronically ill, and especially common in the elderly population.

As the rest of the skin, the scalp and hair are exposed to noxious environmental factors. While UV radiation (UVR) and cigarette smoking are well appreciated as major factors contributing to extrinsic aging of the skin, their effect on the condition of hair and the natural course of androgenetic alopecia have only later attracted the attention of the medical community.

While the consequences of sustained UVR on unprotected skin are well appreciated, mainly photocarcinogenesis and solar elastosis, the effects of UVR on the evolution of androgenetic alopecia have largely been ignored. However, some clinical and morphological observations, as well as theoretical considerations, suggest that UVR has some negative effect:

Camacho et al. reported a peculiar type of telogen effluvium following sunburn of the scalp after 3 to 4 months with hairstyles that left areas of scalp uncovered during prolonged sun exposure. The clinical features were increased frontovertical hair shedding along with a trichogram that disclosed an increase of telogen hairs and dystrophic hairs. In women the hairs on the frontal region appeared unruly and the frontovertical alopecia showed loss of the frontal hair implantation line.

Ultimately, elastosis is regularly found histopathologically in scalp biopsies, especially in alopecic conditions, but so far has largely been ignored. Up to date, no controlled study has been performed on the degree of scalp elastosis in relation to the pace of development, duration, or grade of androgenetic alopecia, though it would seem to be a good marker for exposure to UVR penetrating the skin.

In 1996, Mosley and Gibbs originally reported a significant relationship between smoking and premature gray hair in both men and women and between smoking and baldness in men. Since the number of alopecia in women was very small, no corresponding calculation could be carried out for hair loss in women.

Eventually, a population-based cross-sectional survey among Asian men 40 years or older showed statistically significant positive associations between moderate or severe androgenetic alopecia and smoking status, current cigarette smoking of 20 cigarettes or more per day, and smoking intensity. The odds ratio of early-onset history for androgenetic alopecia grades increased in a dose–response pattern. Risk for moderate or severe androgenetic increased for family history of first-degree and second-degree relatives, as well as for paternal relatives.

Finally, a history of sexual risk behavior and drug abuse may be relevant with respect to hair loss due to syphilis or HIV infection.

The well-recognized psychological effects of alopecia and our society's veneration of youth and its attributes seem to offer a good opportunity for prevention or cessation of smoking by increasing public awareness of the association between smoking and hair loss.

After decreasing drastically with the availability of penicillin for treatment in the 1940s, rates of syphilis infection have increased since the turn of the millennium, often in combination with human immunodeficiency virus. This has been attributed partly to unsafe sexual practices among men who have sex with men, increased promiscuity, prostitution, and decreasing use of condoms.

The literature on the subject of hair loss due to stressful life events has been more confounding than helpful. The presence of emotional stress is not indisputable proof of its having incited the patient's hair loss. The relationship may also be the inverse. Nevertheless, it has long been recognized that psychosomatic factors play a role in dermatologic conditions. According to the psychosomatic theory, an organ system is vulnerable to psychosomatic ailments when several etiologic factors are operable. These include:

- Emotional factors mediated by the central nervous system
- Intrapsychic processes such as self-concept, identity, or eroticism
- Specific correlations between the emotional drive and the target organ, i.e., social values and standards linked with the organ system
- Constitutional vulnerability of the target organ

Ultimately, the issue of overvalued ideas in relation to the condition of the hair is not always easy to resolve; however, it is important to control stress as a complication of hair loss or fear of hair loss. For this purpose, strong psychological support is essential to help limit patient anxiety, and patients need to be educated about the basics of the hair cycle. Information about the hair cycle can be useful to explain why considerable patience is required for effective cosmetic recovery.

The best way to alleviate the emotional distress caused by hair disease is to eliminate the hair disease that is causing the problem. For a successful encounter at an office visit, one needs to be sure that the patient's key concerns have been directly and specifically solicited and addressed.

2.2 Examination Techniques

The skin and hair are gratifying for diagnosis. One has but to look and recognize, since everything to be named is in full view. Looking would seem to be the simplest of diagnostic skills, and yet its simplicity lures one into neglect. To reach the level of artistry, looking must be a skilful active undertaking. The skill comes in making sense out of what is seen, and it comes in the quest for the underlying cause, once the disorder has been named. The first look is best made without prejudices of former diagnoses and without bias of laboratory data. In many instances a specific diagnosis is made in a fraction of a second if it is a simple matter of recognition. The informed look is the one most practiced by dermatologists; it comes from knowledge, experience, and visual memory.

Where the diagnosis doesn't come from a glance, the diagnostic tests come in, i.e., the dermatological techniques of examination and the laboratory evaluation. Access to the following diagnostic tools and facilities may be required for diagnosis:

- Clinical examination (scalp, complete skin, nails, mucous membranes, pattern recognition)
- Dermatological techniques (black and white felt examination, assessment of hair part width, hair pull, and hair feathering test)
- Dermoscopic examination of hair and scalp (trichoscopy)
- Hair pluck (trichogram)
- Microscopic hair analysis (light and polarization)
- Scalp biopsy for histopathology and immunofluorescence studies
- Wood lamp examination
- Mycology, including KOH preparation and fungal cultures
- Other microbiological services
- Photographic methods (global photographic assessment, phototrichogram)
- Blood test facilities (phlebotomy and laboratory services)
- Access to non-dermatological clinical disciplines
- Effective communication with nonmedical hair professions for referrals

The naked eye is right for the global look, but for close inspection, the additional use of a magnifying glass is practiced. The handheld, single-lens magnifier is the simplest and least expensive, most commonly used by dermatologists, usually at a magnification of 3× to 4×. Although the pathologist lives in a world magnified 100–1000 times, the clinician doesn't benefit from a highly magnified view of the patient, lest he performs dermoscopy (10×) and is knowledgeable of the clinicopathologic correlations.

Dermoscopy is a noninvasive diagnostic tool that permits recognition of morphologic structures not visible to the naked eye. Dermatologists involved in the management of and scalp disorders have discovered dermoscopy to also be useful in their daily clinical practice. Scalp dermoscopy or trichoscopy is not only helpful for the diagnosis of hair and scalp disorders, but it can also give clues about the disease stage and progression.

Studies suggest that the use of dermoscopy in the clinical evaluation of hair and scalp disorders improves diagnostic capability beyond simple clinical inspection and reveals novel features of disease, which may extend our clinical and pathogenetic understanding. Therefore, dermoscopy of hair and scalp (trichoscopy) is gaining popularity in daily clinical practice as a valuable tool in differential diagnosis of hair and scalp disorders. This method allows viewing of the hair and scalp at high magnifications using a simple handheld dermatoscope (Heine Delta 20®, DermoGenius®, DermLite II PRO HR®, or DermLite DL3®), with alcohol as the interface solution. It can be combined with photography and digital imaging (Fig. 2.1).

Using dermoscopy, signature patterns are seen in a range of scalp and hair conditions. Some predominate in certain diseases; others can even help making a diagnosis in clinically uncertain cases.

Ultimately, examination of the scalp by dermoscopy can reassure patients with hair loss that they have received a thorough scalp examination, since patients with hair loss are very distressed and often feel that they are not properly examined.

The trichogram or hair pluck test is a semi-invasive technique for hair analysis on the basis of the hair growth cycle. It involves the forceful plucking of 50–100 hairs with a forceps from specific sites of the scalp and microscopic examination of the hair roots (Fig. 2.2a, b). A major objective of trichogram measurements is to evaluate and count the status of individual hair roots and to establish the ratio of anagen to telogen roots.

Following the original description of the hair growth cycle by anatomist Mildred Trotter (1899–1991), studies on the dynamics of the follicular cycle have largely depended on the microscopic evaluation of plucked hairs with quantitative measuring of the number of individual hair roots. Subsequently, the trichogram technique was developed and standardized to serve as a diagnostic tool for evaluation of hair loss in daily clinical practice. For this purpose it is simple to perform, repeatable, and reasonably reliable under standardized conditions.

Since in 95 % of cases, hair loss is due to a disorder of hair cycling, trichogram measurements serve as a standard method for quantifying the hair in its different growth cycle phases as it relates to the pathologic dynamics underlying the loss of hair. The percentage of hair roots in anagen, catagen, or telogen reflects either synchronization phenomena of the hair cycle or alterations in the duration of the respective growth cycle phases. Finally, the presence of dystrophic hair roots signalizes a massive damage to anagen hair follicles, either by toxins or drugs in higher concentrations, or a severe alopecia areata.

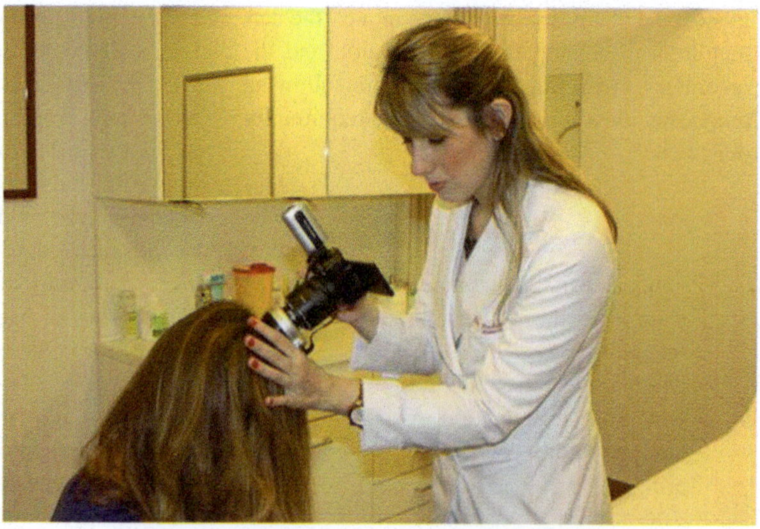

Fig. 2.1 Trichoscopic examination with photography (DermLite Photo®)

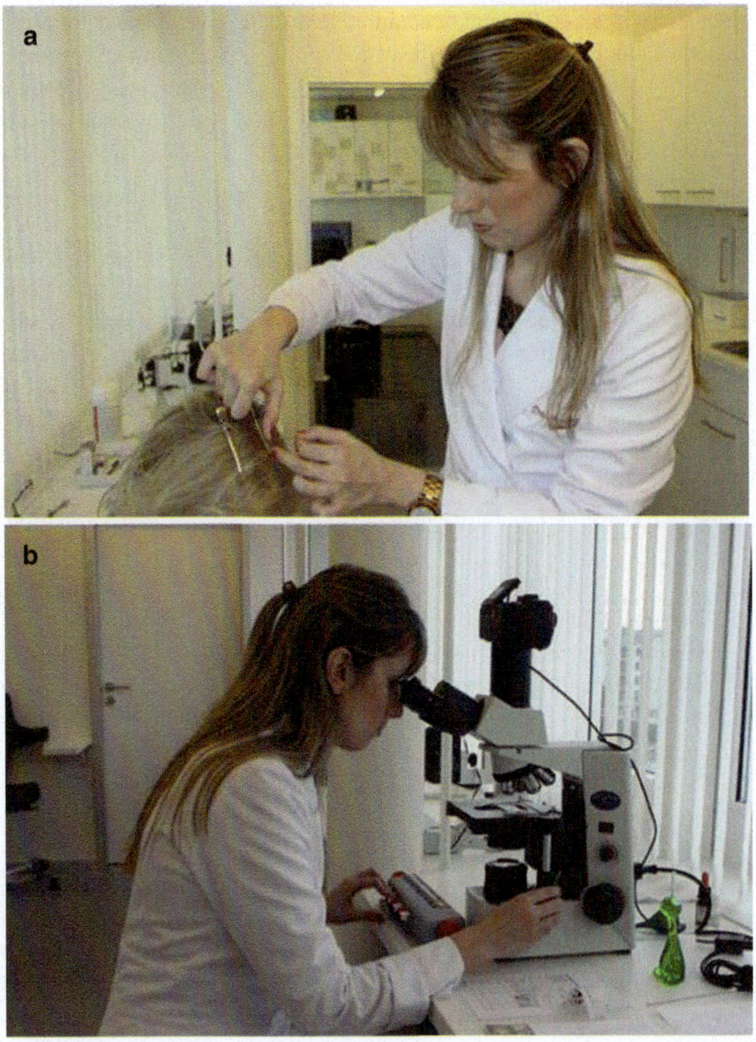

Fig. 2.2 (a) Plucking hair for trichogram. (b) Evaluating plucked hairs by light microscopy

> The trichogram technique provides reliable results under the condition that hair samples are obtained under a standardized procedure.

In case of complaint of hair breakage or a pathologic hair feathering test or if there is a high percentage of broken-off hairs in the trichogram, light microscopic examination of the hair shaft is indicated. In general, the patient with a hair shaft disorder presents with an abnormality or change in hair texture, appearance, manageability (so called unruly hair), or ability to grow long hair. Paramount to the clinical evaluation is to determine whether there is increased fragility or not by performing a hair feathering test. An algorithmic approach to narrow the differential diagnosis is to classify hair shaft disorders into congenital or acquired conditions and in to those with (which consequently give rise to alopecia) and those without increased hair fragility. Finally, a systematic patient history and total clinical examination of the patient with emphasis on the teeth, nails, and sweat glands are needed, especially in the congenital disorders.

Usually, a hair mount and examination of shafts provides important clues to the diagnosis. Using the light microscope and polarization the great majority of congenital or acquired hair shaft disorders can be diagnosed in the office.

Many hair shaft abnormalities can also be recognized by dermoscopy.

Laboratory tests are useful when the probability of a disease being present is neither high nor low, since high degree of clinical certainty overrides the uncertainty of the laboratory data. Clinical suspicion is the determinant, and knowledge of clinical dermatology is the prerequisite for combining medical sense with economic sense in requesting laboratory tests.

The greater the number of different tests done, the greater the risk of getting false positive or irrelevant leads. The possibilities for laboratory errors increase in the automated multiple-screen procedures. Therefore, laboratory testing must be kept sharply focused.

Hair analysis refers to the chemical analysis of a hair sample. Its most widely accepted use is in the fields of forensic toxicology and, increasingly, environmental toxicology. Hair analysis is also used for the detection of recreational drugs, including cocaine, heroin, benzodiazepines, and amphetamines, and detection of the presence of illegal drugs. Chemical hair analysis may prove particularly useful for retrospective purposes when blood and urine are no longer expected to contain a particular contaminant, typically a year or less.

On the other hand, an increasing number of commercial laboratories are committed to providing multielemental hair analyses in which a single test is used to determine values for many minerals simultaneously. This type of analysis used by several alternative medicine fields with the claim that hair analyses can help diagnose a wide variety of health problems and can be used as the basis for prescribing natural chelation therapy, mineral, trace elements, and/or vitamin supplements. However, these uses remain controversial for a number of reasons:

Most commercial hair analysis laboratories have not validated their analytical techniques by checking them against standard reference materials.

Hair mineral content can be affected by exposure to various substances such as shampoos, bleaches, and hair dyes. No analytic technique enables reliable determination of the source of specific levels of elements in hair as bodily or environmental.

The level of certain minerals can be affected by the color, diameter and rate of growth of an individual's hair, the season of the year, the geographic location, and the age and gender of the individual.

Normal ranges of hair minerals have not been defined.

For most elements, no correlation has been established between hair level and other known indicators of nutrition status. It is possible for hair concentration of an element to be high even though deficiency exists in the body, and vice versa.

Microbiological studies are mandatory in inflammatory conditions of the scalp with scaling, crusting, and/or pustulation. While in children fungal infections (tinea capitis) predominate, in the adult, bacterial infection with *Staphylococcus aureus* is the most prominent. Diagnosis of fungal and bacterial skin infections requires swabs and test systems for direct visualization of pathogens (KOH preparation, Gram's stain), cultures and special tests for species identification, and the availability of the appropriate laboratory infrastructure (Fig. 2.3).

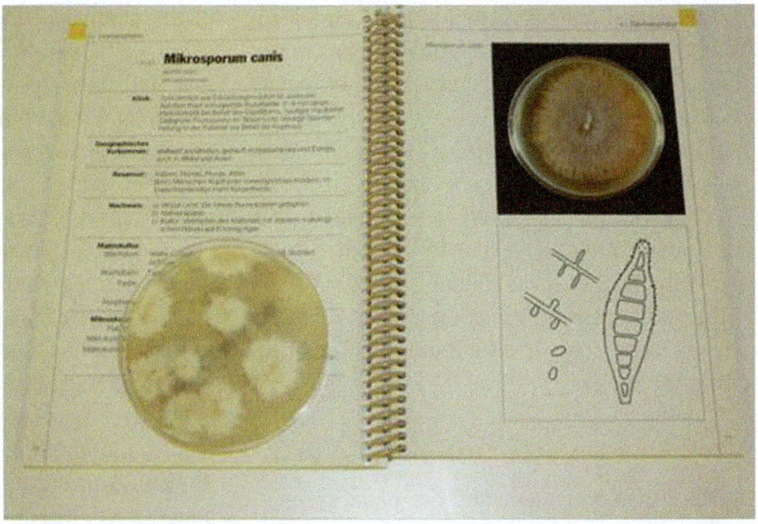

Fig. 2.3 Reading mycological culture: positive dermatophyte culture identified as *Microsporum canis*

At times, repeated microbiological studies are recommended, since with prolonged antibiotic treatments, typically in folliculitis decalvans, new and resistant pathogens may emerge, e.g., Gram-negative folliculitis.

In some cases of alopecia, a diagnosis cannot be made based on results of physical examination, diagnostic hair techniques, and laboratory studies. This is particularly the case in the scarring alopecias. In these cases, a scalp biopsy may provide the specific diagnosis. In addition, it must be kept in mind that two types of alopecia may coexist within the same patient.

In all cases of scarring alopecia, a scalp biopsy is mandatory.

By definition, scarring alopecia is characterized by a visible loss of follicular ostia due to a destruction of the hair follicle on histopathological examination. The biopsy will help to identify the cause and rule out infiltrating malignant disease.

In the non-cicatricial alopecias where the follicular ostia are intact, a scalp biopsy is optional for morphometric studies on transverse sections (hair follicle density, anagen/telogen ratio, terminal/vellus hair ratio) or to detect specific findings for a particular diagnosis, such as trichomalacia in trichotillomania and the peribulbar lymphocytic infiltrate in alopecia areata.

In the inflammatory scarring alopecias with active inflammation, the type of inflammatory infiltrate (lymphocytic, neutrophilic, mixed, granulomatous), the pattern of inflammation, and its relation to the hair follicle usually enable a specific diagnosis. Where active inflammation is missing, an elastin stain will help to identify the scarring process and its pattern.

In a study of 136 scalp biopsies obtained for histopathology and direct immunofluorescence (DIF) studies at the Department of Dermatology, University Hospital of Zurich, a definitive diagnosis was made in 126 of 136 biopsies. In 97 % the definitive diagnosis was made on the basis of histopathology alone. Characteristic DIF patterns for lichen planopilaris and cutaneous lupus erythematosus showed high specificity (98 %) but low sensitivity (34 %) for lichen planopilaris and high specificity (96 %) and sensitivity (76 %) for lupus erythematosus.

The diagnostic yield of DIF studies performed on scalp biopsies is highest when the diagnosis of cutaneous lupus erythematosus is in question.

Frequent problems related to the scalp biopsy are the reluctance of many dermatologists to perform a scalp biopsy and therefore lack of experience with the proper procedure and the lack of familiarity of many pathologists with scalp histopathology. Scalp biopsies are often inadequately performed: superficial (without subcutaneous tissue), small, often tangential to the hair follicle, and with crush artifacts. Finally, the hair follicle and its derangements are complex and dynamic, while a biopsy only gives a momentary snapshot of the pathology.

Nevertheless, if done and examined properly, the scalp biopsy should be an easy, relatively painless, and bloodless procedure that represents an invaluable adjunct for confirming or establishing the diagnosis of a specific type of alopecia, whether scarring or non-scarring.

For an in-depth discussion of the diagnostic techniques, the reader is encouraged to refer to the respective textbooks.

2.3 Quantifying Hair Loss

Reliably assessing the actual shedding of hair is a crucial diagnostic point in trichological practice. To fulfil office requirements, the test should be easy, noninvasive, and not time-consuming. Many methods have been proposed, but all need standardization.

The hair pull represents a poorly sensitive method, while telogen percentage in the trichogram does not correlate with severity of hair loss.

Daily hair counts are done by the patient at home to provide a *quasi* quantitative assessment of the number of hairs shed daily. For this purpose, the patient is instructed to collect all hairs that fall out during the morning grooming, including hairs on the pillow, sink, comb, brush, and shoulders as well as all hairs that come out with the morning shampoo. Placing a piece of nylon netting or gauze over the drain will help secure hairs otherwise lost during washing. The entire morning's collection is placed in a clear, smooth, plastic bag. The date and information on whether the hair has been shampooed or not is written on a label placed on the bag. The patient is also asked to count every hair in the bag and to record the total count on the label as well. Typically, hair collection is done for fourteen consecutive days, and all fourteen bags are brought to the physician's office. It is more practical, to ask patients to collect and count the hairs on the five to seven days prior to the trichogram (daily hair counts) and after washing the hair following the trichogram (hair wash test).

The amount of normal hair shed may vary from 35 to 180 hairs, depending on the amount of scalp hair and seasonal factors. The number is usually higher on the day of shampoo, especially when the hair is not shampooed daily. In diffuse telogen effluvium and anagen effluvium, the number of hairs shed daily is in the 100s, while in androgenetic alopecia, it may well be less than 100.

Therefore, it is not wise to trust in rules of thumb, such as a daily hair count of up to 100 is normal, when evaluating hair loss.

While the daily hair count is a cumbersome procedure, it has been proposed that the wash test is probably the best method to adopt. In the wash test, the patient, five days after the last shampoo, washes the hair in the sink with its drain covered by gauze. The hairs entrapped in the gauze are then counted. In one study assessing hair shedding in children, the wash test proved to be reliable, with a cutoff point of normality close to 11. Wash test values increase with age. Age-dependent normal values in adults do not exist.

In an attempt to find a simple method to evaluate reliably the diagnosis and activity of androgenetic alopecia and telogen effluvium, Guarrera et al. adopted the modified wash test, which accomplishes such a task through the assessment of the number of shed hair and the vellus percentage. The collected hairs after washing are counted and divided into ≤3 cm and ≥5 cm in length. The technique has originally been adapted to differentiate telogen effluvium from female androgenetic alopecia. The test demonstrated that in female androgenetic alopecia, 58.9 % of hair is vellus, whereas in chronic telogen effluvium only 3.5 %.

Eventually, measurement of the effects of treatment needs to be quantified reliably. The method should be more sensitive than the wash test and capable of analyzing relevant parameters of hair growth, which are hair density, hair diameter, hair growth rate, and anagen/telogen ratio. For this purpose, computer-assisted image analysis has been proposed: Some patents have been filed and publications followed since the 1980s. However, it soon became clear that hair is a tricky material for automated computer-assisted image analysis and that numbers might not all be considered as reflecting hair measurements. Physical properties of hair, that is, the object and the variability of the skin, and their background are very complex. The multilayered fiber is composed of a nonpigmented cuticle, a cortex with presence or absence of pigment granules, and a medulla filled with proteinaceous material or air cavities. On top, its organization and orientation at the exit point from the skin must also be taken into account. A follicular unit comprising a number of hair follicles (occasionally up to 5) may exit from a single orifice at the skin surface, and it may be difficult to count individual hair fibers. Some attempts have suggested that use of fully automatic systems may be an option, but this has not been made available to the public.

A software named TrichoScan® combining epiluminescence microscopy with digital image analysis has been proposed and marketed for automated image analysis of scalp hair. This method requires the use of hair dyes for improved detection of less pigmented and thinner hair. Advocates for the method declare that a system must be able to analyze the biological parameters that constitute hair growth, which are (1) hair density (n/cm^2), (2) hair diameter (μm), (3) hair growth rate (mm/day), and (4) anagen/telogen ratio. Intra-class correlation of approximately 91 % within the same operator and an interclass correlation of approximately 97 % for different operators suggested that the method was very precise and reproducible.

Using standardized photographic equipment and calibrated processing for contrast-enhanced phototrichogram (CEPTG) analysis, van Neste established a protocol that was equally sensitive as scalp biopsies for hair detection and growth staging. Taking this as a reference method, a study was performed to evaluate the advantages and limits of TrichoScan® for human hair growth analysis. The study was prompted by a number of variations that were unexpected after considering the original claims for accuracy promoting the TrichoScan® method for hair growth measurement. The investigation did not corroborate these claims. With the available software, numbers were displayed for hair counts (all fibers detected by the software in the target area and those that touched the border of the target area). This number is also split into resting hair (telogen) and those considered growing, that is, in anagen phase of the hair growth cycle. The commercially available software provided to dermatologists and hair clinics originally did not display the thickness of hair fibers and the hair growth rate. Although cumulative thickness may be an indirect way to approach the hair thickness measurement, it provides a global measure that depends on hair cycle duration. Also, it was challenged that TrichoScan® measures growth accurately. First, there are no growth rates on the data display. Second, the precision of anagen hair detection is not optimal. Indeed, the anagen percentage was underestimated (difference >5 %) in two out of four scalp sites as well as in the beard area, but it was overestimated when thinning was more important (overestimation of 32 % anagen hair proportion in the vertex). A number of these errors (especially with thin hair detection) have been described by others using the TrichoScan® method in normal scalp sites, especially a density that was underestimated by 22 % and the lack of detection of thinner hair. As thinning is a phenomenon associated with androgenetic alopecia, published documents and our experimental study clearly documented that especially thin hair counts as well as growth staging generated by the TrichoScan® method may not be considered as reliable. Therefore, it was concluded that TrichoScan® in the present form would not qualify as a test method for quantification of hair loss according to the internal and other standards particularly in patients with androgenetic alopecia.

Ultimately, Guarrera et al. assessed the reliability of TrichoScan® in comparison with the modified wash test. They studied 41 female subjects complaining of hair loss due to androgenetic alopecia or telogen effluvium and compared the results obtained with TrichoScan® versus the modified wash test. The concordance between the clinical diagnosis and that of the modified wash test was found to be fair and that between clinical diagnosis and TrichoScan® fair enough, though less satisfactory. TrichoScan® and the modified wash test were concordant in only 17/41 patients (41 %). The modified wash test proved better in general and especially at detecting telogen effluvium. The authors concluded that clinical observation should be assisted by the modified wash test and dermoscopy, leaving the scalp biopsy for very difficult cases. TrichoScan® proved less useful and may be even misleading in telogen effluvium.

> Computerized methods require further optimization. Ease of use and fast image processing, as pointed out by others, are certainly appreciated. Nevertheless, albeit speed is considered smart in our culture, customers, that is, clinicians, patients, and pharmaceutical or cosmetic companies, deserve the highest standard and a better service than merely a fast one. All should be given the best possible and clinically most relevant information about hair measurements—both qualitatively and quantitatively—that have diagnostic, prognostic, and therapeutic relevance.

Finally, global photographic assessment has successfully been established as a standard method for objectively monitoring hair growth in the course of the finasteride trials in men since 1992. Since its introduction the technique has proven to be essential for follow-up of hair loss patients undergoing long-term treatment in daily clinical practice as well.

For clinical study purposes the method is used in tandem with the phototrichogram technique. While the latter yields a quantitative measure of the hair number (n), hair density (n/cm^2), ratio of anagen to telogen phase hairs (%), hair thickness (μm), and linear hair growth rate (mm/day) within a defined area of the scalp, the former reflects the overall clinical changes in the patient over time in a standardized manner.

> Global photographs can be combined with any other quantitative hair growth method complementing clinical data. For office-based clinical practice, a combination of global photography with trichoscopic examination and photography is recommended.

Global photographs represent head shots taken at short distance from the patient and are therefore different from the close-up photographs used in the phototrichogram technique. For this purpose, the patient's head is positioned in a stereotactic device in which the patient's chin and forehead are fixed and on which a given camera and flash device are mounted, ensuring that the view, magnification, and lighting are the same at consecutive visits, thus enabling precise follow-up of the same scalp area of interest (Fig. 2.4). The stereotactic camera device can be converted

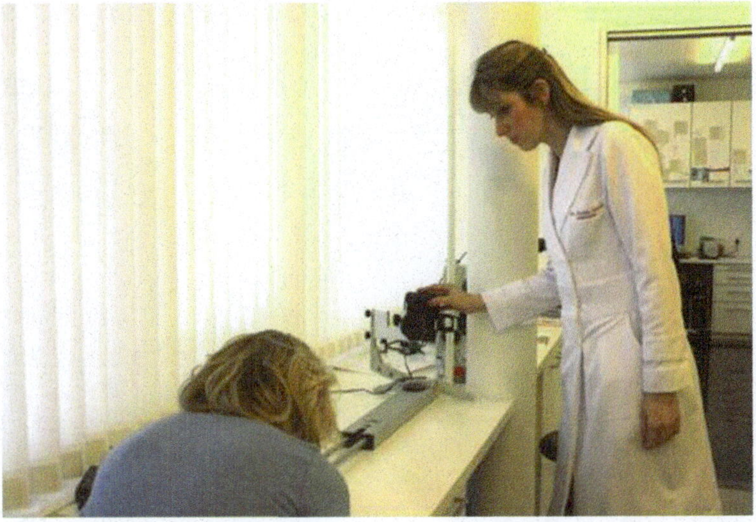

Fig. 2.4 Global photographic assessment using stereotactic device with mounted camera

to the scalp area of interest with frontal and vertex (center of the scalp whorl) views. The original supplier of this kind of equipment is Canfield Scientific.

The length, color, shape, and combing of the hair must remain as constant as possible throughout follow-up. Patients must be informed not to change their hairstyle much, as different hairstyles can change how the hair looks. They should also not use cosmetic treatments like having a perm and coloring or use hair thickening products. Patient's hair should be washed on the morning of photography and no hairstyling products, such as mousse, gel, or spray, should be used. No water should be applied to the hair during hair preparation for the photograph, since this affects the appearance of hair density, especially when the hair is thin. Usually, the hair is neatly parted in the middle.

The result of global photographs is easily falsified, if photographs are taken with different degrees of flash lighting for each photograph. More light reflectance on the skin and hair can give the impression of less hair, while correspondingly less lighting can give the impression of more hair (Fig. 2.5a, b). As a result, photographs taken without fixing the photographic system and maintaining consistency in the way the photographs are taken can look very different and bias the results.

2.4 Communication Skills

Communication is an important part of patient care and has a significant impact on the patient's well-being.

Successful communication is the main reason for patient satisfaction and treatment success, while failed communication is the main reason for patient dissatisfaction, irrespective of treatment success.

Communication skills are not a question of talent. Communication skills can be improved through training and through experience, though traditionally, communication in medical school curricula is incorporated informally as part of rounds and faculty feedback but without a specific focus on skills of communication.

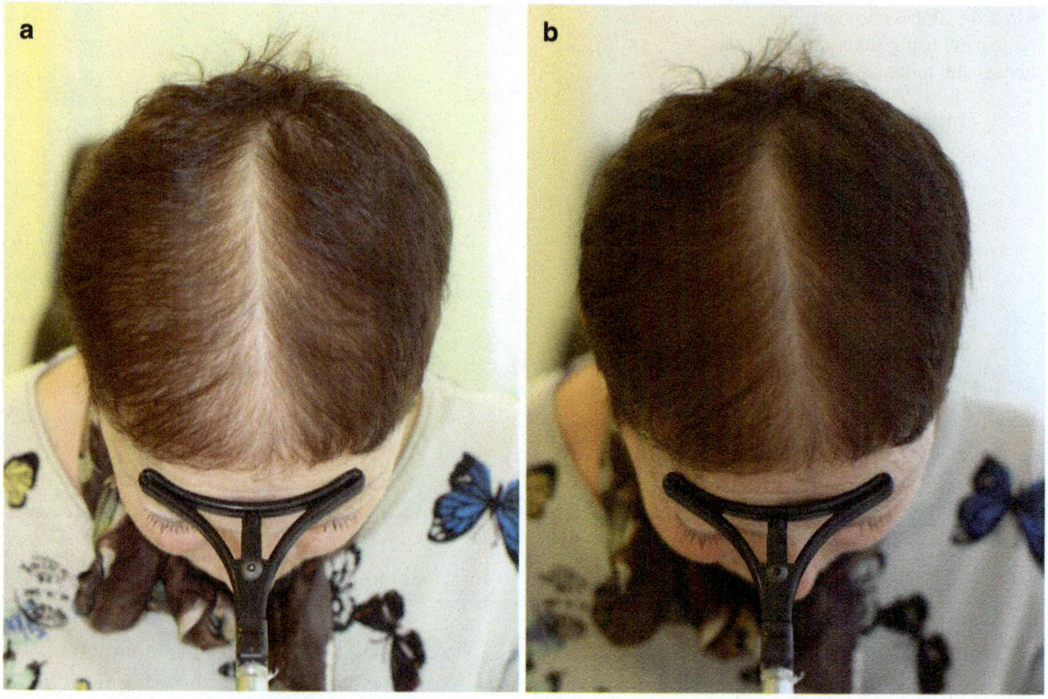

Fig. 2.5 (**a**, **b**) Effect of lighting in global photographic assessment: (**a**) More light reflectance can give the impression of less hair. (**b**) Less lighting can give the impression of more hair

> Communication skills require a genuine interest in the problem of hair loss on the technical level and a genuine interest in the patient on the psychological level.

The motivation for developing patient-centered communication stems from a desire to enhance the quality of patient care, fulfil professional competence requirements, reduce medical errors, and improve health outcomes and patient satisfaction, without significantly prolonging office visits.

The physician attending patients with hair loss faces unique challenges, such as managing complex psychosocial issues associated with the problem of hair loss while upholding high standards of care within the time period allotted to each visit.

The study by Renzi et al. suggests that dermatologists who do not communicate effectively with their patients might not understand how skin disease impacts the patient's daily lives. Moreover, the communication challenges are unique, in that hair loss patients often face frustrations over a condition that usually can be controlled but cannot be cured.

Under time pressure, some physicians tend to rush through the patient encounter without eliciting the full spectrum of concerns and clarifying ambiguous information provided by the patient.

> Nevertheless, patient-centered communication adds minimal timc to officc visits while leading to increased efficiency.

Communication with the patient has to include:

- Listening to the patient
- Understanding the patient
- Informing the patient on diagnostic procedures, diagnosis, therapeutic considerations, and prognosis
- Convincing the patient
- Giving the patient hope
- Leading the patient to take personal responsibility
- Jointly rejoicing over therapeutic progress

Avoid:

- Precipitance/hecticness
- Personal dominant behavior
- Stereotype prejudices

Do:

- Take time to review a patient's chart and prepare to pay attention before entering the examination room.
- Sitting instead of standing is an appropriate way to convey full attention to the patient.
- Ensure that the patient does not feel ignored while you interface with health information technology. Maintain eye contact, verbalize your actions, and try to engage the patient as much as possible. Increase physician–patient interactions by engaging patients in relevant parts of the computer screen.
- Don't interrupt the patient's initial statement. A landmark study found that, on average, patients are interrupted after 18 s. Once interrupted, patients almost never raise additional concerns. Another study revealed that if the patient is allowed to finish the initial statement of concerns, the visit is only prolonged by 6 s.
- Encourage patients to provide more information about their ideas and feelings. The biggest challenge at this moment is to take the time to listen to the answer received. Use *reflective listening* (the act of repeating what you have heard) to verify information provided by the patient and to show that you have been actively listening.
- General principles of a patient-centered approach to communication encourage understanding the patient's story while guiding the interview through the traditionally taught process of diagnostic reasoning.
- Finally, studies have indicated that patient satisfaction with an office visit is increased when there is a brief period of informal nonmedical conversation. That is a way the physician can show that the patient is a person and not only a medical case.
- The closing phase of a visit provides an opportunity to make sure that all patient concerns have been elicited. This can be accomplished by asking: "What other questions do you have?" giving the patient the possibility to voice any remaining issues.

Communication in special situations:

- If the patient becomes *angry*, acknowledge this feeling and explore its cause before attempting to defend your own position.
- If the patient shows *disappointment*, say something like "I wish things were different" to create an alliance.
- *Unrealistic expectations* can frustrate both patients and physicians. Listen first and find out exactly how much patients already know about their condition, and then fill in the appropriate knowledge in the gaps. Provide

patients with an approximate timeline describing when to expect what therapeutic effects. Although most patients are hopeful for a cure, the merits of disease control can still appeal to those receiving appropriate counseling.

tion, and help him make accurate sense of it. Provide or direct the patient to the information he is seeking.

From: Stone MS, Bronkesh SJ, Gerbarg ZB, Wood SD. Improving Patient Compliance. Strategic Medicine, January 1998.

Communication skills are prerequisites for patient confidence and motivation, which are at the heart of patient compliance and treatment success. Based on health communication research, four steps have been suggested to help establish the right conditions for patient adherence to treatment:

1. *Begin from the patient's perspective*: Use the patient's story as the starting place. Listen for the patient's meanings, language, and values as he tells his story. Use the patient's language as much as possible. Translate biomedical terms into terms the patient understands.
2. *Include feelings in the discussion*: Ask the patient how he feels about his situation. Actively listen, using the patient's terms to reflect on what he is saying. Show the patient you care by expressing your feelings about his progress, problems, etc.
3. *Base treatment goals on the patient's values*: Ask the patient how much he prefers to participate in medical decision making. Allow the patient to participate to the extent that he is willing. Guide the patient to set goals, establish steps she is willing to take, and identify barriers to self-care based on his own needs and values.
4. *Support patient learning*: Ask the patient what other sources he has consulted for information about his condi-

The difference between the terms compliance and adherence is not just semantic; it is at the heart of the physician's relationship with patients: while compliance implies an involuntary act of submission to authority, the physician needs to influence patients to become and remain adherents of good self-care. To do this, three key conditions need to be established in the communication with patients—shared values, shared language, and mutual respect.

The following open-ended questions, developed by the Bayer Institute for Health Care Communications, can help gain the patient's adherence under various circumstances:

To clarify the patient's expectations and meanings:
"What were you hoping I would be able to do for you today?"
"You have quite a bit of experience with doctors, what works best for you?"
"Why did you come to see me at this time?"

To clarify what you need from the patient:
"I'd like to be your doctor and to help you with this problem/condition. For me to be effective, though, I'm going to need your help. Would you be willing to []?"

To acknowledge differences in values or points of view:
"I find it difficult to proceed knowing that you have a different view of the situation than I do."

"I'm wondering if we are working together as well as we might be able to."

To encourage problem solving:

"I want to solve this problem we seem to be having. My thoughts about the situation are []. What are your thoughts?"

"Is there something that I can do at this point to help us work together more effectively?"

To express empathy:

"That must be very difficult for you. I'm sorry."

To acknowledge the patient's difficulty:

"This appears to be difficult for you to talk about. Is there some way I can make it easier?"

"I understand that you are scared at the thought of surgery. Let's talk more about it."

To agree on a diagnosis:

"I've arrived at one explanation of what the difficulty is. [Provide the explanation.] How does that fit in with what you have been thinking?"

2.5 Avoiding Mental Traps

"Learning is the only thing the mind never exhausts, never fears, and never regrets" said universal genius Leonardo da Vinci (1452–1519). Dr. Melanie Macpherson from Lima, Peru, did a trichology traineeship at the Center for Dermatology and Hair Diseases from November 1 through 28, 2014, and upon my invitation to make a testimonial, she provided me with the above quote of Leonardo da Vinci and her personal interpretation putting the prerequisites to successful trichological practice in a nutshell: "Exhaustion is not admitted when you are committed and passionate for what you do. Fear only ignorance and the lack of ability to keep learning new things. When the right choice is made, even if the outcome is not what you expected, do not regret it, but keep an open mind for new possibilities" (www.derma-haarcenter.ch/news).

Regardless of a systematic patient history and examination techniques, there remain some subtle mental traps that may lead physicians astray, leading to misdiagnosis.

Different doctors have different styles of practice, and different approaches to problems, but all are susceptible to the same types of mistaking in their thinking.

In his publication "How Doctors Think" (2007), Jerome Groopman, from Harvard Medical School, focuses on the thinking errors in medicine that make up for an estimated 80 % of medical mistakes, while only 20 % are due to technical mishaps. Snap judgment, stereotypical thinking, premature conclusion, and herd instinct are only a few of the subtle traps that dangerously narrow the vision of the physician.

William Osler (Canadian physician, 1849–1919) said "If you listen to the patient, he is telling you the diagnosis." How a doctor asks questions and responds to his patient's emotions are key to patient activation and engagement. The way a doctor poses his questions, gives the patient the feeling that the doctor is really interested in hearing what he has to say, and structures the patient's answers. But doctors, like everyone else, run the risk of being led astray by stereotypes that are based on an individual's appearance, emotional state, or circumstances. Most of us especially dislike patients whom we stereotype as neurotic and anxious. These patients pose one of the greatest challenges to even the most caring among physicians. Moreover, these patients often relate their story in a scattershot way and make it difficult for the doctor to focus his mind.

Doctors who dislike their patients regularly cut them short during the recitation of symptoms and complaints and prefer to fix on a convenient diagnosis and treatment.

This skewing of the physician's thinking potentially leads to poor care. For the worse, patients who pick up on the physician's negativity rarely understand its effect on their medical care and seldom change doctors because of it. Groopman describes this kind of "attribution error" in the case of a nervous young woman who kept losing weight even when prescribed a high-calorie diet. Her doctors, convinced that she was double-dealing about her food intake, attributed her symptoms to suspected anorexia or bulimia, while in fact her problem turned out to be celiac disease, diagnosed only after years of ill health.

This type of error is frequently made in women with a full head of hair complaining of hair loss that is attributed to imaginary hair loss, while in fact the underlying problem is (usually) initial female pattern hair loss.

The statement "Nothing is wrong with you" is dangerous on two accounts: first, it denies the fallibility of all physicians and, second, it splits the mind from the body.

Studies show that while it usually takes twenty to thirty minutes in a didactic exercise for the senior doctor and students to arrive at a working diagnosis, an expert clinician typically forms a notion of what is wrong with the patient within twenty seconds. In "representative error" the doctor's thinking is guided by a prototype, so he fails to consider possibilities that contradict the prototype.

Physicians should caution themselves to be not so ready to match a patient's complaints against their mental templates or clinical prototypes.

"We all tend to be influenced by the last experience we had or something that made a deep impression on us," Groopman states. So if it's winter and you have just seen a series of patients with the flu, the next patient to show up with muscle aches and a fever is most likely to be diagnosed to have the flu, while in a fact it could also be a reaction to a tetanus shot that was forgotten to be mentioned.

Typical trichological examples would be postoperative pressure alopecia and temporary radiation-induced epilation following neuroradiologically guided embolization procedure mistaken for alopecia areata on the basis of clinical and dermoscopic findings, while just asking into the patient's history prior to the hair loss would reveal the underlying cause relationship.

Patient templates may serve as a solution to organizing clinical information. But templates, as well as clinical algorithm, are based on a typical patient with a typical condition. Clinical algorithms may be useful for the average diagnosis and treatment, but they fail when a doctor needs to think outside of their boxes, when symptoms are vague, multiple, or confusing, and when test results are inconclusive. This type of error is also called "vertical line failure."

Algorithms discourage physicians from thinking independently and with creativity.

Doctors who turn down their own thinking on the authority of classification schemes and algorithms have a statistic way of looking at people. But, statistics embody averages, not individuals. Numbers can only complement a physician's personal experience. Sometimes "lateral thinking" that breaks out of the ordinary is vital. Creativity and imagination, rather than adherence to the obvious, are needed in a situation where the data and clinical findings do not all fit neatly together.

"Common things are common" is another cliché. Doctors who "hunt zebras" are often ridiculed by their peers for being obsessed with the esoteric while ignoring the mainstream.

This type of thinking could delay the diagnosis of pemphigus foliaceus or Langerhans cell histiocytosis with seborrheic dermatitis-like clinical presentation on the scalp.

Much has been made of the power of intuition, but relying on intuition alone again has its perils. Clinical intuition is a complex sense that becomes refined over years of practice, and most important, remembering when you were wrong.

> Expertise is largely acquired not only by sustained practice but also by receiving feedback that helps you understand prior technical errors and misguided decisions.

There are aspects to human biology and physiology that just aren't predictable. Doctors, like everyone else, display certain psychological characteristics in the face of uncertainty. There is the overconfident mind-set: people convince themselves they are right because they usually are. But biology, particularly human biology, is inherently variable. One would think that primary care physicians, such as general practitioners, grapple most with uncertainty. The truth is that specialization in medicine often confers a false sense of certainty.

When physicians shift from a theoretical discussion of medicine to its practical application, they do not acknowledge the uncertainty inherent in what they do.

> The denial of uncertainty, the inclination to substitute certainty for uncertainty, is one of the most remarkable human psychological traits. It is both adaptive and maladaptive and therefore guides and risks to misguide.

Physician's denial of awareness of uncertainty serves similar purposes: it makes matters seem clearer, more understandable, and more certain than they really are; ultimately it aims at making action possible.

> Another defense against uncertainty is the culture of conformity and orthodoxy.

Nor are doctors taught to keep an open mind. In both, doctors are educated for dogmatic certainty, for adopting one school of thought or the other.

A typical example is the two schools relating to hair growth in women and ferritin levels: while one school maintains that ferritin levels >70 μg/L ("Rushtonians") are necessary for hair growth, the other claims that levels of 20 μg/L ("Sinclairians") are sufficient.

When queried by patients, some physicians will be uneasy, others even angry, because they may not provide all the answers. Latin and Greek terms may take on unwarranted authority. On the bottom line, the kind of response illuminates how much the doctor really knows.

> Arrogance is a product of narrow vision and ignorance.

The perfect is the enemy of the good. Nothing we do is perfect. Everything is a compromise. In some ways, we are victims of our own success. Some doctors hardly examine patients or take histories anymore.

Ultimately, taking uncertainty into account can enhance a physician's therapeutic effectiveness, because it demonstrates his honesty, his willingness to be more engaged with his patients, and his commitment to the reality of the situation rather than resorting to evasion, half-truth, and even lies. And it makes it easier for the doctor to change course if the first strategy fails, to keep trying.

> Uncertainty sometimes is essential for success.

Thinking is inseparable from acting. Inaction is not what is expected from a physician nor what a physician expects from himself. Doctors typically prefer to act even when in doubt about the nature of the problem. Groopman named this type of error "commission bias." The tendency toward action rather than nonaction again is more likely to happen with a doctor who is overconfident, whose ego is inflated, but it can also occur when a physician is desperate and gives to the urge to "do something," often sparked by pressure from the patient. "Don't just do something. Stand there," one of Groopman's mentors told him years earlier when he was uncertain of a diagnosis. This buys a doctor time to think.

A typical example is the frequent practice of indiscriminately prescribing topical minoxidil solution to a female patient complaining of hair loss and suffering of chronic telogen effluvium in the absence of evidence of female pattern hair loss.

Observation and analysis vary widely among doctors. "Search satisficing" is the tendency to stop searching for a diagnosis once you find something.

> Finding something may be satisfactory, but not finding everything is suboptimal. It is a natural cognitive tendency to stop searching, and therefore stop thinking, when one makes a significant finding.

Doctors are taught at medical school and in residency to be parsimonious in their thinking, to apply Ockham's razor (William of Ockham, English Franciscan friar and philosopher, 1287–1347), and to seek one answer to a patient's complaints. Usually this turns out to bet the correct approach, but not always. The question about multiple causes for a given problem should trigger the doctor to cast a wider net.

A typical example of this error is reducing the treatment of hair loss to iron supplementation in a female with iron deficiency who at the same time is suffering from female androgenetic alopecia and is on an oral contraceptive with proandrogenic action.

We value highly information that fulfils our desires and fail by confirming what we expect to find by selectively accepting or ignoring information.

> The true expert, though, having learned about bias and search satisfaction, consciously tries to keep his mind open so that he sees beyond his preconceptions.

Many doctors have deep feelings of failure when dealing with diseases that resist their therapy. In such cases they become frustrated, because their work seems in vain. So they stop trying. It requires a level of self-awareness by the doctor about his own feelings.

> If you are taking care of someone and he is not getting better, then you have to think of a new way to treat him, not just keep giving him the same therapy. You also have to wonder whether you are missing something.

Given the difficulties in perception and cognition, could computer-aided diagnostic systems replace the specialist? The power of technology, particularly computer based, may shake the confidence of a specialist in his initial diagnosis. Nevertheless, machines cannot replace the doctor's mind, his thinking about what he sees and what he does not see. Ultimately, while modern medicine is aided by a dazzling array of technologies, language is still the bedrock of clinical practice.

> Attention to language can make perception and analysis better.

Just as a clinician needs to choose his words carefully in communicating with patients, he must tailor the language of his request to the lab. If the physician doesn't give us a full history, just the one question in his mind, then he will technically tailor the exam to that one question and risk missing something else that is important.

Many dermatologists don't read a histopathologist's description of observations on scalp biopsies, but want a diagnosis. Typically, androgenetic alopecia with histological evidence of follicular microinflammation and fibrosis is erroneously diagnosed by the histopathologist as lichen planopilaris or folliculitis necrotica as folliculitis decalvans.

> There is great pressure on us to come to a conclusion, and we have to resist that, because sometimes you can't make an exact diagnosis. The best you can do is to describe what you see.

Complicating things is that in medical terminology, sometimes different terms mean different things to different doctors or a single term can guide thinking in different directions.

A typical example is the concept of central centrifugal cicatricial alopecia. The condition with its predilection for female African-Americans represents a USA-specific perspective of Degos' pseudopeladic state due to peculiarities of African-American hair anatomy and hair grooming habits. French dermatologist Robert Degos (1904–1987) defined the pseudopeladic state as the nonspecific end stage of a variety of different types of primary and secondary cicatricial alopecias. Also, it should not be confused with classical pseudopelade of Brocq.

> At length, the way a physician phrases his recommendations can powerfully sway a patient's choice.

There is nothing in biology and medicine that is so complicated that, if explained in clear and simple language, cannot be understood by any layperson. Patients frequently become preoccupied with side effects when they are reluctant to undergo treatment, and some doctors also overestimate side effects. Paradoxically, people are more likely to worry about the well-defined side effects of a therapy than about the uncertainty and seemingly boundless suffering from an illness.

> You have to deal with the problem at hand. Patients must adopt a broad perspective, the long view, not a vision narrowed by fear. The real concern should be the underlying medical condition, but that is often displaced in the patient's mind by fear of the treatment.

The physician's role is to help the patient figure out what he really wants and then to use the power of persuasion to show the patient the way there.

> Even if he says nothing, what the doctor thinks can affect treatment outcomes: the information leaks out, in mannerisms, affect, eyebrows, and nervous smiles.

While you cannot predict a specific outcome for any particular patient, you need to be candid and not paint too rosy a scenario. Each of us is unique in our biology; there can be important differences in both the side effects we suffer and the benefits we gain from the same medication. We can share a single illness but not share its remedy, despite receiving the same drug or undergoing the same procedure. This requires an uncommon degree of honesty, uncommon because it demands a certain deflation of the physician's ego. Such honesty is not rewarded in today's society.

Patients shop for doctors; some doctors are keen to market themselves, knowing that it's easier to make the sale if they present their work as top of the line.

> As a basic principle, the doctor's choice has to be consistent with the patient's philosophy of living.

This particularly pertains to the prescription of oral finasteride for treatment of male pattern hair loss, where a choice must be made for long-term systemic medication with known (sexual side effects, gynecomastia) and unknown risks (post-finasteride syndrome, breast cancer) for treatment of a basically cosmetic condition.

Finally, the question on the role of faith arises: one school of thought holds that religion makes people passive. Such patients transfer their personal responsibilities for choices and actions to a supposed power outside themselves, further infantilizing their part in a paternalistic relationship with their doctor. This view is consistent with Karl Marx's (1818–1883) notorious assertion that religion "is the opium of the people."

> Alternatively, faith can make a person a productive partner in the uncertain world of medicine. Faith, a well-recognized source of solace and of strength to endure, can also give people the courage to recognize uncertainty, acknowledge not only their own fallibility but also their physicians', and thereby contribute to the search for solutions.

Further Reading

Caserio RJ (1987) Diagnostic techniques for hair disorders part III: clinical hair manipulations and clinical findings. Cutis 40:442–448

Patient History

Bi MY, Cohen PR, Robinson FW, Gray JM (2009) Alopecia syphilitica-report of a patient with secondary syphilis presenting as moth-eaten alopecia and a review of its common mimickers. Dermatol Online J 15:6

Boyd AS, Stasko T, King LE et al (1999) Cigarette smoking-associated elastotic changes in the skin. J Am Acad Dermatol 41:23–26

Camacho F, Moreno JC, Garcia-Hernández MJ (1996) Telogen alopecia from UV rays. Arch Dermatol 132:1398–1399

Carlini P, Di Cosimo S, Ferretti G et al (2003) Alopecia in a premenopausal breast cancer woman treated with letrozole and triptorelin. Ann Oncol 14: 1689–1690

Cho M, Cohen PR, Duvic M (1995) Vitiligo and alopecia areata in patients with human immunodeficiency virus infection. South Med J 88:489–491

Daneschfar A, Davis CP, Trüeb RM (1993) Trichomegaly in HIV infection. Schweiz Med Wochenschr 123:1941–1944

Ellis JA, Stebbing M, Harrap SB (2001) Polymorphism of the androgen receptor gene is associated with male pattern baldness. J Invest Dermatol 116:452–455

Finner AM (2013) Nutrition and hair: deficiencies and supplements. Dermatol Clin 31:167–172

Grover RW (1956) Diffuse hair loss associated with selenium (Selsun) sulfide shampoo. J Am Med Assoc 160:1397–1398

Gummer CL (1985) Diet and hair loss. Semin Dermatol 4:35–39

Haley NJ, Hoffmann D (1985) Analysis for nicotine and cotinine in hair to determine cigarette smoker status. Clin Chem 31:1598–1600

Iyengar B (1998) The hair follicle: a specialized UV receptor in the human skin? Biol Signals Recept 7:188–194

Johnson KA, Bernard MA, Funderberg K (2002) Vitamin nutrition in older adults. Clin Geriatr Med 18:773–799

Kullavanijaya P, Gritiyarangsan P, Bisalbutra P (1992) Absence of effects of dimethicone- and non-dimethicone-containing shampoos on daily hair loss rates. J Soc Cosmet Chem 43:195–206

Liu CS, Kao SH, Wei YH (1997) Smoking-associated mitochondrial DNA mutations in human hair follicles. Environ Mol Mutagen 30:47–55

Mirmirani P, Hessol NA, Maurer TA et al (2003) Hair changes in women from the Women's Interagency HIV Study. Arch Dermatol 139:105–106

Mosley JG, Gibbs CC (1996) Premature grey hair and hair loss among smokers: a new opportunity for health education? BMJ 313:1616

Nikolic DS, Viero D, Tijé VC, Toutous-Trellu L (2014) Alopecia universalis associated with vitiligo in an 18-year-old HIV-positive patient: highly active antiretroviral therapy as first choice therapy? Acta Derm Venereol. 94:116–117

Orentreich N, Berger RA (1964) Selenium disulfide shampoo. It's influence on hair growth and the follicular cycle. Arch Dermatol 90:76–80
Osawa Y, Tochigi B, Tochigi M et al (1990) Aromatase inhibitors in cigarette smoke, tobacco leaves and other plants. J Enzyme Inhib 4:187–200
Ostlere LS, Langtry JA, Staughton RC, Samrasinghe PL (1992) Alopecia universalis in a patient seropositive for the human immunodeficiency virus. J Am Acad Dermatol 27:630–631
Piérard-Franchimont C, Uhoda I, Saint-Léger D, Piérard GE (2002) Androgenetic alopecia and stress-induced premature senescence by cumulative ultraviolet light exposure. Exog Dermatol 1:203–206
Reeves JRT, Maibach HI (1977) Drug and chemical induced hair loss. In: Marzulli FN, Maibach HI (eds) Advances in modern toxicology, vol 4. Hemisphere Publishing Corp., Washington/London, pp 487–500
Riedel-Baima B, Riedel A (2008) Female pattern hair loss may be triggered by low oestrogen to androgen ratio. Endocr Regul 42:13–16
Rockey D, Cello J (1993) Evaluation of the gastrointestinal tract in patients with iron-deficiency anemia. N Engl J Med 329:1691–1695
Rushton DH (2002) Nutritional factors and hair loss. Clin Exp Dermatol 27:396–404
Sadick NS (1993) Clinical and laboratory evaluation of AIDS trichopathy. Int J Dermatol 32:33–38
Sawin CT, Geller A, Herschman JE (1979) The aging thyroid: increased prevalence of elevated serum TSH levels in the elderly. JAMA 242:247–250
Sereti I, Sarlis NJ, Arioglu E, Turner ML, Mican JM (2001) Alopecia universalis and Graves' disease in the setting of immune restoration after highly active antiretroviral therapy. AIDS 15:138–140
Severi G, Sinclair R, Hopper JL et al (2003) Androgenetic alopecia in men aged 40-69 years: prevalence and risk factors. Br J Dermatol 149:1207–1213
Smith KJ, Skelton HG, DeRusso D, Sperling L, Yeager J, Wagner KF, Angritt P (1996) Clinical and histopathologic features of hair loss in patients with HIV-1 infection. J Am Acad Dermatol 34:63–68
Starcher B, Pierce R, Hinek A (1999) UVB irradiation stimulates deposition of new elastic fibers by modified epithelial cells surrounding the hair follicles and sebaceous glands in mice. J Invest Dermatol 112: 450–455
Stewart MI, Smoller BR (1993) Alopecia universalis in an HIV-positive patient: possible insight into pathogenesis. J Cutan Pathol 20:180–183
Su L-S, Chen TH-H (2007) Association of androgenetic alopecia with smoking and its prevalence among Asian men. Arch Dermatol 143:1401–1406
Tosti A, Misciali C, Piraccini BM et al (1994) Drug-induced hair loss and hair growth. Incidence, management and avoidance. Drug Saf 10:310–317
Tosti A, Piraccini BM, van Neste DJ (2001) Telogen effluvium after allergic contact dermatitis of the scalp. Arch Dermatol 137:187–190
Trüeb RM (2003a) Association between smoking and hair loss: another opportunity for health education against smoking? Dermatology 206:189–191
Trüeb RM (2003b) Is androgenetic alopecia a photoaggravated dermatosis? Dermatology 207:343–348
York J, Nicholson T, Minors P, Duncan DF (1998) Stressful life events and loss of hair among adult women, a case-control study. Psychol Rep 82:1044–1046

Examination Techniques

Adya KA, Inamadar AC, Palit A, Shivanna R, Deshmukh NS (2011) Light microscopy of the hair: a simple tool to "untangle" hair disorders. Int J Trichol 3:46–56
Barrett S Commercial hair analysis: a cardinal sign of quackery. http://www.quackwatch.com/01QuackeryRelatedTopics/hair.html
Blume-Peytaivi U, Orfanos CE (1995) Microscopy of the hair – the trichogram. In: Derup J, Jemec GBE (eds) Handbook of non-invasive methods and the skin. CRC Press, London, pp 549–554
Braun-Falco O, Heilgemeir GP (1985) The trichogram. Structural and functional basis, performance, and interpretation. Sem Dermatol 4:40–52
Caserio RJ (1987) Diagnostic techniques for hair disorders part III: clinical hair manipulations and clinical findings. Cutis 40:442–448
Daneshpazhooh M, Asgari M, Naraghi ZS, Barzgar MR, Akhyani M, Balighi K, Chams-Davatchi C (2009) A study on plucked hair as a substrate for direct immunofluorescence in pemphigus vulgaris. J Eur Acad Dermatol Venereol 23:129–131
Daneshpazhooh M, Naraghi ZS, Ramezani A, Ghanadan A, Esmaili N, Chams-Davatchi C (2011) Direct immunofluorescence of plucked hair for evaluation of immunologic remission in pemphigus vulgaris. J Am Acad Dermatol 65:e173–e177
Degos R, Rabut R, Duperrat B, Leclercq R (1954) Pseudopeladic state; comments on one hundred cases of circumscribed cicatricial alopecia, apparently primary, of pseudopelade type. Ann Dermatol Syphiligr (Paris) 81:5–26
Dreuw H (1910) Klinische Beobachtungen bei 101 haarkranken Schulknaben. Monatsh Prakt Dermatol 51:103–118
Dunn PM (1992) Litigation over congenital scalp defects. Lancet 339:440
Elston DM, McCollough ML, Angeloni VL (1995) Vertical and transverse sections of alopecia biopsy specimens. Combining the two to maximize diagnostic yield. J Am Acad Dermatol 32:454–457
Frieden IJ (1986) Aplasia cutis congenita: a clinical review and proposal for classification. J Am Acad Dermatol 14:646–660
Hambidge KM (1982) Hair analyses: worthless for vitamins, limited for minerals. Am J Clin Nutr 36:943–949

Hamilton JB (1951) Patterned loss of hair in man; types and incidence. Ann N Y Acad Sci 53:708–728
Harries MJ, Trüeb RM, Tosti A et al (2009) How not to get scar(r)ed: pointers to the correct diagnosis in patients with suspected primary cicatricial alopecia. Br J Dermatol 160:482–501
Headington JT (1996) Cicatricial alopecia. Dermatol Clin 14:773–782
Hidvégi B (2008) Dermoscopy of hair and scalp disorders. Eur J Dermatol 18:607
Kumaresan M, Rai R, Sandhya V (2011) Immunofluorescence of the outer root sheath: an aid to diagnosis in pemphigus. Clin Exp Dermatol 36:298–301
Lacarrubba F, Dall'Oglio F, Nasca MR, Micali G (2004) Videodermoscopy enhances diagnostic capability in some forms of hair loss. Am J Clin Dermatol 5:205–208
Ludwig E (1977) Classification of the types of androgenetic alopecia (common baldness) occurring in the female sex. Br J Dermatol 97:247–254
Mirmirani P, Huang KP, Price VH (2011) A practical, algorithmic approach to diagnosing hair shaft disorders. Int J Dermatol 50:1–12
Norwood OT (1975) Male pattern baldness: classification and incidence. South Med J 68:1359–1365
Olszewska M, Rudnicka L, Rakowska A et al (2008) Trichoscopy. Arch Dermatol 144:1007
Pierard GE (1979) Toxic effects of metals from the environment on hair growth and structure. J Cutan Pathol 16:237–242
Rao R, Dasari K, Shenoi SD, Balachandran C, Dinesh P (2013) Monitoring the disease activity in pemphigus by direct immunofluorescence of plucked hair: a pilot study. Indian J Dermatol 58:164
Ross EK, Tan E, Shapiro J (2005) Update on primary cicatricial alopecias. J Am Acad Dermatol 53:1–37
Ross EK, Vincenzi C, Tosti A (2006) Videodermoscopy in the evaluation of hair and scalp disorders. J Am Acad Dermatol 55:799–806
Rudnicka L, Olszewska M, Rakowska A et al (2008) Trichoscopy: a new method for diagnosing hair loss. J Drugs Dermatol 7:651–654
Schaerer L, Trüeb RM (2003) Direct immunofluorescence of plucked hair in pemphigus. Arch Dermatol 139:228–229
Sherertz E (1985) Misuse of hair analysis as a diagnostic tool. Arch Dermatol 121:1504–1505
Solomon AR (1994) The transversely sectioned scalp biopsy specimen: the technique and a algorithm for its use in the diagnosis of alopecia. Adv Dermatol 9:127–157
Sperling LC (2001) Scarring alopecia and the dermatopathologist. J Cutan Pathol 28:333–342
Templeton SF, Solomon AR (1994) Scarring alopecia: a classification based on microscopic criteria. J Cutan Pathol 121:97–109
Toncić RJ, Lipozencić J, Pastar Z (2007) Videodermoscopy in the evaluation of hair and scalp disorders. Acta Dermatovenerol Croat 15:116–118
Tosti A (2007) Dermoscopy of hair and scalp disorders with clinical and pathological correlations. Informa Healthcare, Andover
Trachsler S, Trüeb RM (2005) Value of direct immunofluorescence for differential diagnosis of cicatricial alopecia. Dermatology 211:98–102
Whiting DA, Dy LC (2006) Office diagnosis of hair shaft defects. Semin Cutan Med Surg 25:24–34
Zlotken SH (1985) Hair analysis. A useful tool or a waste of money? Int J Dermatol 24:161–164

Quantifying Hair Loss

Canfield D (1996) Photographic documentation of hair growth in androgenetic alopecia. Dermatol Clin 14:713–721
DiBernardo BE, Giampapa VC, Vogel J (1996) Standardized hair photography. Dermatol Surg 22:945–952
Guarrera M, Semino MT, Rebora A (1997) Quantitating hair loss in women: a critical approach. Dermatology 194:12–16
Guarrera M, Cardo PP, Rebora A (2011) Assessing the reliability of the Modified Wash Test. G Ital Dermatol Venereol 146:289–291
Guarrera M, Fiorucci MC, Rebora A (2013) Methods of hair loss evaluation: a comparison of TrichoScan(®) with the modified wash test. Exp Dermatol 22:482–484
Hoffmann R (2001) TrichoScan: combining epiluminescence microscopy with digital image analysis for the measurement of hair growth in vivo. Eur J Dermatol 11:362–368
Ihm CW, Lee JY (1991) Evaluation in daily hair counts. Dermatologica 182:67
Olsen EA (1993) Clinical tools for assessing hair loss. In: Olsen EA (ed) Disorders of hair growth: diagnosis and treatment. McGraw-Hill, New York, pp 59–69
Olsen EA (2003) Current and novel methods for assessing efficacy of hair growth promoters in pattern hair loss. J Am Acad Dermatol 48:253–262
Rampini P, Guarrera M, Rampini E, Rebora A (1999) Assessing hair shedding in children. Dermatology 199:256–257
Rebora A, Guarrera M, Baldari M, Vecchio F (2005) Distinguishing androgenetic alopecia from chronic telogen effluvium when associated in the same patient: a simple noninvasive method. Arch Derm 141:1243–1245
Seung Ho Lee, Oh Sang Kwon, Jun Gyu Oh et al (2004) Phototrichogram: Evaluation of Modified Methods with Bleaching and Trichoscan. Seoul, Korea, poster

presentation at the European Hair Research Society, Berlin, 2004

Trüeb RM, Itin P, Itin and Swiss Trichology Working Group (2001) Photographic documentation of the effectiveness of 1 mg oral finasteride in treatment of androgenic alopecia in the man in routine general practice in Switzerland. Praxis (Bern 1994) 90:2087–2093

Van Neste D, Trüeb RM (2006) Critical study of hair growth analysis with computer-assisted methods. J Eur Acad Dermatol Venereol 20:578–583

Communication Skills

Hong J, Nguyen T, Prose NS (2013) Compassionate care: enhancing physician-patient communication and education in dermatology. Part II: patient education. J Am Acad Dermatol 68:364–373

Keller V, White MK, Carroll JG, Segal E (1995) "Difficult" physician-patient relationships workbook. Bayer Institute for Health Care Communication, West Haven

Neumann M, Scheffer C, Tauschel D, Lutz G, Wirtz M, Edelhäuser F (2012) Physician empathy: definition, outcome-relevance and its measurement in patient care and medical education. GMS Z Med Ausbild 29:Doc11

Ngoh LN (2003) Health literacy: a barrier to pharmacist-patient communication and medication adherence. J Am Pharm Assoc 49:e132–e146

Nguyen T, Hong J, Prose NS (2013) Compassionate care: enhancing physician-patient communication and education in dermatology. Part I: patient-centered communication. J Am Acad Dermatol 68:353–360

Renzi C, Abeni D, Picardi A et al (2001) Factors associated with patient satisfaction with care among dermatological outpatients. Br J Dermatol 145:617–623

Stone MS, Bronkesh SJ, Gerbarg ZB, Wood SD (1998) Improving patient compliance. Strategic Medicine. www.patientcompliancemedia.com/Improving_Patient_Compliance_article.pdf

White MK, Keller V, Carroll JG (1995) Physician-patient communication workbook. Bayer Institute for Health Care Communication, West Haven

Avoiding Mental Traps

Groopman J (2007) How doctors think. Houghton Mifflin Company, Boston/New York

3 Patient Expectation Management

It is easier to write a prescription than to come to an understanding with the patient.

Franz Kafka (1883–1924), A Country Doctor

Hair loss is a common dermatologic problem, and few dermatologic problems carry as much emotional overtones as the complaint of hair loss. Adding to some patient's worry may be prior frustrating experiences with physicians, who tend to trivialize complaints of hair loss or dismiss them completely. This attitude on the part of physicians is related either to lack of comprehension of the impact of hair loss on quality of life or to lack of confidence in the treatment of alopecia.

> Treatment options are available, though limited, both in terms of indications and of efficacy. Success depends not only on comprehension of the underlying pathology but also on unpatronizing sympathy from the part of the physician.

3.1 Listening to the Patient

For a successful encounter at an office visit, one needs to be sure that the patient's key concerns have been directly and specifically solicited and addressed. To be effective, the physician must gain an understanding of the patient's perspective on his/her illness. Patient concerns can be wide ranging, including fear of hair loss and disfigurement; apprehension of scalp symptoms; distrust of the medical profession or of pharmacologic agents; concern about loss of wholeness, role, status, or independence; denial of reality of medical conditions; grief; and other uniquely personal issues. Patient values, cultures, and preferences need to be explored. Gender is another element that needs to be taken into consideration. Ensuring key issues are verbalized openly is fundamental to effective patient–doctor communication. Appropriate reassurance or pragmatic suggestions to help with problem solving and setting up a structured plan of action may be an important part of the patient care that is required.

> Psychological research confirms a negative effect of visible hair loss on social perceptions and body image satisfaction. Therefore, a thorough evaluation, a specific diagnosis, effective treatment, and appropriate counseling can be expected to have some psychological efficacy.

R.M. Trüeb, *The Difficult Hair Loss Patient: Guide to Successful Management of Alopecia and Related Conditions*, DOI 10.1007/978-3-319-19701-2_3

Table 3.1 Percentage of men attributing specific effects to the occurrence of androgenetic alopecia

	Extent of hair loss	
Reported experience	Low	High
Cognitive preoccupation		
Wish for more hair	52	84
Notice bald/balding men	54	82
Spend time looking in the mirror at hair/head	54	69
Wonder what others think	47	67
Negative socio-emotional events		
Get teased by peers	45	79
Feel self-conscious	42	78
Look older than actual age	40	55
Worry that others will notice	39	56
Feel helpless about baldness	37	56
Worry about aging	37	46
Feel less attractive	31	51
Envy good-looking men	33	34
Behavioral coping		
Try to improve hairstyle	63	66
Try to improve physique	41	36
Dress more nicely	26	45
Wear hats or caps	23	41
Seek reassurance about looks	23	39
Grow beard or mustache	18	36

From Cash TF (1992) The psychological effects of androgenetic alopecia in men. *J Am Acad Dermatol* 26:926–931

In 1992, Cash examined psychological effects of androgenetic alopecia in men and found that although most men regard hair loss to be an unwanted, distressing experience that diminishes their body image, bald men actively cope and generally retain the integrity of their personality functioning (Table 3.1).

Subsequently, Cash compared psychological effects of androgenetic alopecia on women with balding men and found that androgenetic hair loss was clearly a stressful experience for both sexes, but substantially more distressing for women. Relative to control subjects, women with androgenetic alopecia possessed a more negative body image and a pattern of less adaptive functioning (Table 3.2).

Patients' psychological reactions to hair loss are less related to physicians' ratings than to patients' own perceptions of the extent of their hair loss. Even in women with slight hair loss, that loss is imbued with considerable emotional meaning that the physician should not ignore.

Table 3.2 Descriptions of female androgenetic alopecia patients' specific effects attributed to hair loss

Effects attributed to hair loss	%
Adverse effects	
Wish I had more hair	98
Think about my hair loss	97
Try to figure out if I am losing more hair	95
Feel frustrated or helpless about my hair loss	93
Spend time looking at my hair in the mirror	92
Worry about my looks	92
Feel self-conscious about my looks	92
Have negative thoughts about my hair	91
Worry about whether others will notice my hair loss	90
Worry about how much hair I am going to lose	89
Notice people who are balding	83
Think about how I used to look	78
Notice what other people look like	78
Have the thought, "why me?"	75
Think I am not as attractive as I used to be	72
Wonder what other people think about my looks	71
Have thoughts that I am unattractive	68
Try to think what I would look like with more hair loss	67
Feel depressed or despondent	63
Worry about getting older	62
Worry that my spouse or partner will find me less attractive	60
Feel embarrassment	55
Feel envious of good-looking people of my sex	53
Feel sensitive to personal criticism	50
Am conscious of how others react to me	43
Feel I look older than I am	42
People comment about my hair loss	36
Get friendly teasing or kidding from others	20
Behavioral coping	
Try to figure out what to do about my hair loss	98
Try to hide my hair loss	94
Talk to my hairstylist about my hair loss	82
Try to improve my hairstyle	79
Do things to improve my looks	75
Talk to friends of my own sex about my hair loss	71
Spend time on my appearance	70
Talk to my partner about my hair loss	64
Seek reassurance about my looks	62
Try to improve my figure or physique	44

From Cash TF, Price VH, Savin RC. Psychological effects of androgenetic alopecia on women: comparisons with balding men and with female control subjects. *J Am Acad Dermatol* 1993;29:568–575

Physicians should recognize that androgenetic alopecia goes well beyond the simple physical aspects of hair loss and growth.

Ultimately, androgenetic alopecia is not uniform in its psychological impact. Among men, Cash identified several variables predictive of greater androgenetic alopecia-related distress:

- Younger men (under 26 years old) with earlier-onset hair loss
- Romantically unattached men
- Those who view their alopecia as socially noticeable and expect it to progress
- Men with a heightened social (public) self-consciousness, a vulnerable sense of self-acceptability, and a higher psychological investment in their appearance

Often, hair loss may first become apparent at particularly demanding periods of life, such as during the period of mate selection or at the onset of a challenging career. At such times, the afflicted may find hair loss especially upsetting and even use it as a scapegoat for a lack of satisfaction in other areas of life.

Left to their own resources, individuals with androgenetic alopecia engage in a number of strategies to cope with the unwanted conditions, such as:

- Styling the remaining scalp hair to conceal thinning areas.
- Using cosmetic products to camouflage hair loss.
- Wearing caps or hats to conceal the condition.
- Avoiding situations that aggravate distress by making the hair loss more socially recognizable, e.g., wet hair and windy or brightly lit environments.
- Compensating for the diminished body image by growing a beard or improving grooming and physique.
- Paradoxically shaving the entire head to hide hair loss.

Patients who have concluded that the above strategies, or over-the-counter treatments, are insufficient to abate their distress finally consult professionals for medical or surgical solutions.

With the advent of pharmacologic agents, such as topical minoxidil solution and oral finasteride, and improved surgical hair transplantation procedures for effective treatment of androgenetic alopecia, the options for managing androgenetic alopecia and androgenetic alopecia-related distress have expanded.

In 1991, van der Donk et al. conducted a prospective study of the psychological changes in men who received either 2 % topical minoxidil solution or placebo and found favorable changes in psychological adjustment and self-image among responders to topical minoxidil solution compared to placebo recipients, but only in the group aged above 35 years.

In a study of 1,495 men aged 20–40 years who suffered from androgenetic alopecia and were subjected to treatment with 5 % topical minoxidil solution in the setting of two private dermatologic practices, Mapar and Omidian found that almost all the patients gradually avoided continuing the treatment. Only in a few patients was the cessation of medication due to adverse effects. The causes of discontinuation in the majority of patients were the low effect of medication and an aversion to this topical treatment method. The authors concluded that the insignificant cosmetic effect of minoxidil solution caused discontinuity of treatment among almost all patients.

Therefore, treatment of male androgenetic alopecia in the 20 to 40 years age group with oral finasteride would seem to be more reliable than topical minoxidil.

In 2011, a study was performed in Japan by Tsuboi et al. in order to ascertain whether treatment with 1 mg oral finasteride can improve the quality of life of male patients with androgenetic alopecia. Patients aged 19–76 years (average, 33.8) answered Visual Analogue Scale (VAS), Dermatology Life Quality Index (DLQI), WHO/QOL-26, and State-Trait Anxiety Inventory (STAI) questionnaires before and after administration of oral finasteride for 6 months. The changes in these indices before and after treatment were statistically analyzed, and the improved values of the indices in the high treatment responders (excellent or good) and the low treatment responders (moderate or no change) from baseline were compared. There was a statistical difference in the VAS and DLQI indices before and after administration of oral finasteride, while no significant change was found for the WHO/QOL-26 and STAI indices. Interestingly, comparison of high and low responders failed to reveal any statistical difference in the improvement of VAS and DLQI scores. The authors concluded that oral finasteride improves the quality of life of men treating androgenetic alopecia and VAS and DLQI are useful for the evaluation of patients' quality of life. However, oral finasteride failed to improve the patients' anxiety, nor did its efficacy correlate with the level of reported anxiety.

3.2 Educating the Patient

Patient understanding and involvement are central to optimal treatment selection and active patient role in treatment. This maximizes patient benefit and safety.

Patient education is more than a simple transfer of information. Printed material, visual and audio aids, and staff trained to interact and educate patients are all helpful. But the physician should also directly review information with patients to confirm the effectiveness of the communication and appropriateness of patient expectations. Such a review also enhances rapport and communicates a sense of caring that fosters trust.

Understanding, emotion, satisfaction, rapport, and empathy are among the factors involved. In talking with a patient, a physician should attempt to learn what the patient expects and help shape those expectations to match the physician's intention. If the patient forms different expectations than those the physician is attempting to communicate, the physician needs to direct the dialogue to eliminate this expectation gap.

> Every time a patient says, "I didn't know...," one has an opportunity to consider how to better communicate the information in the future.

Finally, patients read the unspoken language of physicians: Does the doctor look them in the eye or stare at the computer screen? Is he or she standing up or sitting down when addressing the patient? Does he or she frequently look to the door? If patients are asking the receptionist questions that they should be asking the physician, the doctor needs to find out why. Perhaps a change in body language or improved communication with the patient is needed. To ensure that communication goals are achieved, the physician must also pay attention to the patient's nonverbal cues. Listening to the patient must be active—acknowledging and encouraging while sharing agreement and disagreement in an empathic manner.

A patient's hopes and wishful thinking introduce an unconscious dissonance between the patient's understanding of what the physician says and the patient's expectation of the outcome.

> Although it may appear that efforts to communicate more effectively may demand more time, mindful communication that picks up on cues from the patient could result in less time spent reviewing information. It is not so much a matter of more time as it is of using and tailoring the time for each patient's need.

3.3 Creating Reasonable Expectations

Patient expectation management is the art of supporting patients in knowing how to be right and when to be satisfied. Managing expectations is a process of creating the structure that is necessary for achieving trust and confidence from the patient and, ultimately, patient satisfaction.

Patients expect two sorts of value from their attending physicians: *rational value* and *emotional value. Rational value* results from appointment management, the process of examination, technical procedures, and follow-up scheduling. *Emotional value* is the way the patient feels about having been cared for.

How does a patient develop expectations? Patients learn from a number of sources: from family, friends, and others who have experienced treatment, from conventional news sources, and from Internet sites with information of variable quality, potential bias, and sensationalism. Finally, the patient's own past experience contributes significantly to future expectations.

Remember, probably the most frequent cause for difficult patient encounters are prior negative patient experiences with physicians, who tend to trivialize the complaint of hair loss and its treatment.

Both, the understanding of the patient and his or her values, and the patient's apprehension of the attending physician as an individual, rather than as a professional, contribute to emotional value. One way to deliver emotional value is to provide information about oneself before meeting the patient: for example, a website and brochure declaring one's philosophy of care are convenient vehicles for this purpose. Also, public appearance and the social media may be highly effective in directing information to patients. All forms of communication create expectations from patients. Finally, the patient's understanding depends not only on the material received but also on the way the patient assimilates that information and translates into actionable beliefs, based upon cultural and individual values as well as past experiences.

Patients' expectation, not ours, is the yardstick by which our patients measure the course of recovery, occurrence of complications, and the outcome.

The Latin maxim tuto, celeriter, et iucunde stands for "safely, swiftly, and gladly" and was originally coined by Asclepiades of Bithynia (124–56 BC), personal physician and near friend of notable personalities of Ancient Rome, such as Cicero and Mark Antony. While the foreign Greek physicians were originally encountered with much distrust by ancient Romans and especially its aristocracy, Asclepiades managed to convince through his high learning, brilliant medical achievements, and worldly wisdom. Above all, he was always attentive and sympathetic to the individual needs of his patients.

Asclepiades was born in Prusa. He travelled much when young and at first settled at Rome as a rhetorician. Though he did not succeed in that profession, he eventually acquired great reputation as a physician. Asclepiades began by vilifying the principles and practices of his predecessors and by asserting that he had discovered a more effective method of treating diseases than had been before known to the world. His remedies were directed to the restoration of harmony. A part of the great popularity which Asclepiades enjoyed depended upon his attending to every need of his patients and indulging their inclinations. Finally, Asclepiades advocated humane treatment of mental disorders. His teachings are surprisingly modern; therefore, Asclepiades is considered to be a pioneer physician in both the medical sciences and psychotherapy.

The same way Asclepiades won the Roman populace and aristocracy for his cause, the physician must advance to build up his reputation and to secure the confidence of his patients.

3.4 Satisfaction Survey

Also, satisfaction survey questions help create expectations. It is in one's best interest to distribute and review surveys to patients. At the next team meeting, team members should be asked to complete the patient satisfaction survey themselves as they believe most patients would. When the actual survey results are received, they should be compared with the team's predicted results to identify expectation gaps and what changes would be needed to improve your scores.

The patient satisfaction survey verbatim responses provide information about how patient expectations are met. One should take the time to review those comments, since they will reinforce the emotional and rational value of one's care for patients.

Just as providing a checklist for patients is helpful in encouraging follow-through, a checklist for one's proper practice may also be a valuable prompt for enhanced performance. One should consider developing a checklist to increase adherence to the standards created by the satisfaction surveys.

Asking for feedback is a way to identify gaps. Asking for feedback can satisfy a patient's need to let one know that something needs improvement. The patient who is given that opportunity may be less likely to vent frustration in an online chat room.

Having patients verbalize their expectations and guiding them should be a part of any communication; a conscious effort will improve effectiveness. With these efforts, a patient is less likely to feel abandoned in any case of perceived failure.

3.5 Special Patient Groups

Although testing medical interventions for efficacy had existed since Avicenna (Latinate form of Ibn-Sīnā, Persian polymath regarded as one of the most significant thinkers of the "Islamic Golden Age" and described as the "Father of Early Modern Medicine," 980–1037), it was only in the twentieth century that this effort evolved to impact almost all fields of healthcare and policy. Evidence-based medicine (EBM), as established by Alvan Feinstein (American physician and mathematician, 1925–2001) and Archie Cochrane (Scottish physician, 1909–1988) in the 1970s, aims at applying the best available evidence to clinical decision making, using techniques from science, engineering, and statistics, such as systematic review of medical literature, meta-analysis, risk–benefit analysis, and randomized controlled trials (RCTs). Ultimately, EBM aims for the ideal that healthcare professionals should make conscientious, explicit, and judicious use of current best evidence in everyday practice.

However, EBM guidelines do not remove the problem of extrapolation to different patient populations, specifically, certain groups have been historically under-researched, such as special age groups, ethnic minorities, and people with comorbid conditions, and thus the literature is sparse in areas that do not allow for generalizing.

3.5.1 Children

Biologically, a child is a human between birth and puberty. The legal definition of child refers to a minor, otherwise known as a person younger than the age of majority. Recognition of childhood as a state different from adulthood began to emerge only in the sixteenth and seventeenth centuries, when society began to relate to the child not as a miniature adult but as a person of a lower level of maturity needing adult protection, love, and nurturing.

Pediatrics is the branch of medicine that deals with the medical care of children (and adolescents) with the age limit ranging from birth up to 18 years. Pediatrics is a relatively young medical specialty, developing only in the mid-nineteenth century. Abraham Jacobi (1830–1919) is regarded as the father of pediatrics.

The body size differences are paralleled by maturational changes. The smaller body of a neonate, infant, or child is substantially different physiologically from that of an adult.

Congenital defects, genetic variance, and developmental issues are of greater concern to pediatricians than they often are to adult physicians.

Another major difference between pediatrics and adult medicine is that children are minors and, in most jurisdictions, cannot make decisions for themselves. The issues of guardianship, privacy, legal responsibility, and informed consent must always be considered in every pediatric procedure.

In a sense, physicians dealing with children often have to treat the parents and, sometimes, the family, rather than just the child.

Finally, the issues of pediatric nutrition and pediatric dosage in pharmacotherapy are to be taken into consideration. Pediatric nutrition refers to the maintenance of a proper well-balanced diet consisting of the essential nutrients and the adequate caloric intake necessary to promote growth and sustain the physiologic requirements at the various stages of a child's development.

Nutritional needs vary considerably with age, level of activity, and environmental conditions, and they are directly related to the rate of growth.

Pediatric dosage relates to the determination of the correct amount, frequency, and total number of doses of a medication to be administered to an infant or child. Various formulas have been devised to calculate pediatric dosage from a standard adult dose, although the most reliable method is to use one of the formulas to calculate the proportional amount of body surface area to body weight.

Such variables as the ability of the child to absorb, metabolize, and excrete the medication must be considered, as well as the expected action of the drug, possible side effects, and potential toxicity.

Specifically, children are at higher risk of cardiovascular adverse effects of minoxidil solution, from both topical application and accidental ingestion. Claudet et al. reported a case of significant intoxication after the ingestion of topical minoxidil solution. A 7-year-old girl, who accidentally ingested a teaspoon of minoxidil solution (Alopexy®, Laboratoires Pierre Fabre, SA, Switzerland), presented to the pediatric emergency ward with emesis, a blood pressure of 86/56 mmHg, and a pulse of 149 beats per minute. Hypotension lasted 40 h with the lowest value 24 h after ingestion (79/33 mmHg). Infusion of 20 mL/kg of normal saline fluid had no hemodynamic effect. Her blood pressure normalized on day 2. The authors concluded that topical minoxidil solution is an unsafe product for children and therefore should be strictly kept out of reach of children. Moreover, manufacturers should enhance child-resistance security of packaging.

Generalized hypertrichosis is a common side effect of oral minoxidil treatment for hypertension. However, hypertrichosis is uncommon after treatment with topical minoxidil for alopecia and normally only occurs in areas close to the site of application. González et al. reported a 16-year-old girl who developed generalized hypertrichosis 3 months after applying topical minoxidil for treatment of alopecia in doses greater than prescribed. Four months after discontinuing treatment, the abnormal hair gradually diminished and disappeared.

Alopecia in childhood is a source of high concern, frustration, and anxiety.

Young children usually lack self-awareness and it may be the parents who, projecting their own concerns onto the child, most acutely feel any associated anxiety. In addition, parents of a child with an inherited hair condition may feel guilt, and siblings can develop unsupported fears that they may be affected. Hair loss for the older child can lead to low self-esteem, depression, and humiliation. Ultimately, hair loss in children can have psychological effects that interfere with a child's normal development.

> Delineating types of alopecia and those that are chronic or potentially related to underlying medical problems is important.

The proportion of children under the age of 10 years among patients complaining of hair loss in a dermatologic clinic is 5 %. Pediatric alopecia is caused by a number of conditions, and patterns are different from those seen in adults. A thorough understanding of normal hair development enables accurate assessment of the child with hair loss. Knowledge of the normal range and variation observed in children's hair additionally enhances this assessment. Examples are transient neonatal hair loss (Fig. 3.1), trichoglyphics (hair-slope patterns), such as the cowlick (Fig. 3.2) and ridgeback anomaly (Fig. 3.3), scalp whorls (Fig. 3.4), and to some extent short anagen syndrome.

Hair and scalp disorders in children may originate from the hair itself, scalp skin, or infectious causes and be congenital or acquired.

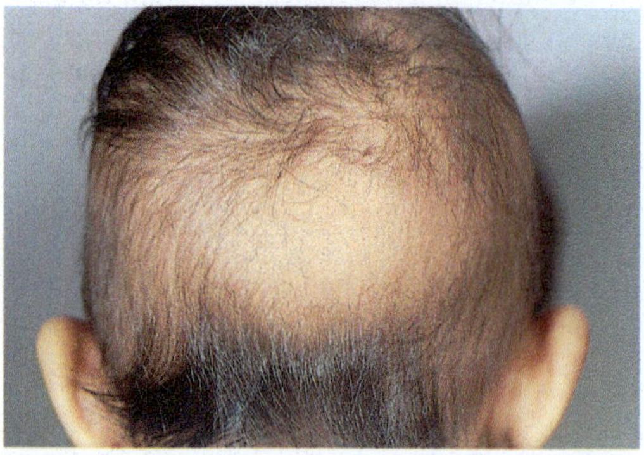

Fig. 3.1 Transient neonatal hair loss

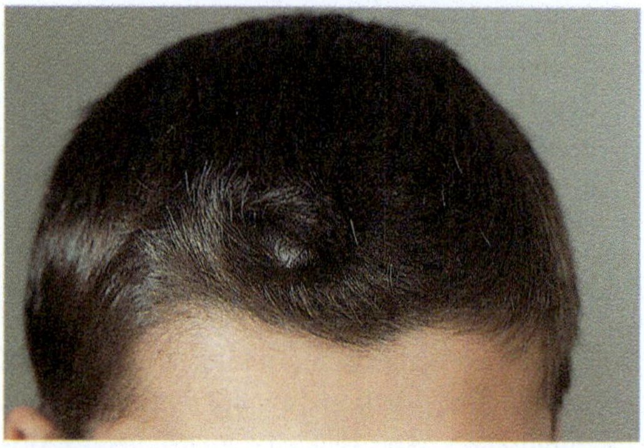

Fig. 3.2 Cowlick

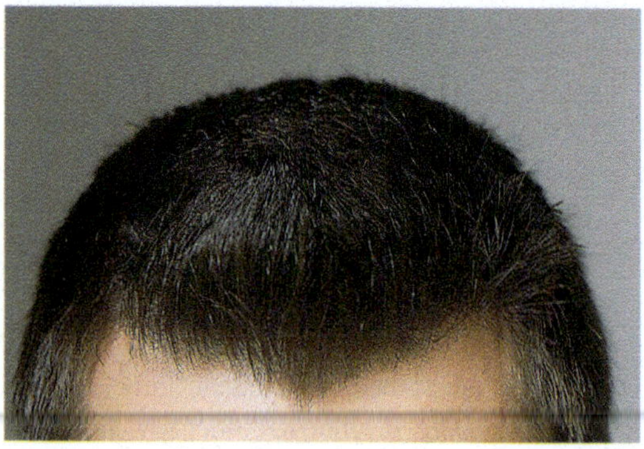

Fig. 3.3 Ridgeback anomaly

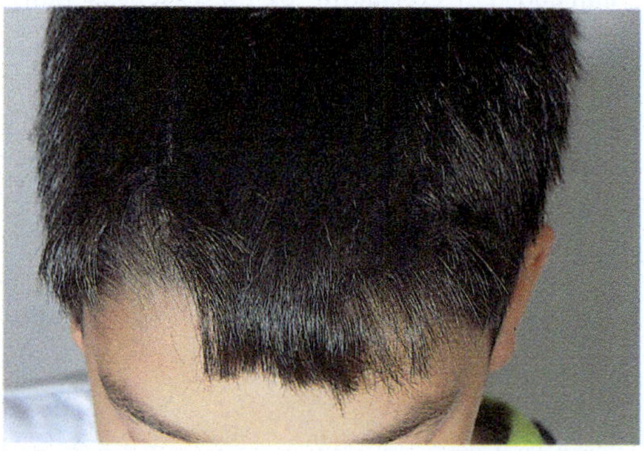

Fig. 3.4 Scalp whorls

> The differential diagnosis of alopecia in the pediatric age group is simplified by the fact that 90–95 % of cases are caused by four major entities: alopecia areata, tinea capitis, telogen effluvium, and trichotillomania. Sometimes clinically more elusive

conditions such as congenital triangular alopecia, or premature androgenetic alopecia, may be responsible for hair loss. Finally, conditions peculiar to the pediatric population are the loose anagen and the short anagen syndromes.

Hereditary and congenital hypotrichosis or atrichia and hair shaft abnormalities have no effective treatment. It should be remembered that congenital abnormalities may exist as a feature of a clinical syndrome. Congenital lesions should also be considered in areas of localized alopecia occurring at birth. Especially, atrophic midline bald patches may be associated with developmental defects.

Tinea capitis responds readily to the appropriate medical therapy, provided it is started before scarring has lead to permanent hair loss.

There is a variety of treatment options for alopecia areata, premature androgenetic alopecia, and trichotillomania, with limited success depending on the extent and duration of disease.

In telogen effluvium underlying medical problems, specifically nutritional deficiencies, should be identified and treated.

Finally, the loose and the short anagen syndromes represent self-limiting conditions with age. Education and reassurance of parents are in the center of management.

3.5.2 Women of Childbearing Age, Pregnancy, and Lactation

Dermatologists are frequently faced with questions about the safety of commonly prescribed topical and systemic medications during pregnancy and lactation from women of childbearing age considering pregnancy, who are pregnant, or who are breastfeeding. Medications are commonly used during pregnancy. In fact, female patients take an average of 2.9 medications during pregnancy. Due to this high prevalence, malpractice litigation poses a high legal risk to dermatologists who prescribe medications to female patients who are or may become pregnant.

No database for determination of precise risk of drug use during pregnancy and lactation is available. There are, however, educated opinions concerning the advisability of use of a drug during the childbearing years from manufacturers, the FDA, various teratologists, the American Academy of Pediatrics, and the WHO. Not all medications are absolutely contraindicated during pregnancy and lactation. Some drugs have been extensively used without apparent adverse effects in the mother or infant. When it is necessary to select a medication for use during pregnancy or lactation, the medication should have minimal risk.

The safety of topical minoxidil for treatment of female pattern hair loss during pregnancy has not been systematically studied, and there have been single case reports of adverse effects: Smorlesi et al. reported on a 28-year-old white pregnant woman who daily applied minoxidil 2 % to her scalp for treatment of hair loss. At the 22nd gestational week, after a routine ultrasound test showing significant brain, heart, and vascular malformations of the fetus, pregnancy was interrupted. The placenta had numerous ischemic areas and a discrepancy between gestational age and villi maturation. In the villi, capillaries were increased in number, significantly enlarged, and excessively marginalized. The fetus' heart was increased in volume and had a globose shape, and the aorta had a distal stenosis. The sigmoid colon was significantly increased in length and a mesentery commune was present. The brain had enlarged ventricles and abundant hemorrhages. Histological examination showed areas of demyelinization with gliosis, signs of excessive and inappropriate angiogenesis, and capillary rearrangement.

Rojansky et al. reported on a fetus with extreme hypotrophy of the caudal body pole, aplasia of the lower spine, and complete renal agenesis (caudal regression syndrome, CRS) diagnosed in the second trimester by ultrasound. While the exact etiology of CRS is unclear, maternal diabetes, genetic factors, teratogens, and vascular anomalies altering blood flow have been hypothesized to play a role in its pathogenesis. Maternal history revealed the use of minoxidil solution for preventing hair loss for 4 years prior to and during gestation. Also, the mother had taken trimethoprim–sulfamethoxazole during the first trimester for treatment of upper respiratory disease. No maternal diabetes or history of familial genetic diseases was evident. In an extreme form of CRS consisting of complete aplasia of the lower body pole and viscera and additional malformations, a possible drug-related etiology was suggested but should be confirmed by more studies.

Finally, Veyrac et al. reported on a hairy infant following cutaneous application of minoxidil during pregnancy.

> Therefore, further knowledge on minoxidil-induced fetal toxicity would be beneficial before allowing its use in pregnant women.

Meanwhile, the use of topical minoxidil during lactation has recently been cleared by the American Academy of Dermatology.

> Due to teratogenicity for the male fetus, oral finasteride and dutasteride are contraindicated for use in premenopausal women.

3.5.3 Elderly

Aging is the process of becoming older. It results from the accumulation of changes in a person over time. Aging in humans represents a multidimensional process of physical, psychological, and social changes. Ultimately, aging is among the largest known health risk factors for most human diseases, ultimately leading to death.

In biology, senescence denotes the state or process of aging. Cellular senescence is a phenomenon where isolated cells demonstrate a limited capacity to divide in culture (the Hayflick limit, discovered by Leonard Hayflick in 1961), while organismal senescence is the aging of organisms. After a period of near perfect renewal between 20 and 35 years of age in humans, organismal senescence is characterized by the declining ability to respond to stress, the increasing homeostatic imbalance, and the increased risk of disease.

Aging hair is characterized by loss of follicle rigor, consistent with age-dependent slowing of other body activities, failure to pigment the hair shaft, decrease in hair growth, and reduction in the diameter of the hair shaft. The condition of the hair depends on hereditary and ethnic factors with great interindividual variability, the condition of the scalp, hair care and hairstyling habits, external factors and hair damage, and the nutritional and overall health status.

Older patients suffer from a variety of conditions that affect the hair: nutritional deficiency, endocrine disorders, psychological problems, and drug-related adverse effects.

> Sometimes, symptoms of overt pathologic conditions are misinterpreted as signs of normal aging, ignored, and left untreated. In taking care of the elderly with hair problems, it is therefore important to be suspicious of the possibility of a more general problem underlying the patient's complaint.

With technologic advances and improvements in medical care, an increasing number of patients survive medical conditions that used to be fatal. This fact combined with the aging of the population means that a growing proportion of patients have multiple concurrent medical conditions. The term "multimorbidity" means several concurrent medical conditions within one person. According to a survey done in Canada in 1998, 30 % of the population reported suffering from more than one chronic health problem, and the percentage increased with age. In the United States, the prevalence of multimorbidity among those 65 and older has been estimated at 65 %. Numerous pharmacological treatments, practice guidelines, and educational programs have been developed for managing chronic diseases. With few exceptions, the interventions address isolated chronic diseases and take little account of the multimorbidity experienced by patients.

The increasing number of chronic conditions per patient and the increasing amount of multimorbidity in the elderly population lead to a more complex approach to successful treatment of hair problems in the elderly.

There is evidence that with age, the needs for types and quantities of nutrients may change, and it has been found that as many as 50 % of older adults have a vitamin and mineral intake less than the recommended dietary allowance and as many as 30 % of the elderly population have subnormal levels of vitamins and minerals. A physiologic decline in food intake is seen in people as they age, regardless of illness, and is often referred to as "anorexia of aging." It probably involves alterations in neurotransmitters and hormones that affect the central feeding drive and the peripheral satiation system. Moreover, sensory decline in both olfaction and taste decreases the enjoyment of food and dietary variety.

Socioeconomic status and functional ability have an important influence on nutritional status. When financial concerns are present, meals are skipped and food that is purchased may not provide a nutritionally adequate diet. Declines in both physical and cognitive functional status affect an individual's ability to shop for food and to prepare meals. Nutritional problems are further compromised by social isolation, which commonly leads to apathy about food and decreased intake.

The older person has experienced change and loss through retirement, disability and death of friends and family, as well as change in financial, social, and physical health status. These changes may lead to depression.

Depression is often unrecognized in older persons. Malnutrition may be a presenting symptom of depression in the elderly.

Ultimately, underlying pathology and medical treatment can cause anorexia and malnutrition. Problems with dentition and disorders of the gastrointestinal system are related to poor intake and malabsorption of nutrients. Many diseases (i.e., thyroid, cardiovascular, and pulmonary disease) lead to an increased metabolic demand and at the same time decreased appetite and caloric intake. Drugs may affect nutritional status through side effects (i.e., anorexia, nausea, and altered taste perception) and through alteration of nutrient absorption, metabolism, and excretion.

Some dimensions of aging naturally grow and expand over time, while others decline. Reaction time, for example, slows with age, while knowledge of world events and wisdom may expand. Steady decline in cognitive processes is seen across the lifespan, accelerating from the twenties or even thirties. Research has focused in particular on memory and has found decline of memory with aging, but not of general knowledge, such as vocabulary definitions, which typically increases or remains steady until the late adulthood.

In fact, research shows that even late in life, potential exists for mental and social growth and development.

Dementia (from "de-" = apart, away + "mens" (genitive: "mentis") = mind) is the progressive decline in cognitive function due to damage or disease in the body beyond what might be expected from normal aging. It represents a nonspecific set of symptoms in which affected areas of cognition may be memory, attention, language, and problem solving. Higher mental functions are affected first in the process, and in the later stages of the condition, affected persons may be disoriented in time, in place, and in person.

Some cases of dementia are due to specific disease processes that may be reversed with treatment. Therefore, routine blood tests are recommended to rule out treatable causes. These include vitamin B12, folic acid, thyroid-stimulating hormone (TSH), C-reactive protein (CRP), full blood count, electrolytes, calcium, renal function, liver enzymes, and syphilis serology.

Also mental illnesses, including depression and psychosis, may produce symptoms of the so-called pseudodementia, which must be differentiated from dementia. Chronic abuse of substances, such as alcohol, can also predispose to cognitive changes suggestive of dementia.

Neglect of hair and hair care in the elderly may be manifestations of dementia or of pseudodementia from depression, psychosis, or chronic alcoholism.

3.5.4 Ethnic Hair (Afro-Textured Hair)

Human hair has been classified into three major groups (African, Asian, Caucasian), as determined by ethnic origin. In these populations, structural and biochemical variations of the hair follicle and shaft are seen, as well as peculiar hair grooming practices. Both structural variations of hair and peculiarities in hair grooming practices are closely linked to specific disorders of the hair and scalp.

Androgenetic alopecia represents the single most frequent cause of hair loss in general, with a prevalence as high as 98 % and as low as 40 % depending on the study definitions.

The global incidence of androgenetic alopecia varies among ethnic groups with the greatest incidence in Caucasians, followed by Asians, African Americans, and Native Americans.

Afro-textured hair is the term used to refer to the natural texture of black African hair that has not been altered by hot combs, flat irons, or chemicals with the purpose of perming, relaxing, or straightening. Each strand of this hair type grows in a tiny, springlike helix shape. The overall effect is such that, despite relatively fewer hair shafts compared to straight hair, Afro-textured hair appears and feels denser than straight hair. The hair forms a mat of tightly interwoven hair shafts. For several reasons, possibly including its relatively flat cross section, this hair type conveys a dry or dull appearance.

A feature of Afro-textured hair is an apparent increased fragility of the hair shaft compared to other ethnic groups.

Using light (LM) and scanning electron microscopy (SEM), Khumalo et al. examined the structure of Afro-textured hair and effects of combing in black African volunteers. Hair samples were collected, by combing, from Africans and compared with those from Caucasian and Asian volunteers. The volunteers had never used chemical treatments, their hair had not been cut for at least 1 year, and grooming had been limited to shampooing, drying, and combing. More than 2,000 hairs in 12 African volunteers were examined by LM. The hairs appeared as a tight coiled springlike structure, and examination of hairs in situ showed interlocking of hair shafts. Many shafts exhibited knots (10–16 % versus 0.15 %) and appeared broken compared with hair shafts from the other ethnic groups. SEM of African hairs showed features consistent with repeated breaks of the shaft.

Since breakage of Afro-textured hair bears certain similarities to that observed in trichorrhexis nodosa from hair weathering and in trichothiodystrophy, a genetic disorder associated with reduced sulfur-rich proteins, Khumalo et al. compared the distribution of cystine-rich proteins in the hair of black Africans to that of Caucasian and Asian volunteers, plus patients with trichorrhexis nodosa and trichothiodystrophy, using transmission electron microscopy and specific silver stains. They found that the silver staining pattern of hair shafts of black Africans was similar to that observed in Caucasians, in Asians, and in individuals with trichorrhexis nodosa. The cuticular cells exhibited an electron-dense A layer and exocuticle, and in the cortex the microfibrils forming the macrofibers were outlined by electron-dense material. This contrasts with the abnormal distribution of the cystine-rich proteins seen in trichothiodystrophy. The study demonstrated no abnormality in the distribution of cystine-rich proteins in black African hair shafts compared to other ethnic groups.

The excessive structural damage observed in the African hair shafts is consistent with physical trauma (resulting from grooming) rather than an inherent weakness of the hair.

Besides hair breakage, the most common hair problems in women of color are traction alopecia (Fig. 3.5) and central centrifugal cicatricial alopecia (Fig. 3.6) and in men acne keloidalis nuchae (also known as dermatitis papillaris capillitii or folliculitis keloidalis nuchae, Fig. 3.7), dissecting cellulitis of the scalp (also known as perifolliculitis capitis abscedens et suffodiens of Hoffman, Fig. 3.8), and pseudofolliculitis barbae (razor bumps, Fig. 3.9).

Differences in the prevalence and severity of peculiar hair and scalp diseases in black Africans are related to structural variations of Afro-textured hair and peculiarities in hair grooming practices.

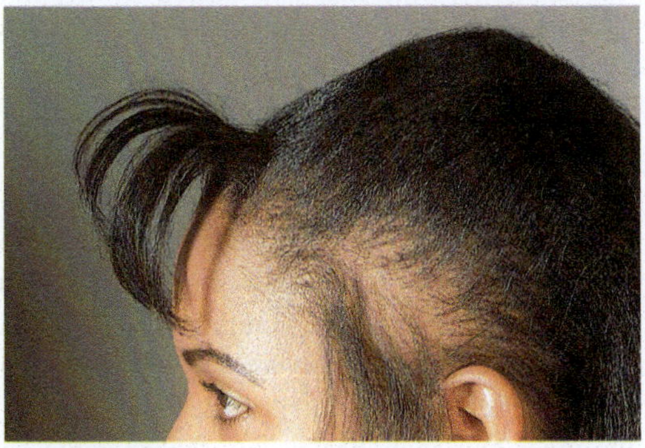

Fig. 3.5 Traction alopecia

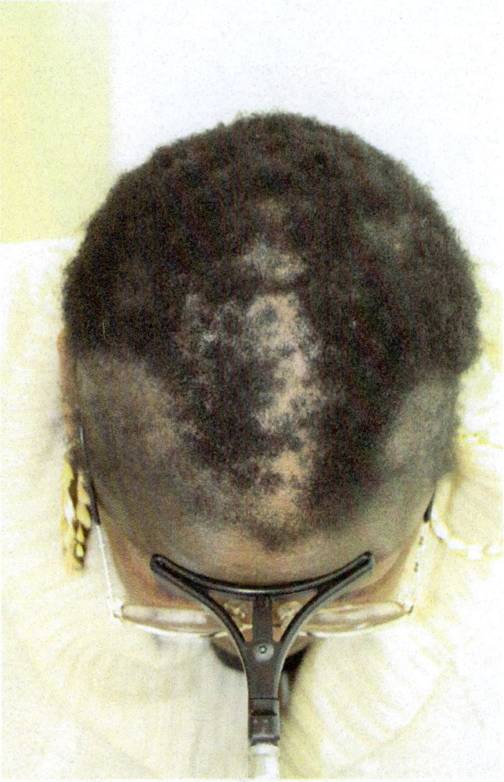

Fig. 3.6 Central centrifugal cicatricial alopecia

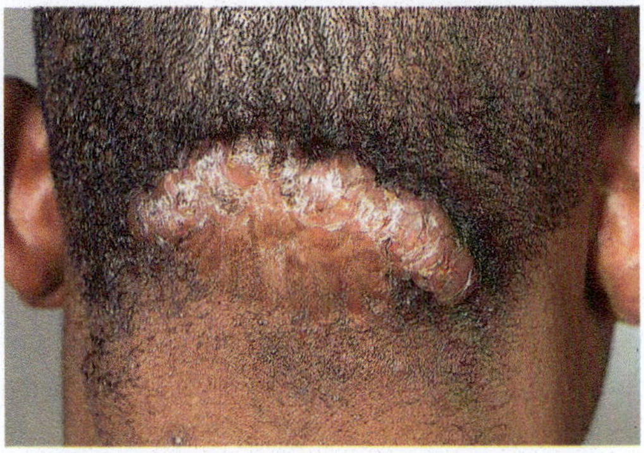

Fig. 3.7 Folliculitis keloidalis nuchae

Khumalo et al. found associations between specific scalp diseases, hairstyles, gender, and age. Therefore, effective treatment and prevention of these disorders involves behavioral modifications besides pharmacologic and procedural interventions.

In a study of 874 African adults in Cape Town, they found a prevalence of acne keloidalis nuchae

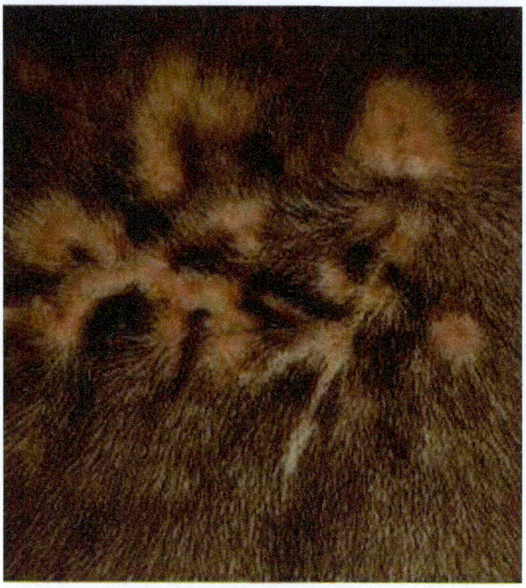

Fig. 3.8 Dissecting cellulitis of scalp

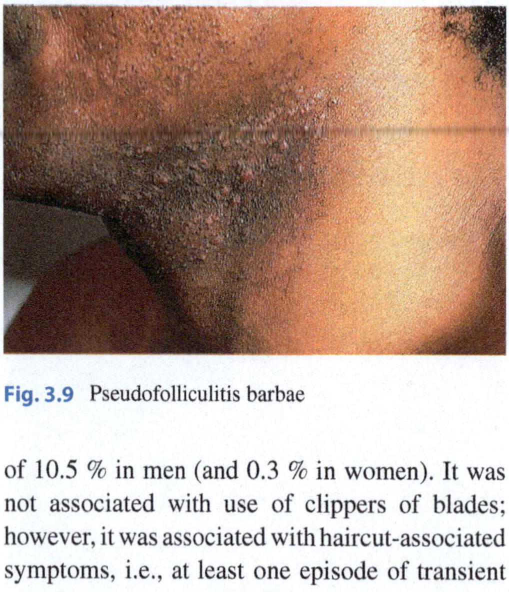

Fig. 3.9 Pseudofolliculitis barbae

of 10.5 % in men (and 0.3 % in women). It was not associated with use of clippers of blades; however, it was associated with haircut-associated symptoms, i.e., at least one episode of transient pimples or crusts and bleeding that were reported in 37 % and 18.9 % of men, respectively. Haircut-associated bleeding raises concern about the potential transmission of blood-borne infections, specifically HIV.

58.7 % of women had chemically treated hair, 49.2 % relaxed, and 9.6 % permed hair (versus 2.3 % men). The prevalences of traction alopecia and central centrifugal cicatricial alopecia were 31.7 % and 2.7 % in women (and 2.2 % and 0 % in men).

Traction alopecia prevalence was highest if the usual hairstyle was extensions attached to relaxed hair.

A cross-sectional study of 1,042 schoolchildren performed by Khumalo et al. included 45 % boys and 55 % girls. The majority of boys, 72.8 %, kept natural hair with frequent haircuts (within 4 weeks). The prevalence of acne keloidalis nuchae was 0.67 % in the whole group and highest (4.7 %) in boys in the final year of high school, all of whom had frequent haircuts.

The majority of girls (78.4 %) had chemically relaxed hair, which was usually combed back or tied in ponytails (versus 8.6 % of boys). Traction alopecia was significantly more common with relaxed than natural hair, with an overall prevalence of 17.1 % in girls, in whom it increased with age from 8.6 % in the first year of school to 21.7 % in the last year of high school. The proportion with traction in participants with a history of braids on natural hair was lower (22.9 %), but not significantly, than among those with a history of braids on relaxed hair (32.1 %). No cases of central centrifugal cicatricial alopecia were identified among schoolchildren.

Prevalence of central centrifugal cicatricial alopecia was highest in women over 50 years (6.7 %). Central centrifugal cicatricial alopecia was originally titled "hot comb alopecia" in 1968 and considered to be associated with excessive use of hot combs, as well as oil pomades and other hair care chemicals. It was thought that the oils applied to the hair and heated by the hot comb would travel down the hair shaft into the hair follicular unit opening and cause inflammation around upper follicles. However, it was later recognized that, while hot combing might elicit the condition in some individuals, central centrifugal cicatricial alopecia can also present in the absence of any cosmetic procedure. With this additional discovery, the condition was retitled "follicular degeneration syndrome" in 1992, and it was believed that premature desquamation of the inner hair root sheath, only recognizable on transversal hair section, was diagnostic of the condition, until in 1995 Gibbons and Ackerman challenged the condition to represent a discrete entity as well as the observation of premature desquamation of the inner hair root sheath to represent nothing more than a fixation artifact. Nevertheless, the condition has again been retitled "central centrifugal cicatricial alopecia" and included by the NAHRS in 2003 in the proposed working classification of primary scarring alopecias in the lymphocytic group.

Central centrifugal cicatricial alopecia tends to present itself in the 20s and progresses over the following 20–30 years.

> One should consider the possibility of central centrifugal cicatricial alopecia in African Americans with what appears to be female pattern hair loss.

The etiopathogenesis of central centrifugal cicatricial alopecia has only been postulated and so far remained elusive. However, one hypothesis involves pressure exerted on the internal root sheath leading to damage, which leads to the recruitment of inflammatory cells and the end result of scarring. African Americans are found to be at increased risk because of the curled hair shaft, distinct styling practices, and chemical processing techniques. Histopathologic features include perifollicular lymphocytic infiltrate, concentric lamellar fibrosis, sebaceous gland loss, and premature disintegration of the internal root sheath. Also, granulomatous inflammation secondary to follicular rupture may be noted.

To investigate medical and environmental risk factors for central centrifugal cicatricial alopecia, Kyei et al. performed a population study involving a quantitative cross-sectional survey of risk factors. A total of 326 African American women participated in the hair study.

> Diabetes mellitus type 2 was significantly higher in those with central centrifugal cicatricial alopecia, as were bacterial scalp infections and hairstyles associated with traction.

Lipedematous scalp (spongy scalp syndrome) represents yet another peculiar condition of the African scalp with or without associated alopecia (lipedematous alopecia). It is characterized by a thick boggy scalp and the complaint of itching, soreness, or tenderness. In one study of 31 cases, the majority of patients were females, suggesting an underlying hormonal pathology. An association with obesity suggested that anatomical differences can be present in lipid distribution. The histological finding of an increase in subcutaneous adipose tissue is notable. Dermal edema and lymphatic dilatation suggested the primary pathology is lymphatic. The etiopathogenesis of lipedematous scalp and alopecia remain unclear. Associated medical problems may be hyperelasticity of the skin and laxity of joints, renal failure, diabetes mellitus, and hyperlipidemia.

3.5.5 Transsexuals

Transsexualism is when an individual identifies with a gender inconsistent or not culturally associated with the assigned sex, i.e., in which a person's assigned sex at birth conflicts with their psychological gender. A medical diagnosis can be made if a person experiences discomfort as a result of a desire to be a member of the opposite sex or if a person experiences impaired functioning or distress as a result of that identification. The terms "gender dysphoria" and "gender identity disorder" were not used until the 1970s; "transsexualism" was replaced in the DSM-IV by "gender identity disorder in adolescents and adults." Male-to-female transsexualism has sometimes been called "Harry Benjamin's syndrome" after the endocrinologist who pioneered the study of dysphoria (Harry Benjamin, German-born, American endocrinologist and sexologist, 1885–1986).

According to DSM-IV (1994) roughly 1:30,000 assigned males seek sex reassignment surgery in the United States. The most frequently quoted estimate of prevalence is from the Amsterdam Gender Dysphoria Clinic. The data, spanning more than four decades in which the clinic has treated roughly 95 % of Dutch transsexual clients, gives figures of 1:10,000 among assigned males.

Sex reassignment therapy (SRT) is an umbrella term for all medical treatments related to sex reassignment of both transgender and intersex people. Psychological techniques that attempt to alter gender identity to one considered appropriate for the person's assigned sex are typically ineffective. The widely recognized standards of care note that sometimes the only reasonable and effective course of treatment for transsexual people is to go through SRT. Individuals make different choices regarding SRT, which can include hormone replacement therapy to modify secondary sex characteristics, sex reassignment surgery to alter primary sex characteristics, facial feminization surgery, permanent hair removal, and treatment of alopecia for trans women.

The need for treatment is emphasized by the high rate of mental health problems, including depression, anxiety, and various addictions, as well as a higher suicide rate among untreated transsexual people than in the general population.

Oral finasteride has been associated with inducing depression and anxiety in both male and female patients, symptoms that are very common in transsexuals, who are already at a high risk.

> As a result, prescription of oral finasteride for treatment of male androgenetic alopecia in male-to-female transsexuals may not be particularly useful or could put them at risk for emotional side effects.

Further Reading

Listening to the Patient

Cash TF (1992) The psychological effects of androgenetic alopecia in men. J Am Acad Dermatol 26:926–931

Cash TF (1999) The psychosocial consequences of androgenetic alopecia: a review of the research literature. Br J Dermatol 141:398–405

Maffei C, Fossati A, Rinaldi F, Riva E (1994) Personality disorders and psychopathologic symptoms in patients with androgenetic alopecia. Arch Dermatol 130:868–872

Mapar MA, Omidian M (2007) Is topical minoxidil solution effective on androgenetic alopecia in routine daily practice? J Dermatolog Treat 18(5):268–270

Neumann M, Scheffer C, Tauschel D, Lutz G, Wirtz M, Edelhäuser F (2012) Physician empathy: definition, outcome-relevance and its measurement in patient care and medical education. GMS Z Med Ausbild 29:Doc11

Nguyen T, Hong J, Prose NS (2013) Compassionate care: enhancing physician-patient communication and education in dermatology. Part I: patient-centered communication. J Am Acad Dermatol 68:353–360

Teutsch C (2003) Patient-doctor communication. Med Clin North Am 87:1115–1145

van der Donk J, Passchier J, Dutree-Meulenberg RO, Stolz E, Verhage F (1991) Psychologic characteristics of men with alopecia androgenetica and their modification. Int J Dermatol 30:22–28

Yamazaki M, Miyakura T, Uchiyama M, Hobo A, Irisawa R, Tsuboi R (2011) Oral finasteride improved the quality of life of androgenetic alopecia patients. J Dermatol 38:773–777

Educating the Patient

Hong J, Nguyen T, Prose NS (2013) Compassionate care: enhancing physician-patient communication and education in dermatology. Part II: patient education. J Am Acad Dermatol 68:364–373

Creating Reasonable Expectations

Jayasankar SJ Patient expectations: how do they matter? American Academy of Orthopedic Surgeons. www.aaos.org/news/aaosnow/mar09/managing6.asp

Keane Baker S Manage risk by managing patient expectations. American Academy of Orthopedic Surgeons. www.aaos.org/news/aaosnow/aug11/managing5.asp

Rawson E (1982) The life and death of Asclepiades of Bithynia. Class Q 1982;32: 358–370. www.wikipedia.org/wiki/Evidence-based_medicine

Satisfaction Survey

Keane Baker S Manage risk by managing patient expectations. American Academy of Orthopedic Surgeons. www.aaos.org/news/aaosnow/aug11/managing5.asp

Special Patient Groups

Abreu-Velez AM, Klein AD, Howard MS (2011) Survivin, p53, MAC, Complement/C3, fibrinogen and

HLA-ABC within hair follicles in central and centrifugal cicatricial alopecia. N Am J Med Sci 3(6):292–295

Alexis A, Heath CR, Halder RM (2014) Folliculitis keloidalis nuchae and pseudofolliculitis barbae: are prevention and effective treatment within reach? Dermatol Clin 32(2):183–191

Al-Fouzan AS, Nanda A (2000) Alopecia in children. Clin Dermatol 18(6):735–743

Al-Refu K (2013) Hair loss in children: common and uncommon causes; clinical and epidemiological study in Jordan. Int J Trichol 5(4):185–189

Altomare G, Capella GL (2002) Depression circumstantially related to the administration of finasteride for androgenetic alopecia. J Dermatol 29:665–669

Antaya RJ, Sideridou E, Olsen EA (2005) Short anagen syndrome. J Am Acad Dermatol 53(2 Suppl 1):S130–S134

Atton AV, Tunnessen WW Jr (1990) Alopecia in children: the most common causes. Pediatr Rev 12(1):25–30

Bodenheimer T (1999) Disease management: promises and pitfalls. N Engl J Med 340(15):1202–1205

Bukhari I, Al Mulhim F, Al Hoqail R (2004) Hyperlipidemia and lipedematous scalp. Ann Saudi Med 24(6):484–485

Butler DC, Heller MM, Murase JE (2014) Safety of dermatologic medications in pregnancy and lactation: part II. Lactation. J Am Acad Dermatol 70:417.e1–417.e10

Callender VD, Onwudiwe O (2011) Prevalence and etiology of central centrifugal cicatricial alopecia. Arch Dermatol 147(8):972–974

Castelo-Soccio L (2014) Diagnosis and management of alopecia in children. Pediatr Clin North Am 61(2):427–442

Claudet I, Cortey C, Honorat R, Franchitto N (2015) Minoxidil topical solution: an unsafe product for children. Pediatr Emerg Care 31(1):44–46

Cutrone M, Grimalt R (2005) Transient neonatal hair loss: a common transient neonatal dermatosis. Eur J Pediatr 164(10):630–632

Daveluy C, Pica L, Audet N, Courtemanche R, Lapointe F (2000) Enquête sociale et de santé 1998, 2nd edn. Institut de la statistique du Québec, Quebec City

Fu JM, Price VH (2009) Approach to hair loss in women of color. Semin Cutan Med Surg 28(2):109–114

Gathers RC, Jankowski M, Eide M, Lim HW (2009) Hair grooming practices and central centrifugal cicatricial alopecia. J Am Acad Dermatol 60(4):574–578

Gathers RC, Lim HW (2009) Central centrifugal cicatricial alopecia: past, present, and future. J Am Acad Dermatol 60(4):660–668

Georgala S, Befon A, Maniatopoulou E, Georgala C (2007) Topical use of minoxidil in children and systemic side effects. Dermatology 214(1):101–102

Gibbons G, Ackerman AB (1995) Resolving quandaries: follicular degeneration syndrome? Dermatol Dermatopathol Pathol Pract Concept 1:197–200

González M, Landa N, Gardeazabal J, Calderón MJ, Bilbao I, Díaz Pérez JL (1994) Generalized hypertrichosis after treatment with topical minoxidil. Clin Exp Dermatol 19(2):157–158

Guerouaz N, Mohamed AO (2014) Minoxidil induced hypertrichosis in children. Pan Afr Med J 18:8

Gupta R, High WA, Butler D, Murase JE (2013) Medicolegal aspects of prescribing dermatological medications in pregnancy. Semin Cutan Med Surg 32:209–216

Hale EK, Pomeranz MK (2002) Dermatologic agents during pregnancy and lactation: an update and clinical review. Int J Dermatol 41:197–203

Harrison S, Sinclair R (2003) Optimal management of hair loss (alopecia) in children. Am J Clin Dermatol 4(11):757–770

Holman H, Lorig K (2000) Patients as partners in managing chronic disease. Partnership is a prerequisite for effective and efficient health care. BMJ 320(7234):526–527

http://en.wikipedia.org/wiki/Afro-textured_hair

http://en.wikipedia.org/wiki/Ageing

http://en.wikipedia.org/wiki/Child

http://en.wikipedia.org/wiki/Transsexualism

Irwig MS (2012) Depressive symptoms and suicidal thoughts among former users of finasteride with persistent sexual side effects. J Clin Psychiatry 73:1220–1223

Janniger CK, Bryngil JM (1993) Hair in infancy and childhood. Cutis 51(5):336–338

Johnson KA, Bernard MA, Funderberg K (2002) Vitamin nutrition in older adults. Clin Geriatr Med 18:773–799

Kelly AP (2001) Pseudofolliculitis barbae and acne keloidalis nuchae. Dermatol Clin 21(4):645–653

Khumalo NP (2005) African hair morphology: macrostructure to ultrastructure. Int J Dermatol 44(Suppl 1):10–12

Khumalo NP (2010) Grooming and central centrifugal cicatricial alopecia. J Am Acad Dermatol 62(3):507–508

Khumalo NP (2012) Folliculitis keloidalis nuchae, bleeding from haircuts, and potential HIV transmission. Int J Dermatol 51(Suppl 1):21–23, 24–26

Khumalo NP, Dawber RP, Ferguson DJ (2005) Apparent fragility of African hair is unrelated to the cystine-rich protein distribution: a cytochemical electron microscopic study. Exp Dermatol 14(4):311–314

Khumalo NP, Doe PT, Dawber RP, Ferguson DJ (2000) What is normal black African hair? A light and scanning electron-microscopic study. J Am Acad Dermatol 43(5 Pt 1):814–820

Khumalo NP, Gantsho N, Gumedze F, Mthebe T (2013) Health risks of the clean-shave chiskop haircut. S Afr Med J 103(7):489–490

Khumalo NP, Gumedze F (2012) Traction: risk factor or coincidence in central centrifugal cicatricial alopecia? Br J Dermatol 2012167(5):1191–1193

Khumalo NP, Gumedze F, Lehloenya R (2011) Folliculitis keloidalis nuchae is associated with the risk for bleeding from haircuts. Int J Dermatol 50(10):1212–1216

Khumalo NP, Jessop S, Gumedze F, Ehrlich R (2007a) Hairdressing and the prevalence of scalp disease in African adults. Br J Dermatol 157(5):981–988

Khumalo NP, Jessop S, Gumedze F, Ehrlich R (2007b) Hairdressing is associated with scalp disease in African schoolchildren. Br J Dermatol 157(1):106–110

Khumalo NP, Pillay K, Ngwanya RM (2007c) Acute 'relaxer'-associated scarring alopecia: a report of five cases. Br J Dermatol 156(6):1394–1397

Kyei A, Bergfeld WF, Piliang M, Summers P (2011) Medical and environmental risk factors for the development of central centrifugal cicatricial alopecia: a population study. Arch Dermatol 147(8):909–914

Leachman SA, Reed BR (2006) The use of dermatologic drugs in pregnancy and lactation. Dermatol Clin 24:167–197

Lencastre A, Tosti A (2013) Role of trichoscopy in children's scalp and hair disorders. Pediatr Dermatol 30(6):674–682

Levy ML (1991) Disorders of the hair and scalp in children. Pediatr Clin North Am 38(4):905–919

LoPresti P, Papa CM, Kligman AM (1968) Hot comb alopecia. Arch Dermatol 98(3):234–238

Macieira-Coelho A (2003) Biology of aging, Progress in molecular and subcellular biology. Springer, Heidelberg, pp 50–52

Mkentane K, Maneli M, Khumalo NP, Davids LM, Freedom G (2014) Relaxers damage hair and increase fragility. Int J Dermatol 53(3):e200–e202

Murase JE, Heller MM, Butler DC (2014) Safety of dermatologic medications in pregnancy and lactation: part I. Pregnancy. J Am Acad Dermatol 70:4011.e1–4011.e14

Nnoruka EN, Obiagboso I, Maduechesi C (2007) Hair loss in children in South-East Nigeria: common and uncommon cases. Int J Dermatol 46(Suppl 1):18–22

Olsen EA, Bergfeld WF, Cotsarelis G et al (2003) Summary of North American Hair Research Society (NAHRS)-sponsored Workshop on Cicatricial Alopecia, Duke University Medical Center, February 10 and 11, 2001. J Am Acad Dermatol 48(1):103–110

Phillips TJ, Demarcay Z, Sahu M (2001) Hormonal effects on skin aging. Clin Geriatr Med 17:661–672

Price VH (1978) Disorders of the hair in children. Pediatr Clin North Am 25(2):305–320

Price VH, Gummer CL (1989) Loose anagen syndrome. J Am Acad Dermatol 20(2 Pt 1):249–256

Reed BR (1997) Dermatologic drugs, pregnancy, and lactation. A conservative guide. Arch Dermatol 133:894–898

Rodney IJ, Onwudiwe OC, Callender VD, Halder RM (2013) Hair and scalp disorders in ethnic populations. J Drugs Dermatol 12(4):420–427

Rojansky N, Fasouliotis SJ, Ariel I, Nadjari M (2002) Extreme caudal agenesis. Possible drug-related etiology? J Reprod Med 47:241–245

Rook A (1975) The clinical significance of abnormal hair-slope patterns-trichoglyphics. Br J Dermatol 92:239–240

Samlaska CP, Benson PM, James WD (1989a) The ridge-back anomaly. A new follicular pattern of the scalp. Arch Dermatol 125(1):98–102

Samlaska CP, James WD, Sperling LC (1989b) Scalp whorls. J Am Acad Dermatol 21:553–556

Sarifakioglu E, Yilmaz AE, Gorpelioglu C, Orun E (2012) Prevalence of scalp disorders and hair loss in children. Cutis 90(5):225–229

Sawin CT, Geller A, Herschman JE (1979) The aging thyroid: increased prevalence of elevated serum TSH levels in the elderly. JAMA 242:247–250

Scheufler O, Kania NM, Heinrichs CM, Exner K (2003) Hyperplasia of the subcutaneous adipose tissue is the primary histopathologic abnormality in lipedematous scalp. Am J Dermatopathol 25(3):248–252

Skelsey MA, Price VH (1996) Noninfectious hair disorders in children. Curr Opin Pediatr 8(4):378–380

Smorlesi C, Caldarella A, Caramelli L, Di Lollo S, Moroni F (2003) Topically applied minoxidil may cause fetal malformation: a case report. Birth Defects Res A Clin Mol Teratol 67:997–1001

Sperling LC, Sau P (1992) The follicular degeneration syndrome in black patients. 'Hot comb alopecia' revisited and revised. Arch Dermatol 128(1):68–74

Stroud JD (1983) Hair loss in children. Pediatr Clin North Am 30(4):641–657

Traish AM, Hassani J, Guay AT, Zitzmann M, Hansen ML (2011) Adverse side effects of 5α-reductase inhibitors therapy: persistent diminished libido and erectile dysfunction and depression in a subset of patients. J Sex Med 8:872–884

Tyler KH, Zirwas M (2013) Pregnancy and dermatologic therapy. J Am Acad Dermatol 68:663–671

van Kesteren PJ, Asscheman H, Megens JA, Gooren LJ (1997) Mortality and morbidity in transsexual subjects treated with cross-sex hormones. J Clin Endocrinol 47:337–343

Veyrac G, Chiffoleau A, Bailly C, Baudot S, Beaudouin S, Larousse C (1995) Cutaneous application of minoxidil during pregnancy: hairy infant. Therapie 50:474–476

Whiting DA, Olsen EA (2008) Central centrifugal cicatricial alopecia. Dermatol Ther 21(4):268–278

Wolff JL, Starfield B, Anderson G (2002) Prevalence, expenditures, and complications of multiple chronic conditions in the elderly. Arch Intern Med 162(20):2269–2276

Yasar S, Gunes P, Serdar ZA, Tosun I (2011) Clinical and pathological features of 31 cases of lipedematous scalp and lipedematous alopecia. Eur J Dermatol 21(4):520–528

The Difficult Dermatologic Condition

4

Wise to resolve, and patient to perform.
Homer

Clinical trichology should represent an integral part of medical training, and the dermatologist participates with the other medical disciplines in the diagnosis and treatment of all types of hair problems relating to systemic disease. On the other hand, hair loss is an important cause of discomfort and disability. The general physician is not always aware of the significance of hair loss and therefore may fail to refer patients with hair disorders to the dermatologist for appropriate management. Too often, the delay of correct diagnosis, and as a result the delay of appropriate therapy, leads to potentially irreversible loss of hair, prolongs the discomfort, and promotes the disfigurement. Knowledge of the main types of hair loss is prerequisite to providing appropriate patient care.

4.1 Congenital Atrichia and Hypotrichosis

By definition, alopecia is the acquired condition of recognizable hair loss. The term derives from Greek with reference to the loss of hair in patches in foxes afflicted with sarcoptic mange. In case of congenital absence or lack of hair, the correct terms are *atrichia* and *hypotrichosis*, respectively: While congenital atrichia is characterized by a total and permanent absence of hair, in congenital hypotrichosis the hair is diffusely thinned, but present.

> Hereditary and congenital hypotrichosis and atrichia are among the most complex areas of disorders of hair growth with several distinctive entities occurring either as an isolated defect or as a feature of a complex hereditary syndrome in association with other ectodermal defects (ectodermal dysplasia).

In 1998, Angela Christiano and coworkers reported the identification of a missense mutation in the zinc finger domain of the hairless (HR) gene (arg620 to gln) on chromosome 8p21.3 underlying *(congenital universal) atrichia with papular lesions*. Almost complete absence of hair associated with papular lesions over most of the body are features of the disorder (Fig. 4.1a). Patients are born with hair that falls out and is not replaced. Histological

R.M. Trüeb, *The Difficult Hair Loss Patient: Guide to Successful Management of Alopecia and Related Conditions*, DOI 10.1007/978-3-319-19701-2_4

studies show cystic malformation of the hair follicles. Although the identification of the HR gene has been shown not to be relevant with respect to the most frequent cause of hair loss and its treatment, androgenetic alopecia and alopecia areata, published estimates of the prevalence of congenital atrichia with papular lesions remain surprisingly low considering pathogenetic mutations of the HR gene have been found in distinct populations around the world.

Some experts have assumed that congenital universal atrichia might be more common than previously thought and frequently mistaken for the autoimmune form of alopecia (areata) universalis and suggested that infants with presumed autoimmune alopecia universalis may warrant testing for HR gene mutations, particularly before embarking on therapeutic modalities that will fail.

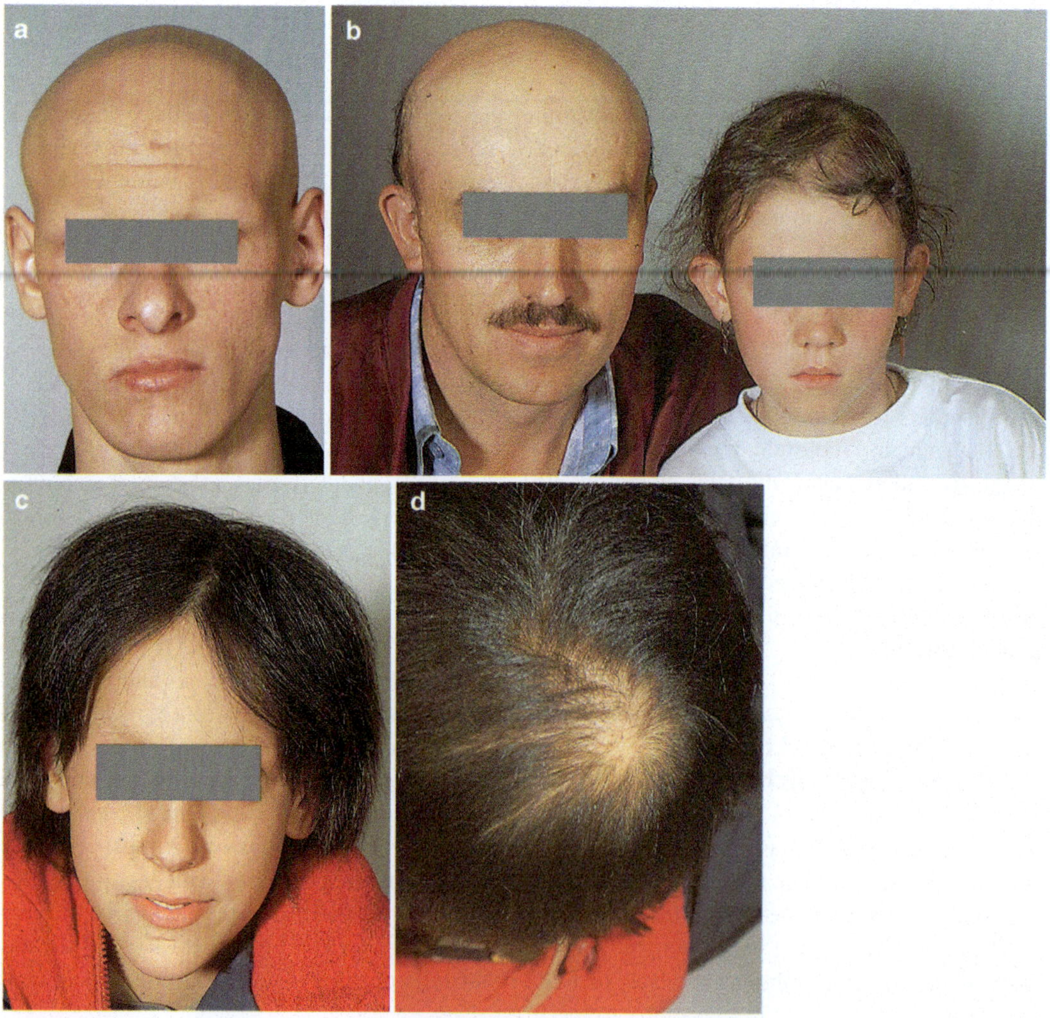

Fig. 4.1 (**a–d**) Congenital atrichia and hypotrichosis: (**a**) Congenital universal atrichia with papular lesions. (**b**) Hereditary hypotrichosis simplex in father and daughter. (**c**) Marie Unna hereditary hypotrichosis, coarse hair, (**d**) and initial vertex alopecia

Hereditary hypotrichosis simplex is a rare form of hereditary hypotrichosis with no associated abnormality or hair shaft anomaly. Affected individuals typically show normal hair at birth, but diffuse hair loss and thinning of the hair shaft start during early childhood and progress with age (Fig. 4.1b).

In contrast, *Marie Unna hereditary hypotrichosis* is distinguished by the presence of a peculiar twisting hair dystrophy. Characteristically coarse, wiry, twisted hair develops in early childhood and is followed by the development of alopecia beginning in the crown area (Fig. 4.1c, d).

Monilethrix represents another monogenic disorder presenting with hair loss. As opposed to hereditary hypotrichosis, loss of hair is due to a hair shaft abnormality with fragility and breakage. It is due to a disorder of hair cortex keratin resulting in brittle hair that tends to fracture and produce varying degrees of alopecia. Individuals with monilethrix have normal hair at birth but, within the first few months of life, sometimes later, develop alopecia. In the mildest forms, only the occipital regions of the scalp are involved, due the friction; however, in severe forms the eyebrows, eyelashes, and secondary sexual hair may also be involved. Follicular hyperkeratosis with predilection for the nape of neck is a consistent feature that is particularly helpful for initially suspecting the diagnosis (Fig. 4.2a). Light microscopic examination is diagnostic and reveals elliptical nodes of normal thickness and intermittent constrictions at which the hair easily breaks (Fig. 4.2b). There may be spontaneous improvement with time, especially during puberty, but the condition never resolves completely.

Localized autosomal recessive congenital hypotrichosis is yet one more form of monilethrix-like, congenital hypotrichosis caused by mutation in the desmoglein 4 gene that has more recently been recognized. The clinical presentation is more severe than in the autosomal dominant form of monilethrix, with more extensive alopecia of the scalp, and body, and a papular rash involving the extremities and periumbilical region.

Associated abnormal features of congenital atrichia or hypotrichosis (with or without hair shaft abnormality) may include dysplastic or brittle fingernails, skin and tooth defects, or other abnormalities that have to be sought for systematically (for an extensive list, see Online Mendelian Inheritance in Man).

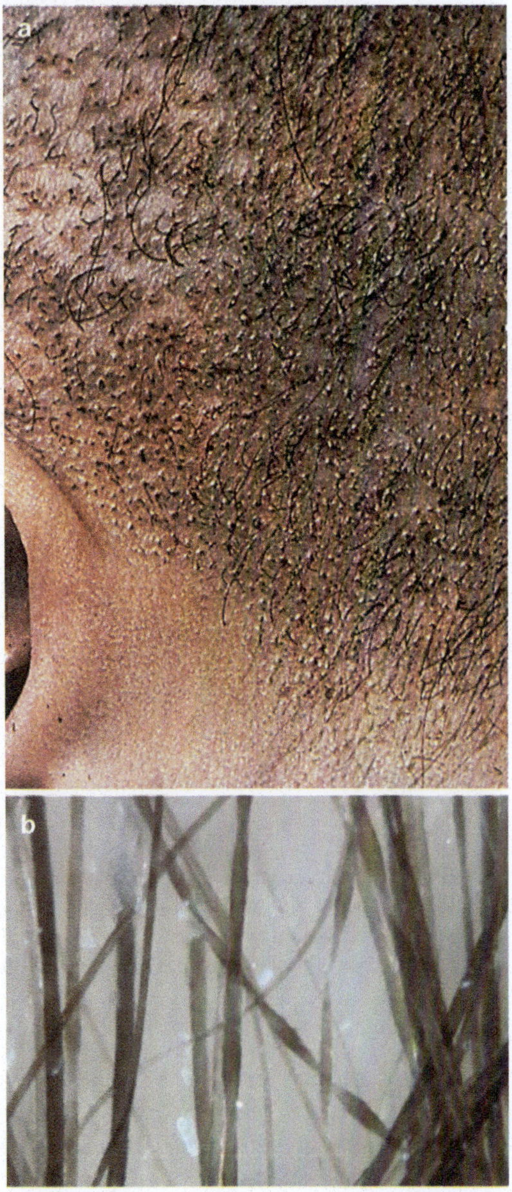

Fig. 4.2 (**a**, **b**) Monilethrix. (**a**) Follicular hyperkeratosis in the nape of the neck. (**b**) Dermoscopy: elliptical nodes of normal thickness and intermittent constrictions

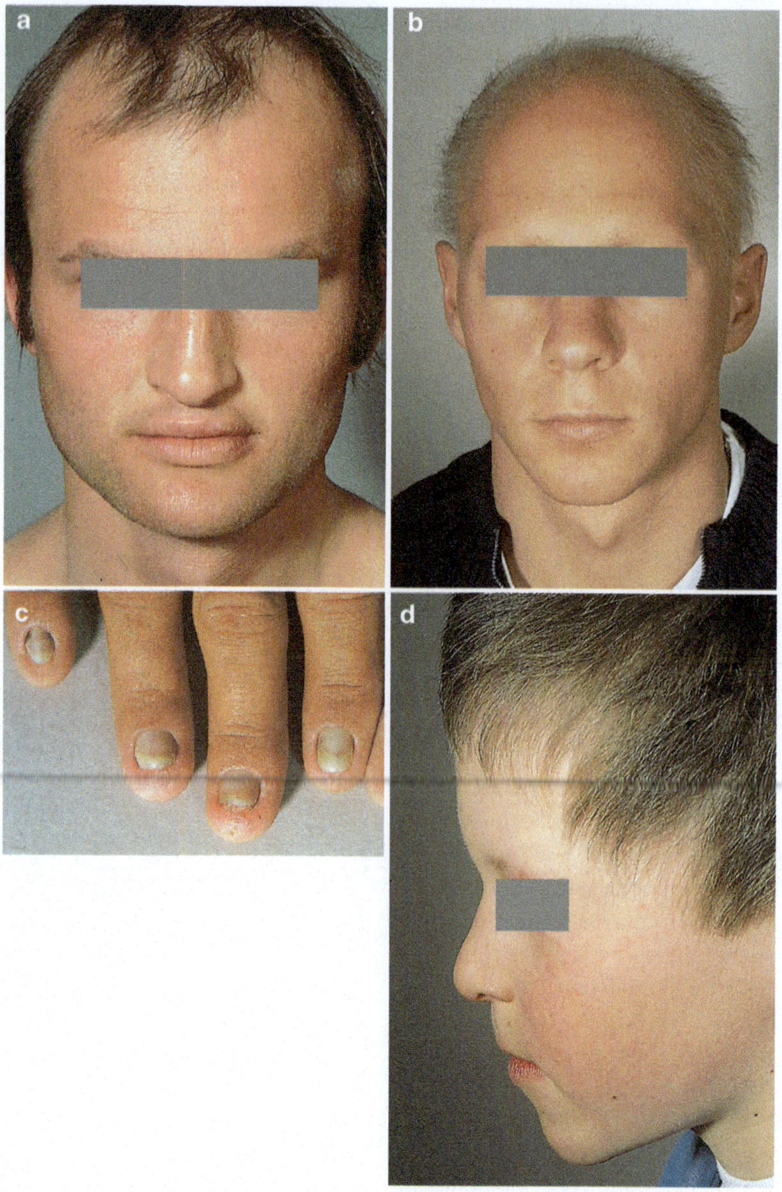

Fig. 4.3 (**a–d**) Ectodermal dysplasia: (**a**) Christ–Siemens–Touraine type (anhidrotic) with typical facies (frontal bossing, midfacial hypoplasia, saddle nose, large chin, and thick lips). (**b**) Clouston-type (hidrotic), with (**c**) associated nail abnormality (milky white in childhood, and gradually become dystrophic, thick, and distally separated from nail bed) (**d**) Rapp–Hodgkin syndrome, with coarse hair and midfacial hypoplasia

Typical examples include *X-linked recessive anhidrotic ectodermal dysplasia of Christ–Siemens–Touraine* (Fig. 4.3a) and *hidrotic ectodermal dysplasia of Clouston* (Fig. 4.3b, c). Also, the *Rapp–Hodgkin/Hay–Wells syndrome* shows characteristic features with coarse and sparse scalp hair, chronic inflammatory dermatitis of the scalp, midfacial hypoplasia, and cleft lip/palate (Fig. 4.3d), and the *trichorhinophalangeal syndrome* with fine and sparse scalp hair, a pear-shaped broad nose, and cone-shaped epiphyses of the middle phalanges (Fig. 4.4a, b).

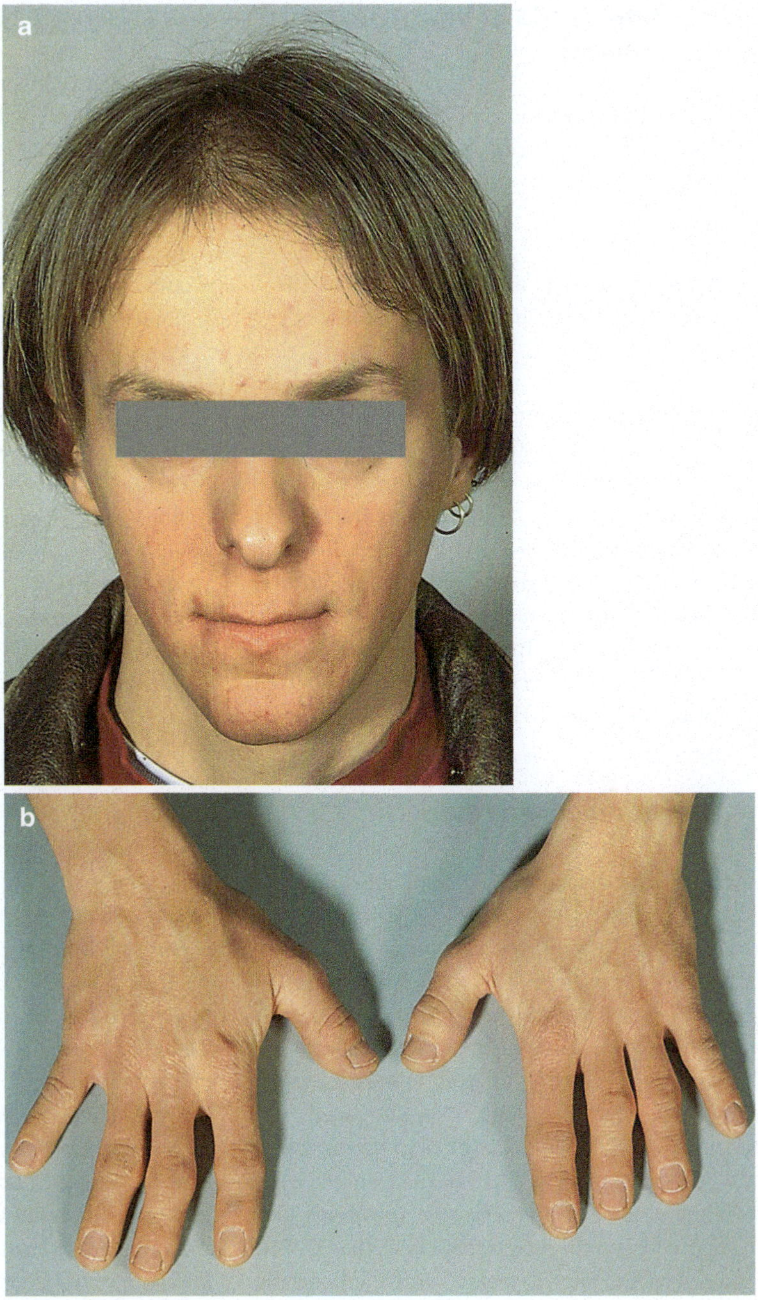

Fig. 4.4 (**a**, **b**) Trichorhinophalangeal syndrome. (**a**) Fine and sparse scalp hair, pear-shaped nose. (**b**) Cone-shaped epiphyses of the middle phalanges

> While in many of the congenital disorders of hair growth and/or structure, little more can be done than making the diagnosis and giving advice on genetic counseling and coping strategies, in others the genetic hair disorder may be a marker of more serious associated anomalies.

Examples are congenital sensorineural deafness associated with pili torti in *Bjornstad syndrome* and arrhythmogenic or dilated cardiomyopathy associated with woolly hair and palmoplantar keratoderma in *Naxos disease* and *Carvajal syndrome*, respectively, to name but a few.

4.2 Challenges in Non-scarring Alopecia

In daily clinical practice, we are usually dealing with the acquired disorders of hair growth and cycling.

> The non-scarring alopecias represent the most frequent cause of acquired hair loss.

While androgenetic alopecia (75 %), telogen effluvium (10 %), and alopecia areata (10 %) represent the most common causes in the adult population, alopecia areata (60 %), tinea capitis (20 %), and trichotillomania (10 %) are among the most frequent in children (in brackets are frequencies determined at the Hair Consultation Clinic of the Department of Dermatology, University Hospital of Zurich, between 1999 and 2010).

4.2.1 Androgenetic Alopecia

Androgenetic alopecia is the single most frequent cause of male and female hair loss. It is understood to represent a hereditary and androgen-dependent, progressive thinning of the scalp hair that follows a defined pattern, though there exist significant differences with respect to frequency, age of onset, and pattern of alopecia between male and female androgenetic alopecia. Androgenetic alopecia affects at least 50 % of men by the age of 50 years and up to 70 % of all males in later life, while estimates of its prevalence in women have varied widely. Recent studies claim that 6 % of women aged under 50 years are affected, increasing to a proportion of 30–40 % of women aged 70 years and over. While male pattern androgenetic is characterized by its typical bitemporal recession of hair and balding vertex, female pattern androgenetic alopecia is set apart by its diffuse thinning of the crown and intact frontal hairline. Nevertheless, 4 % of males may present with the female pattern of androgenetic alopecia, while 13 % of premenopausal women and 37 % of postmenopausal women present with the male pattern of androgenetic alopecia. Androgenetic alopecia that is clinically manifest between the ages of 10 and 20 is called premature alopecia or alopecia praecox. Before puberty it presents in both females and males exclusively with the female pattern.

> The diagnosis and treatment of androgenetic alopecia are relatively straightforward and easy, with 2 or 5 % topical minoxidil solution in men and in women and 1 mg oral finasteride in men having excellent evidence levels for their therapeutic use in androgenetic alopecia (either randomized, double-blind, comparative clinical studies of high quality, e.g., sample size calculation, flow chart of patient inclusion, ITT analysis, sufficient size, or meta-analysis, which includes at least one randomized double-blind, comparative clinical studies of high quality).

Minoxidil promotes hair growth through increasing the duration of anagen. It causes hair follicles at rest to grow and enlarges suboptimal follicles. Minoxidil was serendipitously discovered to be a hair growth-promoting agent, when patient taking the compound orally for treatment of arterial hypertension developed generalized hypertrichosis. Originally developed for treatment of androgenetic alopecia in men, topical minoxidil proves to be more effective in female androgenetic alopecia.

While the drug's action as a vasodilating agent is best understood, its mechanism of action on hair growth remained unclear. Only recently, with the discovery of the mutation underlying *hypertrichotic osteochondrodysplasia* or *Cantu's syndrome*, light has been shed on the molecular basis of the action of minoxidil. In Cantu's syndrome, the hypertrichosis leads to thick scalp hair extending onto the forehead and a general increase in body hair. It is caused by a mutation in the ABCC9 gene that codes for sulfonylurea receptor 2, involved in ATP-sensitive potassium channels, while minoxidil has been understood to be a potassium-channel opener, with evidence that this effect is mediated by sulfonylurea receptor 2B. Both the vasorelaxant and hair growth-promoting effects of minoxidil are due to the actions of its sulfated metabolite, minoxidil sulfate. Minoxidil is sulfated by a group of enzymes known as sulfotransferases, some of which are expressed in the hair follicle with wide interindividual variations in the level of enzyme activity.

> Recent studies have proposed that enzymatic assay of sulfotransferase activity in plucked hair follicles may predict response to topical minoxidil in the treatment of androgenetic alopecia. A subsequent analysis confirmed the clinical utility and validity of a sulfotransferase enzyme test in successfully ruling out 95.9 % of nonresponders to topical minoxidil for the treatment of androgenetic alopecia.

Finasteride is a competitive inhibitor of type 2 5-alpha reductase and inhibits the conversion of testosterone to dihydrotestosterone (DHT). The rationale for the use of finasteride to treat androgenetic alopecia in men is based on the absence of alopecia in men with congenital deficiency of type 2 5-alpha reductase and the presence of increased 5-α reductase activity and DHT levels in balding scalp. While oral finasteride has unanimously been shown to be effective in treatment of hair loss in men, its efficacy in women remains controversial: In a double-blind, placebo-controlled, multicenter trial, Price et al. demonstrated that oral finasteride, 1 mg/day, taken for 1 year did not slow progression of hair loss or promote hair growth nor improve follicular counts in horizontal sections of scalp biopsies in postmenopausal women with androgenetic alopecia. One explanation might be that the different pattern of hair loss in the majority of women from that usually seen in men may be due to differences in the relative levels of 5-α reductase, aromatase, and androgen receptors in scalp hair follicles in women compared with those in men. Thai and Sinclair were the first to report successful oral finasteride treatment of androgenetic alopecia in a postmenopausal woman with androgen levels within normal values. Trüeb et al. also reported successful treatment of androgenetic alopecia with 2.5 or 5 mg/day oral finasteride in 5 normoandrogenic, postmenopausal women. Improvement with growth of hair was observed as early as 6 months of therapy, irrespective of the pattern of hair loss. Efficacy was evaluated by patient and investigator assessments and review of photographs taken at baseline and at months 6, 12, and 18 by an expert panel. Finasteride treatment improved scalp hair by all evaluation techniques. The patients' self-assessment demonstrated that finasteride treatment decreased hair loss, increased hair growth, and improved appearance of hair. These improvements were confirmed by investigator assessment and assessments of photographs. No adverse effects were noted. Shum et al. reported four cases of hair loss with characteristics of both male and female pattern hair loss in women with hyperandrogenism, in which finasteride improved the alopecia. Their patients differed from those in the trial reported by Price et al. in that the patients had increased androgen levels, and finasteride was used in a slightly higher dose (1.25 mg/day) and given for a longer period of time (24–30 months as opposed to 1 year). On the other hand, Carmina and Lobo did not find finasteride, 5 mg/day, to be effective in treatment of alopecia in hyperandrogenic women. In the so far largest series of 37 premenopausal women treated for 1 year with finasteride in doses of 2.5–5 mg daily, Iorizzo et al. showed some improvement in 62 % as assessed by global photography.

> Differences in response of women to oral finasteride have led to the suggestion that not all types of female hair loss have the same pathophysiology, i.e., a distinction should be made between alopecia with early (premenopausal) or late (postmenopausal) onset and with or without hyperandrogenemia.

In an attempt to identify predictive factors for response of women with androgenetic alopecia to oral finasteride therapy, Keen and Goren aimed at analyzing the variant repeat nucleotide sequences in exon 1 of the androgen receptor (AR) gene that have been shown to determine androgen sensitivity in a variety of androgenic conditions in men and women. In a 6-month pilot study of 13 patients, women with greater androgen sensitivity (<24 cytosine, adenine, and guanine (CAG) repeats) were likely to have a significant response to finasteride 1 mg/day compared with patients treated with placebo and compared with patients with normal androgen sensitivity (≥24 CAG repeats) based on epigenetic weighted evaluation of the CAG alleles. Results of the present pilot study support the hypothesis that AR-CAG repeats, in conjunction with epigenetic factors, may help determine which women with hair loss will respond to finasteride therapy.

Finally, more recent studies demonstrated superiority of 0.5 mg oral dutasteride *versus* 1 mg oral finasteride in the treatment of male androgenetic alopecia.

Dutasteride is a dual inhibitor of 5-alpha reductase isotypes 1 and 2 (used for treatment of benign prostatic hyperplasia) and therefore capable of decreasing DHT levels to a greater extent than finasteride. A study performed by Gubelin Harcha et al. demonstrated efficacy and safety of 0.5 mg dutasteride in increasing hair growth and restoration in men with androgenetic alopecia while being well tolerated.

In another study performed by Jung et al., 0.5 mg dutasteride/day also proved to be effective in men with androgenetic alopecia recalcitrant to finasteride.

The plasma half-life time of dutasteride (3–5 weeks) is significantly longer than that of finasteride (age-dependent, from 5 to 8 h).

With respect to possible adverse effects related to therapeutic 5-alpha reductase inhibition, it may therefore be advisable to start patients on oral finasteride, and only if results are unsatisfactory at 6 months and tolerance is good, to switch from finasteride to dutasteride.

Olszewska and Rudnicka originally reported efficacy of 0.5 mg oral dutasteride for treatment of female androgenetic alopecia in a single case report: A 46-year-old female with androgenic alopecia, nonresponsive to minoxidil, who initially benefited from oral finasteride was switched to dutasteride due to only limited improvement under finasteride and persisting profound psychological distress resulting from the alopecia. Clinical evaluation and trichogram were applied for assessment of treatment. Additionally, mean hair diameter was monitored by means of computer-assisted dermoscopy. After 6 months of treatment, the authors noted significant improvement, and after 9 months the pattern hair loss was no longer recognizable. So far, efficacy of oral dutasteride for treatment of female androgenetic alopecia has not been confirmed in larger, and randomized, placebo-controlled trials.

Challenges in androgenetic alopecia are diagnosis and treatment of premature alopecia, early female androgenetic alopecia, androgenetic alopecia with comorbidities, and androgenetic alopecia with follicular microinflammation and fibrosis.

The first case series of premature alopecia in children in the age range from 6 to 10 years was reported by Tosti et al. Clinical examination showed hair loss with thinning and widening of the central parting of the scalp, both in boys and girls. There was a strong family history of androgenetic alopecia in all patients. All had normal physical development. In children and adolescents with early-onset alopecia, it is first important to differentiate if the hair loss is congenital or acquired. The differential diagnosis includes hypotrichosis simplex (without associated abnormalities) and ectodermal dysplasia (with associated delayed physical/psychological development, sweating, dental or nail abnormalities).

Premature androgenetic alopecia is an acquired hair loss with a characteristic pattern distribution and no associated abnormalities.

Therefore, it is important to assess the child's general health status, physical and mental development, and particularly early onset of puberty. Premature androgenetic alopecia without signs of premature puberty is usually not associated with endocrinological abnormalities; nevertheless, referral to a pediatric endocrinologist is recommended.

Efficacy and safety data for topical minoxidil solution are not available before the age of 18 years; therefore, treatment occurs at the discretion of the prescribing physician (off-label use).

> Systemic side effects of topical minoxidil (hypertrichosis and cardiovascular) are observed more frequently in children, especially at higher than the recommended dosages.

Nevertheless, treatment with topical 2 % minoxidil solution (before the age of 12 once daily, thereafter twice daily) is usually very effective.

Recognition of early female androgenetic alopecia may be challenging, when the patient complains of increased hair loss, but a widened hair part is yet not identifiable. At this stage, hair density is relative to the patient's prior assessment of her hair, and only longitudinal observation would reveal the evolution over time.

> Diversity of hair shaft diameter or anisotrichosis is an early diagnostic feature of androgenetic alopecia and is best appreciated in a central hair part with the dermatoscope.

Originally, Tosti et al. suggested that diversity of hair shaft diameter >20 % be diagnostic of androgenetic alopecia. Eventually, Rakowska et al. proposed more sophisticated criteria for diagnosis of female androgenetic alopecia based on dermoscopic findings:

Major criteria were (1) ratio of more than four empty follicles in four images (at 70-fold magnification) in the frontal area, (2) lower average thickness in the frontal area compared to the occiput, and (3) more than 10 % of thin hairs (<0.03 mm in diameter) in the frontal area.

Minor criteria were (1) increased frontal to occipital ratio of single-hair pilosebaceous units, (2) vellus hairs, and (3) peripilar signs.

Fulfillment of two major criteria or of one major and two minor criteria allows diagnosis of female androgenetic alopecia with a 98 % specificity.

Galliker and Trüeb performed a study to evaluate the value of trichoscopy as compared to the trichogram for the diagnosis of female androgenetic alopecia and found that trichoscopy is a valuable and superior method to the trichogram for diagnosis of female androgenetic alopecia, especially in early cases, with the highest yield irrespective of the formerly proposed cutoff of 20 % diversity of hair shaft diameter.

The coexistence of androgenetic alopecia with other morbid conditions may complicate the diagnosis, treatment, and course of androgenetic alopecia.

> It must be borne in mind that hair loss often does not result from a single cause effect, but from a combination of factors that all need to be addressed simultaneously for success.

Particularly in women, the coexistence with iron deficiency, thyroid dysfunction, endocrine disorders, and hormonal treatments (oral contraceptives, replacement treatments) has an impact.

In a landmark study on hormonal diagnostics in female androgenetic alopecia, Moltz investigated 125 women aged 18–68 years with clinically typical androgenetic alopecia. Atypical uterine bleeding, seborrhea, acne, and hirsutism were frequently observed. Pathologic changes of one biochemical parameter was detected in 22.4 %, while 67.2 % revealed deviations of two or more parameters. The incidence rates of pathologic parameters were as follows: ferritin = 42 %, prolactin = 34 %, estradiol (E2) = 34 %, free testosterone (fT) = 29 %, dihydrotestosterone (DHT) = 28 %, sex hormone-binding globulin (SHBG) = 26 %, thyroid-stimulating hormone (TSH) = 20.8 %, DHEA-sulfate (DHEAS) = 19 %, testosterone = 14 %, 17α-hydroxyprogesterone = 11 %, folate = 7 %, Δ_4-androstendione = 6 %, cortisol = 6 %, and vitamin B_{12} = 5 %.

Group and individual case analyses revealed significant correlations between the levels of the various androgens, prolactin, and TSH and the E2, sex hormone-binding globulin, and fT values; these in turn correlated with the occurrence of uterine bleeding anomalies (amount, duration, and interval) and resultant ferritin deficiency.

In a later study aiming at biochemical and trichological characterization of diffuse alopecia in women, Rushton et al. investigated one hundred women who presented with diffuse alopecia and compared them with 20 controls. In 40.9 % hormonal values were within control ranges. A raised DHT was found in 29.5 % and was the most frequently elevated androgenic finding. Thirty-four percent had changes in iron metabolism, while in 72.0 % serum ferritin levels were below the lowest control value. Taking high doses of multivitamins can influence iron absorption. According to Rushton a raised serum folic acid (>40 nmol/L) may indicate an excessive supplement intake. Rushton suggested that raised folic acid and vitamin B12 levels may induce excessive telogen hair shedding. On the other hand, vitamin B12 levels are adversely affected by cyproterone acetate/estradiol (CPA-E2) therapy; therefore, patients treated with CPA-E2 may require concurrent vitamin B12 supplementation in a suggested daily oral dosage of 100–200 µg to maintain their serum concentration levels above ideally 300 ng/L. With quantitative hair data available, no correlation between hormonal levels and any hair value was established.

The authors concluded that the endocrine dependence of diffuse alopecia appears to involve tissue dynamics such as receptor populations and binding protein phenomena, rather than specific levels of circulating hormones.

Diffuse alopecia was not significantly associated with any major endocrine disturbance; therefore, extensive laboratory investigations would seem unnecessary in the majority of women. However, a detailed hormonal profiling may be of value in women with marked bitemporal recession or when acne, hirsutism, or uterine bleeding anomalies coexist.

Finally, Schmidt et al. pointed out that androgen-dependent disorders of hair growth are due to more varied hormonal disturbances than elevated androgen serum levels alone. In view of the complex hormonal interactions between androgens, thyroid hormones, and prolactin, the thyrotropin-releasing hormone (TRH) stimulation test was performed in 38 female patients with androgen-induced alopecia, and the results were compared with those recorded in female control persons. The test is based on feedback mechanisms between hypothalamic TRH and hypophyseal TSH and prolactin and peripheral thyroid hormones. Baseline and stimulated TSH levels were significantly elevated. Therefore, hypothyroidism was recognized to be a significant contributing factor. In the case of prolactin, Schmidt et al. found stimulated levels also to be significantly elevated in the women with androgen-dependent alopecia. Orfanos and Hertel previously pointed out that functional hyperprolactinemia may yet be another cause of hair loss in women.

Hyperprolactinemia is the most frequent abnormality of the anterior pituitary gland. Clinical signs include inappropriate lactation, lack of menses, decreased libido, and infertility. General guidelines for diagnosing prolactin excess (hyperprolactinemia) define the upper threshold of normal prolactin at 25 µg/L for women. However, different methods for measuring prolactin are employed by different laboratories, and as such the serum reference range for prolactin is often determined by the laboratory performing the measurement. Furthermore, prolactin levels vary with age, sex, menstrual cycle stage, and pregnancy. The circumstances surrounding a given prolactin measurement (method and patient condition) must therefore be considered before the measurement can be accurately interpreted.

Diagnostic tests are useful when the probability of a disease being present is neither high nor low, since high degree of clinical certainty overrides the uncertainty of the laboratory data. The greater the number of different tests done, the greater the risk of getting false-positive or irrelevant leads. The possibilities for laboratory errors increase in the automated multiple-screen procedures. Therefore, remaining open-minded for the possibility of a multitude of cause-relationships underlying alopecia on the one hand, laboratory testing must be kept sharply focused on the other hand. Clinical suspicion is the determinant, and knowledge of clinical dermatology is the prerequisite for combining medical sense with economic sense in requesting the appropriate tests.

The most consistent of endocrinological abnormality associated with female androgenetic alopecia is polycystic ovary syndrome (PCOS). Originally described by Irving Stein and Michael Leventhal in 1935 in a case series of seven women with anovulation and polycystic ovaries discovered during surgery, the syndrome has most recently been defined by the Rotterdam criteria (Table 4.1). Given the broad definition described by the Rotterdam criteria, the prevalence of PCOS has been estimated to range from 15 to 18 %.

PCOS represents a complex disorder with several aberrant hormonal and metabolic pathways. Hyperandrogenism is one of the most important clinical features of the syndrome and the most relevant to the role of the dermatologist in

Table 4.1 2003 Rotterdam criteria for the diagnosis of polycystic ovary syndrome (PCOS)

1. *Oligo- or anovulation*
<9 menses a year or missed menses for ≥3 months
2. *Clinical and/or biochemical signs of hyperandrogenism*
Hirsutism, acne, alopecia
Serum levels of androgens, including androstenedione and testosterone, may be elevated. The free testosterone level is thought to be the best measure, with ca. 60 % of patients demonstrating elevated levels. Some other blood tests are suggestive but not diagnostic. The ratio of LH (luteinizing hormone) to FSH (follicle-stimulating hormone), when measured in international units, is elevated. Common cutoffs to designate abnormally high LH/FSH ratios are 2:1 or 3:1 as tested on day 3 of the menstrual cycle
3. *Echogenic evidence of polycystic ovaries and exclusion of other causes of hyperandrogenism and anovulation*
Polycystic ovaries on ultrasound are defined by the presence of >12 follicles in each ovary (each follicle measuring 2–9 mm in diameter) and/or increased ovarian volume of >10 mL
Differential diagnosis of PCOS (laboratory evaluation): pregnancy (elevated serum or urine HCG), premature ovarian failure (elevated FSH and LH, low-normal estradiol levels), hypothyroidism (elevated TSH, low thyroxine levels), hyperprolactinemia (elevated prolactin level), late-onset congenital adrenal hyperplasia (elevated day 5 morning level of 17 hydroxyprogesterone), virilizing ovarian/adrenal tumor (total testosterone >200 ng/dL, DHEAS >700 μg/L, and elevated androstenedione), Cushing's syndrome (elevated 24-h urinary free cortisol level, unsuppressed morning serum cortisol during the low-dose dexamethasone suppression test, and elevated midnight salivary cortisol)
Requires 2 out of 3 for diagnosis of PCOS

diagnosis and management of the condition. Up to 60 % of women with PCOS have hirsutism, frequently seen on the upper lip, chin, areola, chest, back, and lower abdomen. Acne is another common cutaneous manifestation of hyperandrogenism in PCOS. Acne that originates or persists into adulthood and that is refractory to conventional treatment should raise suspicion to underlying PCOS. Compared with pubertal acne, women with PCOS tend to have more inflammatory lesions, especially on the lower face, neck, chest, and upper aspect of the back. Since

19–37 % of women with moderate to severe acne meet the diagnostic criteria for PCOS, these patients need to be investigated for PCOS.

> Among women with PCOS, alopecia is a less frequent manifestation of hyperandrogenism than hirsutism and acne, though it responds less well to topical minoxidil than in female androgenetic alopecia that is not associated with PCOS, and therefore should be treated with combined antiandrogen therapy.

Most importantly, PCOS presents with potentially serious systemic long-term implications, including risks of metabolic syndrome and of endometrial carcinoma. PCOS is associated with several metabolic complications, including obesity, metabolic syndrome, and insulin resistance. Obesity is present in 75 % of women with PCOS, and up to 47 % of women with PCOS have metabolic syndrome. The diagnostic criteria for metabolic syndrome are summarized in Table 4.2.

Insulin resistance is common among patients with PCOS independent of obesity. The cutaneous signs of hyperinsulinemia include acanthosis nigricans and acrochordons. Insulin plays an important role in the development of anovulation and hyperandrogenism, which explains the ability of insulin-sensitizing agents, such as metformin, to lower androgen levels and induce ovulation.

Women with PCOS have an increased risk of cardiovascular disease; however, it is not clear whether PCOS is an independent risk factor or whether cardiovascular disease results from the comorbidities associated with PCOS. In general, patients should be closely monitored and managed for obesity, diabetes, hyperlipidemia, and hypertension.

Table 4.2 Diagnostic criteria for metabolic syndrome (Adult Treatment Panel III)

Requires >3 of the following criteria
Waist circumference >88 cm
Triglyceride level ≥150 mg/dL
High-density lipoprotein (HDL) cholesterol <50 mg/dL
Blood pressure ≥130/85
Fasting glucose level ≥100 mg/dL

Treatment of PCOS includes weight loss, exercise, glucose control, combined oral contraceptives and antiandrogen agents (cyproterone acetate, drospirenone), insulin-sensitizing drugs (metformin), and topical therapies for hair removal (laser hair removal, topical eflornithine), acne (standard dermatologic therapies), and hair growth (topical minoxidil), as needed.

Although combined oral contraceptive pills are widely considered first-line therapy in PCOS, a drawback may be metabolic side effects and risk of thromboembolism. The current recommendation suggests low-dose ethinyl estradiol (<50 μg), avoiding androgenic progestins, and addition of metformin to offset insulin resistance.

> There has been significant recent media discussion regarding venous thromboembolic events in conjunction with drospirenone use.

Relative to nonusers, drospirenone increases venous thromboembolus risk 6.3-fold, levonorgestrel 3.6-fold, gestodene 5.6-fold, cyproterone acetate 6.8-fold, and desogestrel 7.3-fold. The absolute venous thromboembolus risk of drospirenone-containing oral contraceptive pills is 23–137 events/100,000 women-years, and comparatively risk in pregnancy 199.7 events/100,000 women-years.

> The observation that many women show increased shedding of hair from 2 weeks to 3–4 months after they stop taking an oral contraceptive probably simulates that which is commonly seen after parturition.

During the second half of pregnancy, the percentage of anagen hairs increases from the normal 85–95 %, at this time also the percentage of hairs of large shaft diameter is higher than in nonpregnant women of the same age. After partuition the follicles, in which anagen has been prolonged, rapidly enter catagen and then telogen, with an increased shedding of hair evident after 3–4 months (postpartum effluvium). Most women will return to their usual hair growth cycle between 6 and 12 months after birth. Postpartum hair loss usually returns the hair to pre-pregnancy thickness, unless it leads over to female androgenetic alopecia. In case of persistent postpartum effluvium (>12 months), excessive hair loss may be caused by common conditions, such as female androgenetic alopecia, iron deficiency, or hypothyroidism. Lesser common conditions include persistent hyperprolactinemia (Chiari–Frommel syndrome) and postpartum hypopituitarism (Sheehan syndrome) caused by pituitary necrosis due to blood loss and hypovolemic shock during childbirth.

More frequently, contraceptive pills or hormone replacement therapies with progestogens that possess net androgenic activity, such as norethisterone, levonorgestrel, and tibolone, induce hair loss in genetically predisposed women.

It has been proposed that in the presence of a genetic susceptibility, it is the estrogen to androgen ratio that might be responsible for triggering hair loss in women. In the same line is the observation of hair loss induced in the susceptible women by treatment with tamoxifen or with the aromatase inhibitors letrozole, anastrozole, and formestane for breast cancer.

Besides the aforementioned comorbid conditions, lifestyle factors, such as malnutrition, obesity, smoking, exposure to ultraviolet radiation (UVR), and stress, may play an additional role.

The quantity and quality of hair are closely related the nutritional state of an individual. Normal supply, uptake, and transport of proteins, calories, trace elements, and vitamins are of fundamental importance in tissues with a high biosynthetic activity such as the hair follicle. Because hair shaft is composed almost entirely of protein, protein component of diet is critical for production of normal healthy hair. The rate of mitosis is sensitive to the calorific value of diet, provided mainly by carbohydrates stored as glycogen in the outer hair root sheath of the follicle. Finally, a sufficient supply of vitamins and trace metals is essential for the biosynthetic and energetic metabolism of the follicle.

Debate exists regarding protein intake requirements. The amount of protein required in an individual's diet is determined by overall energy intake, the body's need for nitrogen and essential amino acids, body weight and composition, rate of growth of the individual, physical activity level, individual's energy and carbohydrate intake, and presence of illness or injury. Physical activity and exertion as well as larger muscular mass increase the need for protein. Requirements are also higher during childhood for growth and development, during pregnancy and lactation, or when the body needs to recover from malnutrition, trauma, or after an operation. In case of lack of energy through nutrition, the body utilizes protein from the muscle mass to meet energy needs, eventually leading to muscle wasting. If the individual's intake of protein is inadequate, then the muscle will also waste as more vital cellular processes, such as respiration enzymes and blood cells, recycle muscle protein for their proper requirements. Recommended dietary allowance in grams of protein needed per day are listed in Table 4.3.

Table 4.3 Recommended dietary allowance in grams of protein per day

Children ages 1–3 years	13 g of protein per day
Children ages 4–8 years	19 g of protein per day
Children ages 9–13 years	34 g of protein per day
Girls ages 14–18 years	46 g of protein per day
Boys ages 14–18 years	52 g of protein per day
Women ages 19–70+ years	46 g of protein per day
If pregnant or breastfeeding	71 g of protein per day
Men ages 19–70+ years	56 g of protein per day

The generally accepted daily protein dietary allowance, measured as intake per kilogram of

Table 4.4 Micronutrients relevant to the hair and recommended daily allowances

Vitamins
B vitamins
Biotin (vitamin H): 300 µg
Niacin (vitamin B3): 20 mg
Folic acid: 300 µg
Riboflavin (vitamin B2): 1.7 mg
Pantothenic acid (vitamin B5): 5 mg
Pyridoxine (vitamin B6): 1.5 mg
Cyanocobalamin (vitamin B12): 3 µg
Antioxidants
Vitamin A/beta-carotene: 6 mg
Alpha-tocopherol (vitamin E): 10 IU
Trace metals
Iron: depending on age and sex (in men: 8–10 mg)
Zinc: 15 mg
Selenium: 50 µg

body weight, is 0.8 g/kg. However, this recommendation is based on structural requirements but disregards the use of protein for energy metabolism. This requirement is for a normal sedentary person, while several studies have come to the conclusion that active people and athletes may require more elevated protein intake due to increase in muscle mass and sweat loss, as well as need for body repair, and energy source. Suggested amounts vary between 1.6 and 1.8 g/kg, while a proposed maximum daily protein intake would be at least 10 %, but not more than 35 % of energy requirements, i.e., approximately 2–2.5 g/kg.

Micronutrients relevant to the hair and their recommended daily allowances are listed in Table 4.4.

It appears that on a typical Western diet, the hair follicle should have no problem in producing an appropriate hair shaft.

Nevertheless, vitamin and nutritional deficiencies are not uncommonly observed in adolescent females and young women with eating disorders (anorexia and bulimia nervosa) and are especially common in the elderly population.

In general, malnutrition is due to one or more of following factors: inadequate food intake, food choices that lead to dietary deficiencies, and illness that causes increased nutrient requirements, increased nutrient loss, poor nutrient absorption, or a combination of these factors.

Obesity is a risk factor for multiple health problems. In a cross-sectional study conducted in Taiwan, the authors attempted to determine the association between body mass index (BMI) and alopecia severity in men with male pattern androgenetic alopecia. The medical charts and photographs of 189 men with a clinical diagnosis of male pattern androgenetic alopecia were reviewed. The men had a mean age of 30.8 years. In those with male pattern androgenetic alopecia ($n=142$), men with severe alopecia (grades V–VII) had higher BMI than those with mild to moderate alopecia (grades I–IV) (25.1 vs. 22.8 kg/m^2, $p=0.01$). After multivariate adjustments, the risk for severe alopecia was higher in the overweight or obese (BMI ≥24 kg/m^2) subjects with androgenetic alopecia (odds ratio 3.52, $p<0.01$). In early-onset male pattern androgenetic alopecia ($n=46$), the risk for having severe alopecia was also higher in the overweight or obese subjects (odds ratio 4.97, $p=0.03$).

The authors concluded that higher BMI was significantly associated with greater severity of hair loss in men with male pattern androgenetic alopecia, especially in those with early-onset androgenetic alopecia.

Since previous investigations had revealed an association of severe early-onset androgenetic alopecia with ischemic heart disease, Hirsso et al. examined the possible association between early-onset alopecia and low-grade inflammation measured by high-sensitivity C-reactive protein (hs-CRP) that has been recommended for the assessment of the cardiovascular disease risk. The study population consisted of 727 young Finnish men, aged 25–34 years, participating in a national survey. The grade of alopecia was assessed by a trained nurse using the Hamilton–Norwood

Classification Scale. Men with moderate to extensive alopecia (17 %) had a BMI and larger waist, upper arm, hip and waist circumference than those with little to no alopecia ($p<0.05$), and statistically insignificant differences were seen in the waist-to-hip circumference ratio (WHR), diastolic blood pressure, and hs-CRP. With increasing hs-CRP, the mean WHR increased, but only among men with moderate to extensive alopecia ($p=0.043$).

The authors concluded that there is a relation between moderate to extensive alopecia and low-grade inflammation, a predictor of a future cardiovascular disease, especially combined with central obesity, among men younger than 35 years.

Ultimately, a study was performed to analyze the presence of cardiovascular risk factors included in the Adult Treatment Panel III criteria for metabolic syndrome, the prevalence of carotid atheromatosis, hormonal (aldosterone, insulin, testosterone, and sex hormone-binding globulin) factors, and acute phase reactant (C-reactive protein, fibrinogen, D-dimers, erythrocyte sedimentation rate) variables in male and female patients with androgenetic alopecia and in a control group and to analyze differences among the groups. The case–control study included 154 participants, 77 with early-onset androgenetic alopecia (40 males and 37 females) and 77 healthy control subjects (40 males and 37 females) from the Department of Dermatology at a University Hospital in Granada, Spain. Metabolic syndrome was diagnosed in 60 % of male patients with androgenetic alopecia (odds ratio [OR] = 10.5, 95 % confidence interval [CI] 3.3–32.5), 48.6 % of female patients with androgenetic alopecia (OR = 10.73, 95 % CI 2.7–41.2), 12.5 % of male control subjects, and 8.1 % of female control subjects ($p<0.0001$). Atheromatous plaques were observed in 32.5 % of male patients with androgenetic alopecia (OR = 5.93, 95 % CI 1.5–22.9) *versus* 7.5 % of male control subjects ($p=0.005$) and 27 % of female patients with androgenetic alopecia (OR = 4.19, 95 % CI 1.05–16.7) *versus* 8.1 % of female control subjects ($p=0.032$). Aldosterone and insulin levels were significantly higher in the male and female patients with androgenetic alopecia *versus* their respective control subjects. Mean values of fibrinogen were significantly higher in male patients with androgenetic alopecia, whereas values of fibrogen, C-reactive protein, and D-dimers were significantly higher in female patients with androgenetic alopecia *versus* their respective control subjects. The authors concluded that the determination of metabolic syndrome and ultrasound study of carotid arteries may be useful screening methods to detect risk of cardiovascular disease in male and female patients with early-onset androgenetic alopecia and signal a potential opportunity for early preventive treatment.

Finally, Starka et al. suggested that premature androgenetic alopecia and insulin resistance are a clinical constellation that may represent the male homologue or phenotype of polycystic ovary syndrome. Because of its association with metabolic syndrome and altered glucose metabolism, both men and women with early androgenetic hair loss should be screened for impaired glucose tolerance and diabetes mellitus II.

Besides being the single most preventable cause of significant cardiovascular and pulmonary morbidity and an important cause of death in the general population, tobacco smoking has been associated with various adverse effects on the skin and hair. Premature skin aging has attracted the attention of the medical community only since the 1960s, although a relation between smoking and skin complexion was first suggested as early as 1856. In 1996, Mosley and Gibbs originally reported a significant relationship between smoking, premature gray hair, and baldness in patients visiting a general surgical outpatient clinic in the United Kingdom. Subsequently, Trüeb's observation of strikingly dissimilar androgenetic alopecia in a 52-year-old monozygotic male twin pair led to further speculations on the possibility of an association between smoking and hair loss, since studies on the degree of alopecia among monozygotic twins aged over 50 have shown that intrapair differences are negligible in 92 %, slight in 8 %, and striking in none. A salient feature differing the twin brothers in their personal histories was that the balding brother admitted to long-standing, heavy cigarette smoking, while the other was a nonsmoker. Eventually, a population-based cross-sectional survey among Asian men 40 years or older showed statistically significant positive associations between moderate or severe androgenetic alopecia and smoking status, current cigarette smoking of 20 cigarettes or more per day, and smoking intensity. The odds ratio of early-onset history for androgenetic alopecia grades increased in a dose–response pattern. Risk for moderate or severe androgenetic increased for family history of first-degree and second-degree relatives, as well as for paternal relatives.

The mechanisms by which smoking accelerates hair loss have not been examined, but are believed to be multifactorial and related to effects of cigarette smoke on the microvasculature, cutaneous collagen, and elastic tissue, to pro-oxidant effects of smoking, and to increased hydroxylation of estradiol, as well as inhibition of the enzyme aromatase, which converts androgens to estrogens, creating a relative hypoestrogenic state. Evidence of the consequence of impaired circulation and wound healing is a higher complication rate of hair restoration surgery in smokers *versus* nonsmokers. Besides inducing local ischemia, the decreased capillary blood flow in the dermal papilla of the hair follicles may focally shunt more toxic substances. Cigarette smoke contains over 4800 chemicals, many of which are known to be toxic to cells and 69 are known to cause cancer. Both nicotine and cotinine are detected in hair samples of smokers. Smoke genotoxicants metabolized in hair follicle cells may cause DNA damage through the production of DNA adducts, and smoking-associated mitochondrial DNA mutations have been shown in human hair follicles, though the relevance of these for hair follicle pathology is as yet unknown. Since substantial extracellular matrix remodeling is involved in the hair follicle growth cycle, especially during catagen-associated hair follicle regression, it is conceivable that cigarette smoke-induced imbalance in the intra- and perifollicular protease/antiprotease systems controlling tissue remodeling may also affect the hair follicle growth cycle. Finally, smoking-induced oxidative stress and a disequilibrium of antioxidant systems may lead to the release of proinflammatory cytokines from follicular keratinocytes, which by themselves have been shown to inhibit the growth of isolated hair follicles in culture.

The fact that cigarette smoke-associated hair loss is of the androgenetic type indicates that genetic factors contribute. On the other hand, recent studies on the evolution of androgenetic hair loss have focused on oxidative stress: Naito et al. analyzed the effect of the lipid peroxides on hair follicles and observed that the topical application of linolein hydroperoxides, one of the lipid peroxides, leads to the early onset of the catagen phase in murine hair cycles. Furthermore, they found that lipid peroxides induced apoptosis of hair follicle cells. They also induced apoptosis in human epidermal keratinocytes by upregulating apoptosis-related genes. These results indicate that lipid peroxides, which can cause free radicals, induce the apoptosis of hair follicle cells, and this is followed by early onset of the catagen phase.

Ultimately, Bahta et al. cultured dermal hair papilla cells (DPCs) from balding and non-balding scalp and demonstrated that balding DPCs grow slower in vitro than non-balding DPCs. Loss of proliferative capacity of balding DPCs was associated with changes in cell morphology, expression of senescence-associated beta-galactosidase, decreased expression of proliferating cell nuclear antigen and Bmi-1, upregulation of p16(INK4a)/pRb, and nuclear expression of markers of oxidative stress and DNA damage including heat shock protein-27, superoxide dismutase catalase, ataxia-telangiectasia-mutated kinase (ATM), and ATM- and Rad3-related protein.

The finding of premature senescence of balding DPC in vitro in association with expression of markers of oxidative stress and DNA damage suggests that balding DPCs are particularly sensitive to environmental stress.

While the consequences of yet another environmental stress, namely, sustained UVR on unprotected skin, are well appreciated, mainly photocarcinogenesis and solar elastosis, the effects of UVR on the evolution of androgenetic alopecia have only recently found attention.

However, some clinical and morphological observations suggest that UVR has some negative effect on hair growth.

Camacho et al. originally reported a peculiar type of telogen effluvium following sunburn of the scalp after 3–4 months with hairstyles that left areas of scalp uncovered during prolonged sun exposure. The clinical features were increased frontovertical hair shedding along with a trichogram that disclosed an increase of telogen hairs and dystrophic hairs. In women the hairs on the frontal region appeared unruly, and the frontovertical alopecia showed loss of the frontal hair implantation line.

The pathomechanism of this type of telogen effluvium is not clear. It has been proposed that the columns of the cells in the hair shaft act as an efficient fiber-optic-type system, transmitting UV light downward into the hair follicle. Morphologically, the keratinocytes within the hair shaft are arranged in compressed linear columns that resemble the coaxial bundles of commercial fiber-optic strands. Thus, hair follicular melanocytes located in the region of the hair matrix may function as UV biosensors and respond to photic inputs. Depending on the quantity of UVR exposure, it is conceivable that also photodamage may occur at this site, resulting in telogen effluvium.

Histopathologically, elastosis is regularly found in scalp biopsies, especially in alopecic conditions, but so far has largely been ignored. Up to date, no controlled study has been performed on the degree of scalp elastosis in relation to the pace of development, duration, or grade of androgenetic alopecia, though it would seem to be a good marker for exposure to UVR penetrating the skin. Interestingly, UVB irradiation has been found to stimulate the synthesis of elastic fibers by modified epithelial cells surrounding the hair follicle and sebaceous glands in mice.

As a consequence of increased leisure time with a growing popularity of outdoor activities and holidays in the sun, awareness of sun protection has become important. Topically applied chemicals that act as sun protectors are widely utilized and offer the most convenient means of protecting the glabrous skin against acute (sunburn) and chronic pathologic effects of UVR. Out of cosmetic reasons, their use on the hair-bearing scalp is problematic, unless complete baldness is present. Although hats provide the best protection of the scalp from UVR, not all patients find it convenient or acceptable for this purpose.

Ultimately, alternatives have been the focus of more recent investigation to overcome the problems associated with the topical use of sunscreens: studies illustrate photoprotective properties of topical melatonin and of supplemented antioxidants, particularly beta-carotene (pro-vitamin A), α-tocopherol (vitamin E), and L-ascorbate (vitamin C). Topical melatonin has been found to suppress UV-induced erythema and UV-induced reactive oxygen species in a dose-dependent manner. Preclinical studies illustrate photoprotective properties of supplemented antioxidants; however, clinical evidence that these prevent, retard, or slow down solar skin damage is still impending.

Nevertheless, these results suggest the probable utility of combining topical melatonin, supplemented antioxidants, and sunscreens to maximize photoprotection.

Finally, the limited success rate of treatment of androgenetic alopecia with minoxidil and finasteride—even in the absence of comorbid conditions—means that further pathogenic pathways may be taken into account. On histological examination of scalp biopsies, the miniaturization of terminal hairs is frequently associated with perifollicular lymphocytic infiltration and eventually fibrosis. Therefore, it is conceivable that the role of this microscopic follicular inflammation causing fibrosis below the shortened balding follicle has been underestimated, though it seems likely that this would prevent the follicle to reform a terminal hair follicle.

The implication of microscopic follicular inflammation in the pathogenesis of androgenetic alopecia has emerged from several independent studies.

An early study referred to an inflammatory infiltrate of activated T-cells and macrophages in the upper third of the hair follicles, associated with an enlargement of the follicular dermal sheath composed of collagen bundles (perifollicular fibrosis), in regions of actively progressing alopecia. Horizontal section studies of scalp biopsies indicated that the perifollicular fibrosis is generally mild, consisting of loose, concentric layers of collagen that must be distinguished from cicatricial alopecia.

Mahé et al. proposed the term follicular microinflammation, because the process involves a slow, subtle, and indolent course, in contrast to the inflammatory and destructive process in the classical inflammatory scarring alopecias. However, the significance of follicular microinflammation and fibrosis in androgenetic alopecia has remained controversial.

Nevertheless, morphometric studies in male patients with androgenetic alopecia treated with topical minoxidil showed that 55 % of those with microinflammation had regrowth in response to treatment, in comparison to 77 % in those patients without inflammation and fibrosis.

In general, androgenetic alopecia is understood to represent a noninflammatory and non-scarring process that eventually leads to permanent hair loss of the affected scalp. In Zinkernagel and Trüeb's original description of *fibrosing alopecia in a pattern distribution*, patients displayed progressive scarring alopecia in a pattern distribution. Close clinical examination reveals obliteration of follicular orifices, perifollicular erythema, and follicular keratosis limited to the area of androgenetic hair loss (Fig. 4.5a–c). Histological findings of androgenetic alopecia, i.e., increased numbers of miniaturized hair follicles with underlying fibrous streamers, are evident in the majority of patients and associated with a perifollicular lymphocytic infiltrate. A pattern of follicular interface dermatitis targeting the upper follicle is found in early lesions, whereas perifollicular lamellar fibrosis and the presence of selectively fibrosed follicular tracts characterize late lesions.

The pattern distribution and histological findings share features with Kossard's original description of *postmenopausal frontal fibrosing alopecia*. Frontal fibrosing alopecia represents a peculiar condition originally described in women in the postmenopause. The condition presents with a symmetric, marginal alopecia along the frontal and frontotemporal hairline, often with concomitant thinning or complete loss of the eyebrows (Fig. 4.6a). Affected women typically present with the complaint of asymptomatic, progressive recession of their frontal hairline. The affected scalp skin is pale and smooth with loss of follicular orifices; often perifollicular erythema and follicular keratinization are observed marking the underlying inflammatory process. Histopathologic examination of affected scalp shows again a reduced number of hair follicles, which have been replaced by fibrous tracts, and a perifollicular, lymphocytic, lichenoid infiltrate that is typical of lichen planopilaris. Kossard et al. later interpreted this type of alopecia as a frontal variant of lichen planopilaris on the basis of histopathologic and immunohistochemical studies.

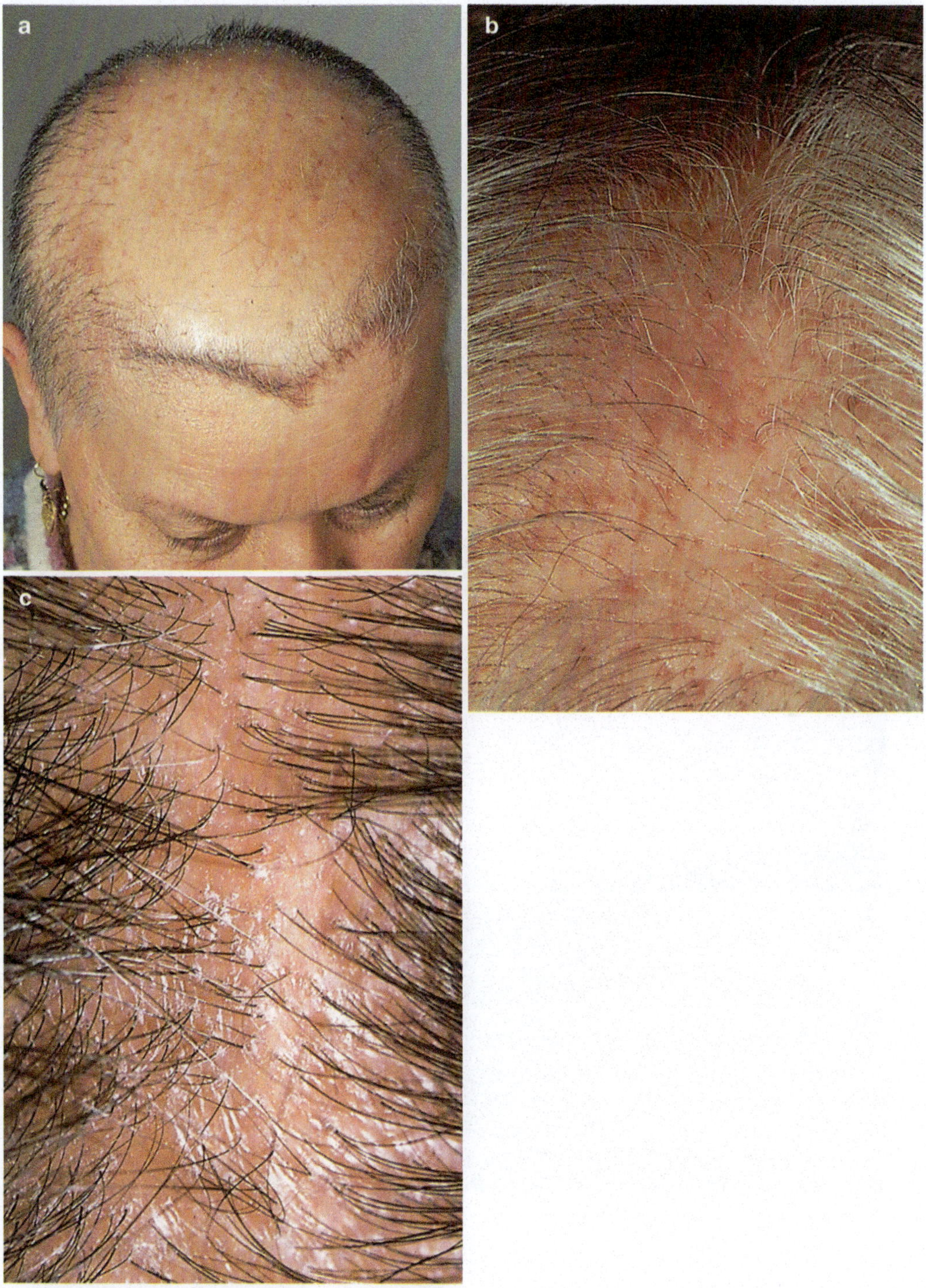

Fig. 4.5 (**a–c**) Fibrosing alopecia in a pattern distribution: (**a**) Patterned scarring alopecia. (**b**) Follicular erythema. (**c**) Follicular keratosis

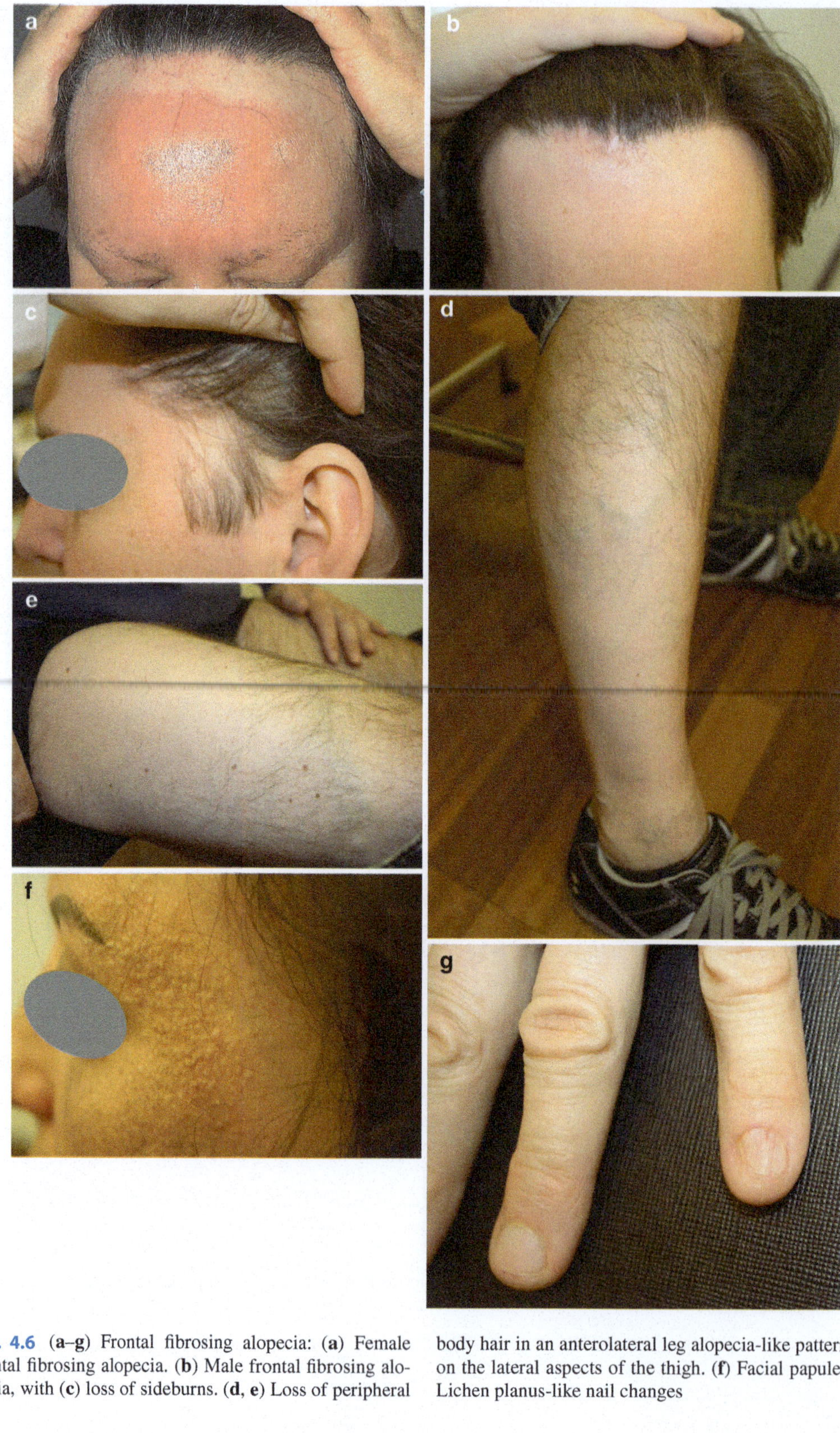

Fig. 4.6 (**a–g**) Frontal fibrosing alopecia: (**a**) Female frontal fibrosing alopecia. (**b**) Male frontal fibrosing alopecia, with (**c**) loss of sideburns. (**d**, **e**) Loss of peripheral body hair in an anterolateral leg alopecia-like pattern and on the lateral aspects of the thigh. (**f**) Facial papules. (**g**) Lichen planus-like nail changes

Since Kossard's original description in 1994, the number of cases of frontal fibrosing alopecia has exploded exponentially worldwide, while its etiology remains obscure. The condition has meanwhile also been described in men with the typical presentation of scarring alopecia of the sideburns (Fig. 4.6b, c). Moreover, it has been recognized to represent a more generalized rather than localized process of inflammatory scarring alopecia, with extension beyond the frontotemporal hair line, and loss of peripheral body hair (Fig. 4.6d, e).

More recently, peculiar facial papules have been reported in association with frontal fibrosing alopecia representing facial vellus hair involvement and described by patients as "roughening" of facial skin (Fig. 4.6f).

Follicular microinflammation and fibrosis, frontal fibrosing alopecia, and fibrosing alopecia in a pattern distribution seem to represent a continuum from microscopic inflammation and fibrosis to localized, more generalized forms of clinically perceptible inflammatory scarring alopecia. Moreover, considerable overlap exists among frontal fibrosing alopecia, lichen planopilaris, and fibrosing alopecia in a pattern distribution: postmenopausal frontal fibrosing alopecia has been described in association with lichen planus elsewhere, including the oral cavity and the nails (Fig. 4.6g), and frontal fibrosing alopecia-type changes as well as facial papules (Fig. 4.7) can also be observed in patients with fibrosing alopecia in a pattern distribution.

Ultimately, Olsen acknowledged existence of clinically significant inflammatory phenomena and fibrosis in androgenetic alopecia and proposed the term *cicatricial pattern hair loss* for these conditions.

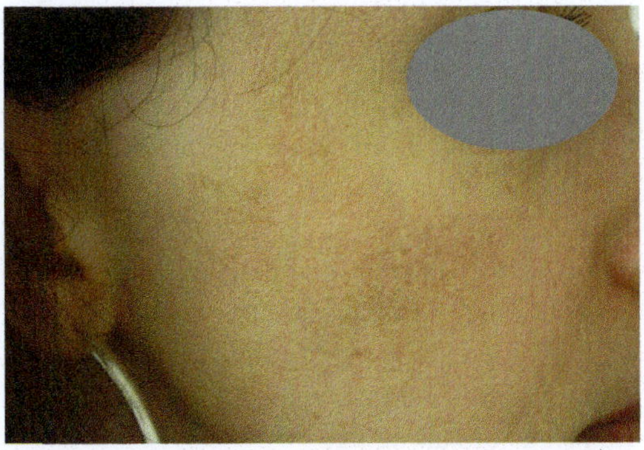

Fig. 4.7 Facial papules in fibrosing alopecia in pattern distribution

4.2.2 Aging Hair

Hair length, color, and cosmetic properties play an important role in people's physical appearance and self-perception. Civilized mankind's ancient preoccupation with hair is heightened as today's increasing life expectancy fuels the desire to preserve youthfulness. This attention reflects a hair care market that is a multibillion dollar enterprise.

The study of hair aging focuses on two main streams of interest: on the one hand, the *esthetic problem* of aging hair and its management, in other words everything that happens outside the skin, and, on the other hand, the *biological problem* of aging hair, in terms of microscopic, biochemical (hormonal, enzymatic), and molecular changes, in other words the "secret life" of the hair follicle in the depth of the skin.

Most literature on age-related hair changes focuses on alopecia, but it is equally important that the hair fibers that emerge from the scalp exhibit significant age-related changes that have an equal impact on the overall cosmetic properties of the hair. It is these changes that are ultimately experience by subjects that have retained their hair as they age.

Aging of hair affects hair color, hair production, and structural properties of the hair fiber with its consequence for manageability and overall appearance of hair. Age-related deterioration of cosmetic properties of hair is related to changes in hair pigmentations (graying), diameter, curvatures, structural properties (stretching, bending, torsional rigidity), lipid composition, and the interdependence of these changes. Depending on the individual's original hair color, quantity, quality, and hair care habits, there is a great variability in the age of onset of first signs of hair aging.

Hair graying is closely related to chronological age, and the age of its onset is largely controlled by genetics. The normal incidence of hair graying is 34 ± 9.6 years in Caucasians and 43.9 ± 10.3 years in Africans. As a rule of thumb, by 50 years of age, 50 % of people have 50 % gray hair. This graying incidence appears irrespective of sex and hair color. In men, graying usually begins at the temples and in the sideburns. Women will usually start around the perimeter of the hairline. Gradually, the gray works its way back through the top, sides, and back of the hair. Finally, the perception of graying is dependent on the original hair color, with the perception of "any gray" occurring earlier in dark hair and later in light hair. Vice versa, the perception of "completely gray" is perceived to occur earlier in light hair and later in dark hair.

> Hair is said to gray prematurely if it occurs before the age of 20 in Caucasians, of 25 in Asians, and of 30 in Africans.

While premature canities most commonly appear without underlying pathology, presumably inherited in an autosomal dominant manner (familial premature graying), it has also been linked to a similar cluster of autoimmune disorders observed in association with vitiligo, i.e., pernicious anemia, and autoimmune thyroid disease, as well as with rare premature aging syndromes (progerias), such as Hutchinson–Gilford and Werner's syndrome.

> Reports—again—linking cigarette smoking with premature hair graying have drawn on the one hand the attention to the role of oxidative stress on hair growth and pigmentation and on the other hand to canities as a marker for the general health status.

A possible explanation of the observation may be that smoking-related diseases increase aging in general, including pigmentation. However, more direct effects, e.g., via smoke genotoxin-induced apoptosis, may also be involved. Wood et al. demonstrated for the first time that human white scalp hair shafts accumulate hydrogen peroxide (H_2O_2) in millimolar concentrations and almost absent catalase and methionine sulfoxide reductase (MSR) protein expression in association with functional loss of methionine sulfoxide repair in the entire gray hair follicle. Accordingly, methionine sulfoxide formation of methionine residues (Met), including Met 374 in the active site of tyrosinase, the key enzyme in melanogenesis, limits enzyme functionality, which eventually leads to loss of hair color. While the entire hair follicle is subject to H_2O_2-mediated stress, it is tempting to assume that, besides tyrosinase and MSR, other proteins and peptides, including anti-apoptotic Bcl-2 protein, are targets for oxidation, which in turn could explain melanocyte apoptosis in the gray hair follicle. Moreover, H_2O_2-mediated oxidation has been documented for many other important regulators of pigmentation, including the proopiomelanocortins a-melanocyte-stimulating hormone (MSH) and β-endorphin, the prohormone convertases, and the synthesis and recycling of the ubiquitous cofactor 6-tetrahydrobiopterin.

> Whether canities, premature or otherwise, is a predictor or risk marker for disease remains controversial, mainly due to poor epidemiologic study design. Moreover, if it exists at all, it is more likely to reflect associated genetic effects rather than direct linkage.

Anecdotal evidence indicates that gray hair becomes coarser and less manageable than pigmented hair. Gray hair is said to often fail to hold a temporary or permanent set and to be more resistant to incorporating artificial color, both of which suggest changes to the underlying substructure of the hair fiber. Gray hair has been found to have increased sensitivity to weathering, increased cysteic acid residues and decreased cystine, and increased fiber reactivity to reducing and oxidizing agents. Moreover, gray hair is more sensitive to UVR. Photochemical impairment of the hair includes degradation and loss of hair proteins as well as degradation of hair pigment. UVB radiation is responsible for hair protein loss, and UVA radiation is responsible for hair color changes. Absorption of radiation in photosensitive amino acids of the hair and their photochemical degradation is producing free radicals. They have adverse impact on hair proteins, especially keratin, while melanin can partially immobilize free radicals and block their entrance in keratin matrix.

Given the close interaction of melanin-transferring melanocytes with hair shaft-forming pre-cortical keratinocytes, it is conceivable that other functions of these cell types are affected by this activity. One possibility is that melanin transfer decreases keratinocyte turnover and increases keratinocyte terminal differentiation. Indeed, white beard hair has been shown to grow up to four times the rate of adjacent pigmented hair. In this way, aging hair follicles may reprogram their matrix keratinocytes to increase production of medullary, rather than cortical, keratinocytes. In fact the medulla is often enlarged and collapsed, forming a central cavity in gray and white hairs.

> An evolutionary basis for the increased medullation of senile white hair may reflect the enhanced insulation provided by these hairs which would confer an important benefit for temperature regulation. In this way, it may compensate for the loss of sunlight-absorbing and thus heat-trapping properties of melanized dark hair.

Hair diameter changes with age are likely to impart the largest impact on overall perception of hair aging. The largest study on female hair diameter in relation to age was performed in 1988 by Otsuka and Nemoto on >18,000 Japanese females aged 10 through 60 years. The study showed that hair diameter *versus* age does not represent a linear relationship, but rather a curvature that increases to a maximum near the age of 40 and thereafter decreases. The second largest study performed more recently by Robbins et al. on 1,099 Caucasian females aged 18 through 66 years with perceived hair loss revealed the age for maximum diameter to be 43–46 years. Several smaller studies on age *versus* diameter were in reasonable agreement with the conclusions of these two large studies, indicating that the age of maximum diameter for females is near the 40s. One exception is the study of Birch et al. on >300 Caucasian females concluding that the age for maximum hair diameter was near the 30s.

Postmenopausal women were shown to have significantly lower hair fiber diameters (lower frontal scalp hair density and lower growth rates) than premenopausal women for the frontal but not the occipital scalp region. This effect was independent of age, together with the co-localization with androgenetic alopecia, suggesting an impact of the hormonal effects of menopause on hair diameter.

In contrast to females, again, Otsuko and Nemoto found in Japanese men scalp hair fiber diameter to increase to a maximum in the late teenage years and then to decrease relatively rapidly with increasing age. Trotter and Dawson found similar effects in a study on 82 male French Canadians. Courtois et al. studied 10 French male subjects aged 25–49 over a period of 14 years and demonstrated that the diameter of hair shafts decreased with increasing age beginning at age 25.

Changes in hair fiber curvature with age has an important effect on almost all important cosmetic properties. Nagase et al. studied curvature of hair from 132 Japanese females aged 10 through 70 years and found an increase in curvature with age. In a different publication by the same authors, *frizziness* was explained as a lack of synchronization in the curvature of neighboring hair fibers in an assembly of hair. Respective data for Caucasian women and men are as yet not available.

Changes in hair fiber diameter and curvature with age also affect *structural properties of hairs* increasing combing forces and therefore breakage. Combing forces have been shown to increase with decreasing fiber curvature and increasing fiber curvature. Therefore, combing forces can be expected to increase with age, leading to increase breakage of hair.

Hair breakage is a multifactorial phenomenon involving bending, stretching, and torsion deformations and including:

- Tangle formation, with hair looped over other hairs
- Knots (trichonodosis)
- Impact breakage or pulling a comb or brush through a tangle
- Physical damage or wear by abrasion from specific grooming devices such as combs, picks, or brushes

Robbins et al. described the effects of diameter and hair density in relation to age and proposed a new metric *relative scalp coverage* for the perception of the amount of hair on one's head. This metric is defined as a two-dimensional parameter as the average of fiber cross-sectional area multiplied by the number of hair fibers per square centimeter. Considering diameter and density, relative scalp coverage was found to peak at age 35, as a result of hair diameter increasing until about age 45, and density peaking in the late 20s. Robbins et al. further proposed that when additional relevant parameters are taken into account for relative scalp coverage, it will provide a multidimensional parameter involving diameter, density, fiber curvature, and color. Ultimately, as the color of hair changes with age, the perception of scalp coverage will change. Also, the graying effect with age will decrease luster.

Finally, hair lipid levels and hair lipid composition change with age: the two major sources of hair lipids are the hair matrix cells (cholesterol, cholesterol sulfate, ceramides, covalent fatty acids, 18-methyl eicosanoic acid) and the hair follicle-associated sebaceous glands (squalene, wax esters, triglycerides, total fatty acids). The amount of sebum produced varies with the size of sebaceous glands, being low before puberty, rapidly increasing at puberty, and remaining at a high level until 45–50 where it declines. The decline is greater in females than in males.

> Age-related lipid changes affect hair greasiness, shine, softness, and smoothness.

At last, basic scientists interested in the biology of hair growth and pigmentation have exposed the hair follicle as a highly accessible and unique model that offers important opportunities also to the gerontologist for the study of aging. Its complex multicell-type interaction system involving epithelium, mesenchyme, and neuroectoderm and its unique cyclical activity of growth, regression, rest, and regrowth provides the investigator with a range of stem, differentiating, mitotic, and postmitotic terminally differentiated cells, including cells with variable susceptibility to apoptosis, for study.

Aging is a complex process involving various genetic, hormonal, and environmental mechanisms. A number of intrinsic and extrinsic modulating factors for hair growth and pigmentation have been identified and are being further tested in vitro.

> Much like the skin, the hair is subject to intrinsic or chronologic aging and extrinsic aging due to environmental factors. Both occur in conjunction with the other and are superimposed on each other.

Intrinsic factors are related to individual genetic and epigenetic mechanisms with interindividual variation. Examples are familial premature graying and androgenetic alopecia. Extrinsic factors include ultraviolet radiation (UVR), smoking, and nutrition.

Senile involutional or senescent alopecia has been defined as non-androgen-dependent hair thinning found in those over 60 years of age. Much like androgenetic alopecia, it involves a progressive decrease in the number of anagen follicles and hair diameter. It frequently occurs together with androgenetic alopecia, further complicating its delineation from the latter.

In their study on aging and hair cycles over an exceptionally long duration of 8–14 years, Courtois et al. found a reduction in the duration of hair growth and in the diameter of hair shafts and a prolongation of the interval separating the loss of a hair in telogen and the emergence of a replacement hair in anagen (latency phase).

These phenomena resemble those observed in the course of androgenetic alopecia, although their development is less marked, suggesting androgenetic alopecia to represent a premature aging phenomenon.

This aging process was evidenced by a reduction in the number of hairs per unit area and deterioration in the quality of scalp hair. The reduction in density was manifested to different degrees in different individuals. It amounted to less than 10 % in 10 years in the individuals with the least alopecia and was much more pronounced in the balding subjects. The maximal length of hair diminished as the subjects aged; in parallel, the hairs became finer. However, among non-balding subjects, there was a tendency for the proportion of thicker hairs to increase. Finally, aging did not appear to follow a perfectly regular course over time. Periods of stability, or even partial remission, alternated with periods of more marked evolution, reflecting perhaps the influence of individual factors such as the subject's general health, lifestyle, and risk factors for accelerated aging.

Recent data comparing androgenetic alopecia and senescent alopecia using microarray analysis have demonstrated significant differences in the gene expression patterns suggesting they represent different entities.

In androgenetic alopecia, genes required for anagen onset (Wnt-beta-catenin, TGF-alpha, TGF-beta, Stat-3, Stat-1), epithelial signal to dermal papilla (PPARd, IGF-1), hair shaft differentiation (Notch, Msx2, KRTs, KAPs), and anagen maintenance (Msx2, Activin, IGF-1) were downregulated, and genes for catagen (BDNF, BMP2, BMP7, VDR, IL-1, ER) and telogen induction and maintenance (VDR, RAR) were upregulated. In senescent alopecia, genes involved in epithelial signal to dermal papilla (FGF5), actin cytoskeleton (DST, ACTN2, TNNI3, PARVB), and mitochondrial function (JAK2, PRKD3, AK2, TRAP1, TRIO, ATP12A, MLL4, STK22B) were downregulated, while oxidative stress and inflammatory response genes were upregulated.

More recently, Nishimura found mouse hair follicles to age through defective renewal of hair follicle stem cells much in the manner as maintenance of melanocyte stem cells becomes incomplete with aging.

Hair production is fueled by stem cells, which transition between cyclical bouts of rest and activity. Aged hair follicle stem cells exhibit enhanced resting and abbreviated growth phases and are delayed in response to tissue-regenerating cues. Ultimately, aged hair follicle stem cells are poor at initiating proliferation and show diminished self-renewing capacity upon extensive use.

Aging-related loss of hair follicle stem cell marker expression starts well before hair follicles have shortened. Using genomic instability syndromes and exposure to ionizing radiation as models, Nishimura proposed an accumulation of DNA damage to be involved in the aging process (oral communication, 7th World Congress for Hair Research, May 4–6, 2013, Edinburgh, Scotland).

Finally, though being exceedingly rare, the progerias (Hutchinson–Gilford and Werner's syndrome), together with other rare conditions associated with premature hair loss, such as the Laron syndrome and myotonic dystrophy

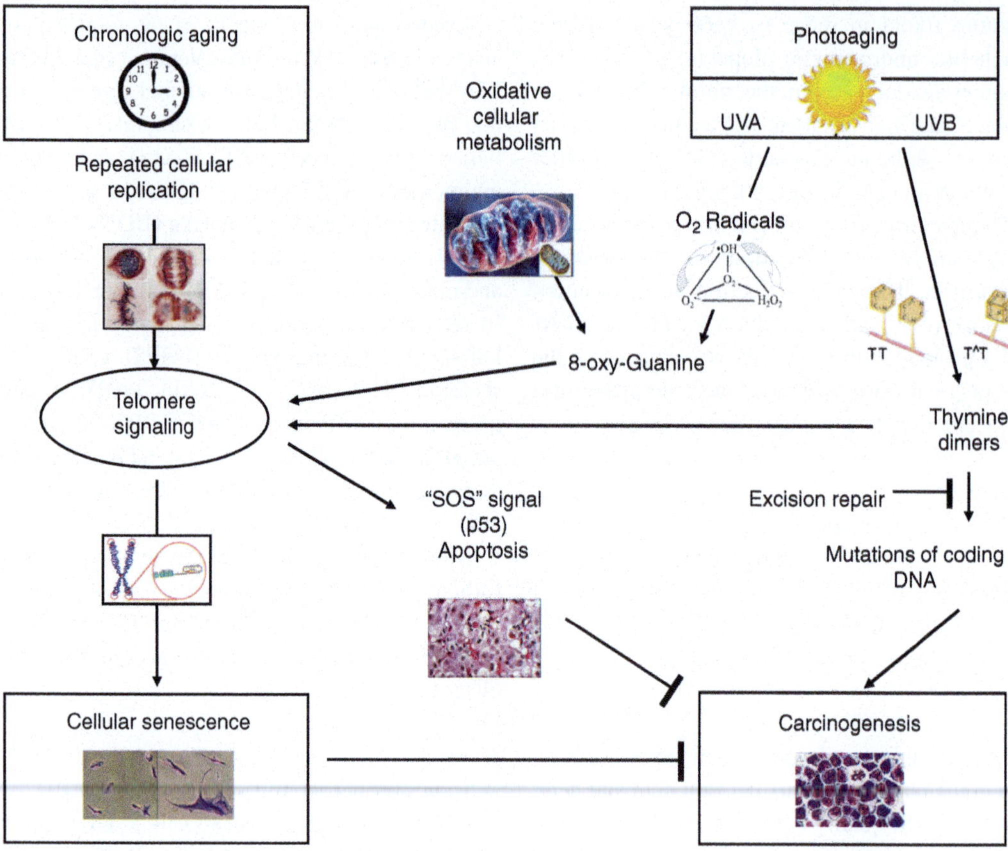

Fig. 4.8 Intrinsic and extrinsic aging, telomere signaling, p53, and senescence *versus* carcinogenesis (From: Trüeb 2006a)

(Curschmann–Steinert), give insights into the roles of telomeres, mitochondrial function, human growth hormone (HGH), and insulin-like growth factor 1 (IGF-1) for the growth and aging of hair.

Telomeres represent repeated TTAGGG DNA sequences that cap the end of the chromosomes. The 3' end strand extends by 75–300 bases beyond the complementary 5' strand of DNA, leaving a single-stranded G-rich overhang at the very end. This overhang forms a loop structure by inserting into the proximal telomeric double helix. With each cell cycle, the DNA polymerase is unable to replicate the outermost end of the DNA, resulting in progressive shortening of telomeres with each new cell division until they shorten to a critical length driving the cell into senescence, in which cell growth diminishes and then cell division stops altogether, or into apoptosis (programmed cell death) via the p53 pathway (Fig. 4.8).

Telomere length and integrity of its loop structure are understood to be crucial in maintaining the stability of the chromosome and viability of the cell, respectively.

When telomere shortening reaches a critical point, signals are produced to induce cell senescence. Therefore, it is believed that the progressive shorting represents the internal clock that determines the onset of senescence of cells and therefore plays a pivotal role in intrinsic aging. Accordingly, older individual's cells have shorter telomeres. In Werner's syndrome, the defective gene product unwinds G-rich DNA structures and is implicated in telomere maintenance.

Environmental factors, on the other hand, play a major role in the process of extrinsic aging. A typical example that has been extensively studied in skin aging is UV radiation, which can lead to oxidative stress (UVA) and to mutations of coding DNA (UVB). Oxidative damage toward the GGG residues, produced through UV radiation, cigarette smoking, or cellular metabolism, may accelerate telomere shortening in order to counteract carcinogenesis. The p53 signaling pathway has many mechanisms of anticancer function: It can activate DNA repair mechanism. It can arrest growth by holding the cell cycle long enough for the DNA repair mechanisms to fix the damage allowing the cell to continue the cell cycle. Ultimately, it can initiate apoptosis if DNA damage proves to be irreparable.

Telomerase is an enzyme with reverse transcriptase activity (TERT) that is capable of adding telomeric sequences to the ends of the telomere, thereby preventing its shortening. In the hair follicle, its degree of activity is highest in the hair rapidly proliferating cells of the hair bulb, while it is low in the region of the hair follicle stem cells. Therefore, any damage to the hair follicle stem cell niche, elicited by any type of genotoxic injury, including UVR and chemotherapy, may lead to telomerase deficiency, resulting in shortened telomeres and cellular senescence. The importance of telomerase is underlined by the observation of premature hair graying, alopecia, and decreased wound healing in mice deficient of telomerase, a phenotype with analogies to progeria in humans. Vice versa telomerase is expressed in 90 % of all tumors. Therefore, telomerase appears to be stringently repressed in normal human somatic tissues but reactivated in cancer, where immortal cells are likely required to maintain tumor proliferation.

Mitochondrial damage, particularly as a result of oxidative injury, contributes to changes, such as deletions or mutations, in mitochondrial DNA. Analysis of plucked hair from participants ranging in age from 5 days to 91 years has revealed an increase in the incidence of a specific mitochondrial deletion over time, with 4,977 base-pair deletions by year 91. Moreover, smoking-associated mitochondrial DNA mutations have also been identified in human hair follicles.

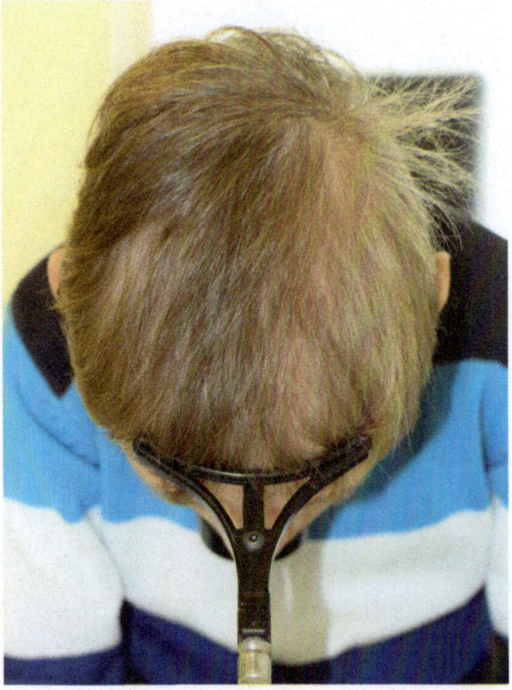

Fig. 4.9 Hair loss in primary growth hormone deficiency

The *Laron syndrome (primary growth hormone insensitivity)* sheds light on the role of HGH and IGF-1 for hair growth. The syndrome represents an autosomal recessive disorder characterized by insensitivity to growth hormone, caused by a variant of the growth hormone receptor. The principal feature of the syndrome is abnormally short stature (dwarfism). The hair of patients with Laron syndrome is thin and easy to pluck. Young adults have various degrees of alopecia, more pronounced in males. Accordingly, Olszeska et al. originally reported in their publication on methods of hair loss evaluation in patients with endocrine disorders, hair loss to be a symptom in growth hormone deficiency (Fig. 4.9). Not unexpectedly, scalp hair loss has been reported both with octreotide therapy for acromegaly and after transsphenoidal adenomectomy in patients with acromegaly. Finally, in the course of hormonal anti-aging protocols containing recombinant human growth hormone (hGH) at the Palm Springs Life Extension Institute, Chein claims improvement of hair thickness and structure in 38 % of patients, darkening of hair in some, and increased hair growth in few.

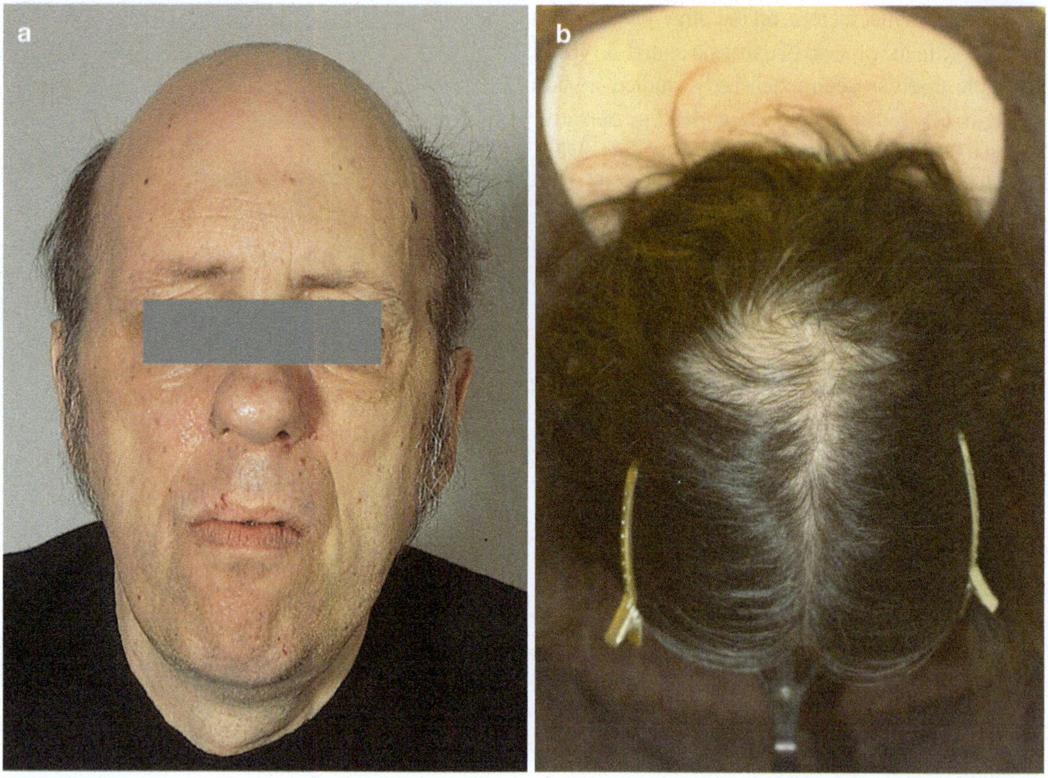

Fig. 4.10 (**a**, **b**) Myotonic dystrophy Curschmann–Steinert. (**a**) Frontal alopecia and myopathic facies in an affected male. (**b**) Vertex alopecia in an affected female

Curschmann–Steinert's myotonic dystrophy is an autosomal dominant disorder of trinucleotide repeat characterized by wasting of the muscles (muscular dystrophy), cataracts, heart conduction defects, endocrine changes, and myotonia. Myotonia is the designation for a peculiar form of muscle disorder characterized by delayed relaxation (prolonged contraction) of the skeletal muscles after voluntary contraction or electrical stimulation. Although early frontoparietal alopecia is one of the most common symptoms in myotonic dystrophy (Fig. 4.10a. b), it has not received the deserved attention.

> Altering the delicate balance between cellular senescence and cellular proliferation and carcinogenesis by manipulating the respective signaling pathways with the aim to prevent or reverse aging seems rather precarious.

IGF-1 has shown some interesting results in studies examining its use as a hair growth-promoting agent. IGF-1 regulates cellular proliferation and migration during the development of hair follicles and is known to be regulated by androgens, and its deficiency is related to premature alopecia in the Laron syndrome. Dermal papilla cells from balding scalp follicles have been found to secrete significantly less IGF-1 than their non-balding counterparts, and the expression of IGF-1 in follicular dermal papillae has been shown to correlate with the therapeutic efficacy of finasteride in androgenetic alopecia.

Currently, commercial products containing IGF-1 exist for transdermal application using a dermaroller, usually in combination with other growth factors, such as bFGF (basic fibroblast growth factor), and VEGF (vascular endothelial growth factor), copper peptide, hyaluronic acid, coenzyme Q, vitamins B3, B6, and B5, and amino acids (arginine and lysine).

However, their efficacy has as yet not been sufficiently substantiated in clinical studies published in peer-reviewed scientific publications.

Alternatively, liposomal IGF-1 and VEGF in topical gel formulation to promote hair growth have been studied in the hamster (*Mesocricetus auratus*): efficacy was determined by dermatoscopic analysis of hair density and microscopic analysis of hair diameter. Hair was found to grow faster and thicker in the 3 % liposomal IGF-1 and VEGF groups than in the respective 1 % or control groups.

Finally, another potential signaling pathway involved in the aging of hair as it relates to hair cycling is the bone morphogenic protein (BMP)-/calcium-regulated nuclear factor of activated T-cell c1 (NFATc1) pathway. Although the complex mechanisms underlying hair cycling and stem cell proliferation in humans remains ill-defined, the role of BMP and NFATc in hair growth and cycling has been unravelled in the mouse. NFATc1 is activated by BMP signaling, in turn leading to quiescence of stem cells. Transcriptional profiling presents differences consistent with defects in aged hair follicle stem cell activation. Notably, NFATc1 becomes recalcitrant to its normal downregulating cues. Given these findings, prolonged telogen phase in aging hair may be the result of increased expression of the NFATc1 transcription factor. Given the propensity for NFATc1 to put off stem cell proliferation, an inhibition of BMP signaling and/or NFATc1 results in increase of hair growth in the mouse model due to a decrease in the time that the stem cells spend in the quiescent state.

For the time being, current available treatment modalities for age-related hair loss remain topical minoxidil, and oral finasteride, though with some limitations. Moreover, older patients often suffer from a variety of conditions that may affect the hair: nutritional deficiency, endocrine disorders, psychological problems, and drug-related adverse effects. Therefore, one must remain suspicious of the possibility of a more general problem underlying the patient's complaint in taking care of the elderly with hair problems.

It has been known for over 30 years that minoxidil stimulates hair growth, and clinical trials with topical 2 or 5 % minoxidil solution in male and female hair loss have all shown remarkably rapid increase in hair growth, measured by hair counts or hair weight: The increase is evident within 6–8 weeks of treatment and has generally peaked by 12–16 weeks.

Local application of minoxidil 2 % twice daily has also proven to be safe and effective for eyebrow enhancement.

However, topical minoxidil has not been studied in the specific perspective of aging and senescent alopecia. In an analysis of clinical trial data in 636 males and 630 females, a therapeutic benefit of topical 2 and 5 % minoxidil solution was compared to age, duration of balding, and diameter of balding vertex area in males and age and duration of hair loss in females: Age was found to be the denominator for predicting treatment success for both males and females. The younger subjects experienced better efficacy than the older subjects.

Nevertheless, clear treatment benefits of topical minoxidil solution are also noted in the older age group that has retained some hair.

Males showed an inverse relationship between effect and duration of balding. Males with duration of balding <5 years showed a significantly better effect than those with duration of balding >21 years. Females, in contrast, showed no correlation with duration of balding. The diameter of vertex balding in men showed an inverse relationship with efficacy of minoxidil. Males with <5 cm diameter vertex balding area showed a better effect of treatment than subjects with diameters >15 cm. Finally, duration of hair loss less than 1 year compared to more than 10 years at onset of treatment resulted in a significantly more effective treatment with respect to stabilization of alopecia and new hair growth.

One milligram oral finasteride daily has also proven to be effective in aging male, though with a lesser degree of efficacy and a higher frequency of sexual adverse effects compared to men between 18 and 40 years.

With respect to menopause and hormonal replacement therapy (HRT), the focus tends to be on the issues recently covered by the Women's Health Initiative. Consequently, many women have become reluctant toward systemic estrogen substitution therapy. Alternatively, topical estrogen supplementation with estradiol has been suggested to be of some benefit. Unfortunately, these studies are relatively small. Also no literature exists comparing efficacy and safety of topical *versus* systemic estrogens in postmenopausal women.

As a general rule, hormone replacement therapies with progestogens that possess net androgenic activity, such as norethisterone, levonorgestrel, or tibolone, should be avoided, since they may precipitate alopecia.

Finally, oral 2.5–5 mg oral finasteride or 0.5 mg dutasteride may be tried in postmenopausal women not responsive or intolerant to topical minoxidil without the teratogenicity issues in premenopausal women, though with mixed results. Adverse effects include dry skin, libido reduction, and breast tenderness.

Thyroid hormones have influence on the growth and differentiation of many tissues and total energy expenditure of the organism and on the turnover of many substrates, vitamins, and other hormones. Thyroid activity affects oxygen consumption, protein synthesis, and mitosis and is therefore essential for the formation and growth of hair. Schell et al. originally demonstrated by means of DNA flow cytometry the influence of thyroid hormones on in vivo cell cycle kinetics of human scalp hair bulbs. Expression of the thyroid hormone receptor beta1 was demonstrated in the human hair follicle, and it was shown that triiodo-L-thyronine significantly enhances human hair survival in vitro.

The impact of thyroid hormone activity on the hair is most notable during deficient (hypothyroidism) or excess (hyperthyroidism) states. Thyroid dysfunction represents a frequent disorder related to hair loss, especially in women: hypothyroidism is about ten times more frequent in women than in men and particularly affects women between the ages of 40 and 60 years. Dull, coarse, brittle hair or diffuse alopecia may be present with particular thinning of the lateral eyebrows. The hair growth rate is slowed, with an increase in the proportion in telogen. The alopecia is of very gradual onset. Such symptoms may easily be overlooked or ascribed merely to aging. Also, there is an increasing prevalence of high levels of TSH with age, particularly in postmenopausal women, while the symptoms of thyroid disease can be similar to postmenopausal complaints. Finally, HRT in women with hypothyroidism treated with thyroxine causes changes in free thyroxine and TSH. Increased binding of thyroxine to elevated thyroxine-binding globulin causes an elevation of TSH by feedback. Since adaptation is insufficient, there is an increased need for thyroxine in women taking HRT.

Long-standing hypothyroidism is often associated with patterned hair loss. The mechanism has been presumed to be due to an increase in plasma-free androgens. While normally, the hair shows a Gauss distribution of shaft diameters with a peak at 80 μm, in both androgenetic alopecia and hypothyroidism, hair shaft diameters are decreased with a bimodal distribution, suggesting that a genetic predisposition to patterned hair loss may be preliminary to the development of alopecia of hypothyroidism.

Currently, thyroid receptor agonists are in development for the treatment of androgenetic alopecia. A thyroid receptor beta subtype-selective thyromimetic 5 was found to be efficacious in both mouse and monkey hair growth models after topical application.

Coenzyme Q10 (CoQ10) has previously been used for its anti-aging effects on aging skin, where it has been theorized that there is an increase in anaerobic metabolism due to a decrease in mitochondrial function as a result of oxidative damage. Expanding the cutaneous application to the hair, it has been shown with quantitative polymerase chain reaction techniques that CoQ10 administration results in an increase in particular keratins in the hair root compared to placebo. Specific keratin and keratin-associated protein levels have been found to be decreased in aged hair compared to fibers from a younger individual. A decrease in keratin levels correlates with a decrease in interactions between the filaments and keratin-associated proteins resulting in a decline in the mechanical strength of the hair fiber.

However, as with all cosmetic anti-aging treatments, the question arises whether and to what extent a quantifiable improvement in a particular parameter measured translates into improvement perceived by the consumer.

The efficacy of hair growth-promoting agents or anti-aging substances in shampoo form is questionable given their dilution with water and short contact time, unless they can be absorbed in effective quantities.

Nevertheless, cosmetic products represent a key integral part of management of aging hair, since they may significantly improve the condition of the hair fiber with more immediate effects, while pharmacologic agents take their time.

Since hair fiber diameter has been recognized to represent another key contributor to hair thinning, a novel leave-on technology has been developed at Procter & Gamble that combines caffeine, niacinamide, panthenol, dimethicone, and an acrylate polymer (CNPDA) to affect the diameter and behavior of individual scalp hair fibers as an approach to improve decreasing fiber diameter. Utilizing laser scan micrometer for assessment of fiber diameter measures and tensile break stress and torsion pendulum testing for assessment of behavioral properties, it was found that CNPDA significantly increased the diameter of individual terminal scalp hair fibers by 2–5 μm, which yields an increase in the cross-sectional area of approximately 10 %. Beyond the increase in hair fiber diameter, the CNPDA-thickened fibers demonstrated enhanced mechanical properties characteristic of thicker fibers, such as increased suppleness/pliability and better ability to withstand force without breaking.

Although cosmetic treatments will not reverse the process of hair aging, new technologies may help to mitigate the effects of age-related thinning of hair.

Finally, there are a number of botanicals with alleged anti-aging effects from both traditional Chinese medicine (TCM) and from Ayurvedic medicine (the literal meaning of Ayurveda is "life-knowledge"). Asia, Korea, China, and Japan have legally adopted the traditional Oriental medical system along with the Western system. A number of traditional herbal drugs including the polypharmacy type of prescription (combination of multiple herbs) are available and widely dispensed. This polypharmacy type of herbal therapy allegedly exhibits holistic effectiveness by exerting multitargeted effects. The Traditional Oriental Medicine Database (TradMed 2000 DB) represents a database of traditional Oriental herbal therapy containing specific information such as formulas, chemical information on ingredients, botanical information on herbal materials, and a dictionary of disease classifications. Using the TradMed 2000 DB, Chang from Seoul National University, Korea, identified more than a dozen herbs with anti-aging effects used in traditional Oriental herbal therapy, of which *Polygonum multiflorum* (Ho Shou Wu: the name literally means "Mr. Ho's hair is black." The name refers to the story of a 58-year-old man named Ho, whose gray hair returned to its black

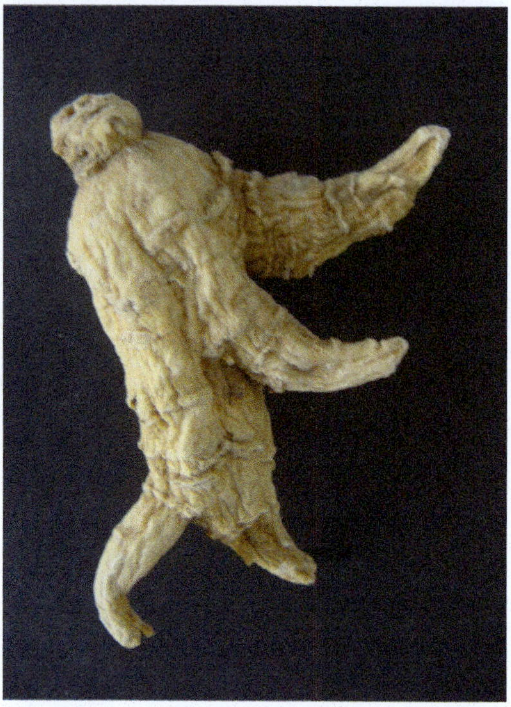

Fig. 4.11 Panax Ginseng. The Ginseng root is among the most prized among traditional Oriental herbal remedies based upon a *similia similibus* type of selection for its anthropomorphic form (Gift from Alexander Navarini, MD, PhD, University Hospital of Zurich)

color after taking the herb. He also became more youthful and was able to father several children. Supposedly he lived to become 160, retaining his black hair), and *Ginseng Radix* (Ren Shen: Fig. 4.11) probably represent the commercially most utilized in hair cosmetics, also on the contemporary Western market.

However, the effective constituents of the traditional herbal remedies have not been fully elucidated, though there is a great opportunity to study them systematically with respect to current research trends in anti-aging.

4.2.3 Telogen Effluvium

Diffuse shedding of hair has originally been called "defluvium capillorum." In 1932 Sabouraud restricted the term to sudden diffuse loss of hair following shortly after a severe emotional shock, while others applied it to all forms of alopecia. In 1961 Kligman revealed the pathodynamics of one common pattern of response of hair follicles to a variety of insults and named it telogen effluvium.

Whatever the cause, the follicle tends to behave in a similar way. To grasp the meaning of this generalization requires understanding of the hair cycle and its derangements.

As originally proposed by Mildred Trotter, the hair follicle is subject to constant turnover in the course of perpetual cycles through phases of proliferation in anagen, involution in catagen, and resting in telogen, with regeneration in the successive hair cycle (Fig. 4.12a).

It is a major characteristic of *anagen* (duration: 2–6 years) that not only the hair shaft is growing but that most epithelial hair follicle compartments undergo proliferation, with the hair matrix keratinocytes showing the highest proliferative activity.

During *catagen* (duration: 2 weeks), hair follicles enter a process of involution that is characterized by a burst of programmed cell death (apoptosis) in the majority of follicular keratinocytes. The resulting shortening of the regressing epithelial strand is associated with an upward movement of the follicle.

In *telogen* (duration: 3 months), the hair shaft matures into a club hair, which is held tightly in the bulbous base of the follicular epithelium, before it is eventually shed. It was unresolved, whether shedding of the telogen hair (*teloptosis*) is an active, regulated process or represents a passive event that occurs at the onset of subsequent anagen, as the new hair grows in.

Cyclic hair growth activity occurs in a random mosaic pattern with each follicle possessing its own individual control mechanism over the evolution and triggering of the successive phases, though systemic factors as

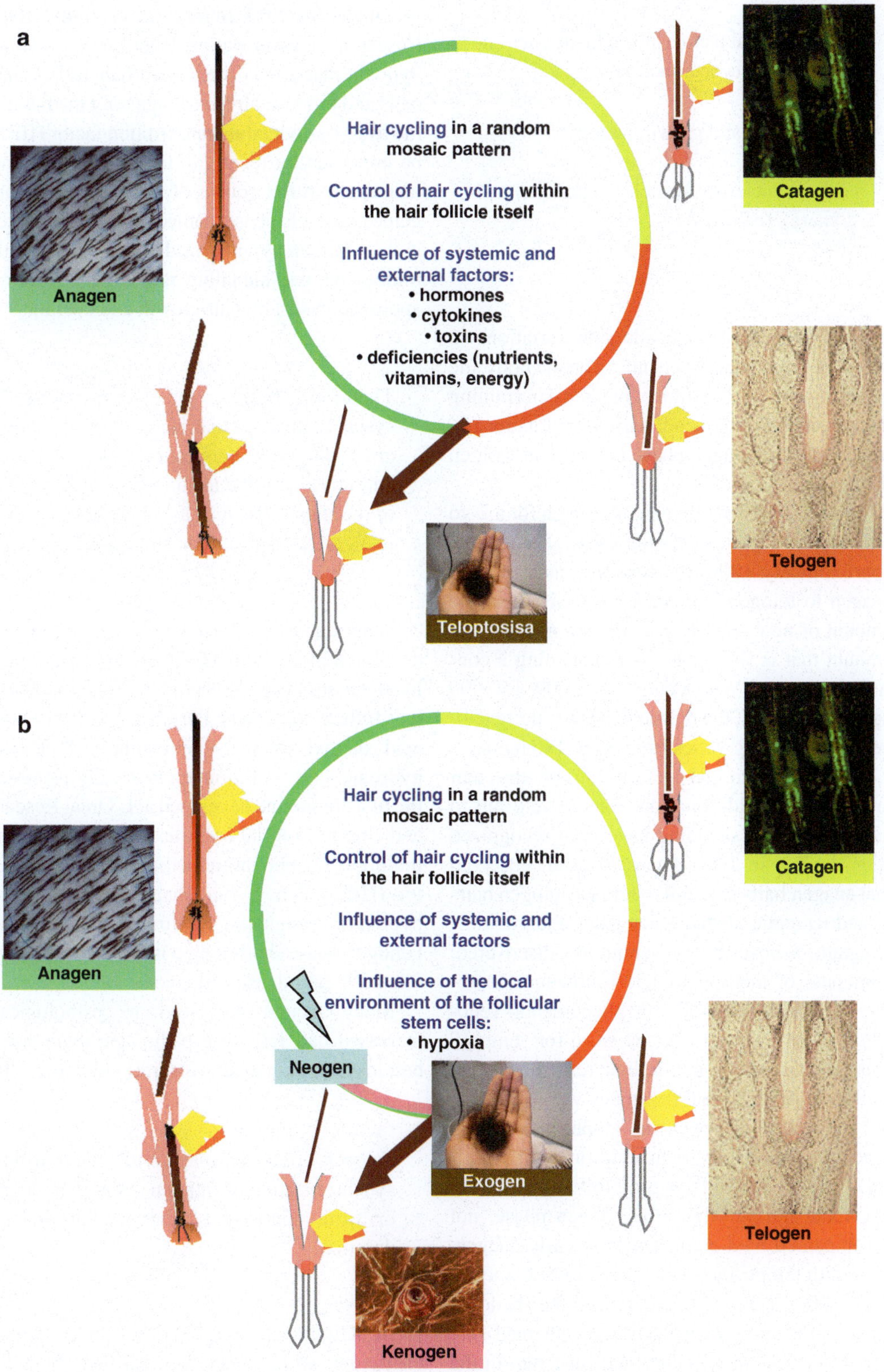

Fig. 4.12 (**a**, **b**) Hair cycle. (**a**) As originally described by Mildred Trotter. (**b**) Extended concept, including kenogen, exogen, and neogen

well as external factors linked to the environment have influence, such as:

- Hormones
- Cytokines and growth factors
- Toxins
- Deficiencies of nutrients, vitamins, and energy (calories)

Finally, there are considerable variations in length of these phases depending on the body site location, with the duration of anagen determining the type of hair produced, particularly its length. In general, the anagen phase is longer in women than in men.

On the scalp, hairs remain in anagen for a 2- to 6-year period of time, whereas that of telogen is approximately 100 days, resulting in a ratio of anagen to telogen hairs of 9:1. On average, the amount of new scalp hair formation matches the amount that is shed, thereby maintaining a consistent covering. With a range of 75,000–150,000 hairs on the head, the reported average daily telogen hair shedding varies from 35 to 180 hairs.

Since the original description of the hair growth cycle, additional phenomena relevant to hair growth and shedding have been recognized (Fig. 4.12b): In 1996, Guarrera et al. observed that anagen hairs may fail to replace telogen hairs in androgenetic alopecia. By using the phototrichogram, a novel phenomenon was discovered: emptiness of the hair follicle following teloptosis. Rebora chose to call this phenomenon kenogen, deriving from the Greek word for "empty." During kenogen, the hair follicle rests physiologically, but duration and frequency were shown to be greater in androgenetic alopecia, possibly accounting for baldness. In addition to the classical cycle, the hair follicle may follow an alternative route during which the telogen phase, not accompanied by a coincident new early anagen, ends with teloptosis leaving the follicle empty.

In 2002, Stenn et al. recognized the shedding phase of the hair growth cycle, then renamed exogen, to be a uniquely controlled final step in the hair cycle involving a specific proteolytic step.

Finally, in 2013 Bernard et al. from L'Oréal Research and Innovation laboratories identified hypoxia markers in the human hair follicle stem cells and proposed hypoxia signaling mediated by the hypoxia-inducible transcription factor HIF1 to be important for reentry of the follicle into a new hair cycle in the course of a novel neomorphogenic hair cycle phase, named neogen. Ultimately, it was further hypothesized that molecules that mimic hypoxic signaling may figure as a new approach to sustain hair growth and cycling.

Therefore, besides the well-recognized systemic and external factors linked to the environment (hormones, cytokines, toxins, and nutrients), the local milieu at the level of the stem cells, such as hypoxia, has been recognized to also impact hair cycling.

Consequently, it seemed conceivable to develop a biomimetic of the effects of a hypoxic local environment to optimize functionality of hair follicle stem cells. Pyridine-2,4-dicarboxylic acid diethyl ester (Stemoxydine®) 5 % in a hydroalcoholic solution applied daily represents the first compound developed at L'Oréal Research and Innovation laboratories as a competitive inhibitor of hypoxia-inducible transcription factor (HIF1) that is functionally able to induce hypoxia-like signaling in vitro and results in hair kenogen phase shortening with an increase in visible scalp hair density in vivo.

Many factors can lead to pathologically increased hair loss. The pathologic dynamics of hair loss can be related to disorders of hair cycling.

Telogen effluvium may result either from synchronization phenomena of hair cycling or from decrease of the anagen phase duration.

In Kligman's original description, telogen effluvium is an acute and diffuse hair loss brought about by a variety of triggers. Clinical experience, however, proves that chronic telogen effluvium also exists. It is defined as diffuse telogen hair loss that persists longer than 6 months.

While a number of attempts have been made with respect to the underlying pathologic dynamics of telogen effluvium and its classification, Headington's original classification of the functional types of telogen effluvium remains unabated the most comprehensive.

On the basis of the changes in different phases of the follicular cycle, Headington proposed further classification of telogen effluvium into five functional types.

> Telogen effluvium is by far the most common cause of hair loss and results from increased shedding of hairs from the telogen phase of the hair cycle. An increase in the percentage of follicles in telogen >20 % leads to a pathological increased shedding of normal club hairs.

In *immediate anagen release*, follicles would normally complete a longer cycle by remaining in anagen prematurely enter telogen. It is a very common form of telogen effluvium, typically occurring after periods of physiologic stress including episodes of high fever. In fever, the pyrogens, basically circulating cytokines, drive the hair follicle keratinocytes into apoptosis initiating catagen with following telogen. Because the shedding is dependent on transition from anagen through catagen and telogen with subsequent release of telogen hairs, hair loss occurs 3–4 months after the inciting event. A host of different triggers has been implicated and identifies the clinical species of the genus, e.g., post-febrile, post-traumatic, post-interventional, psychogenic effluvium, etc. Severe febrile illness, accidental trauma or surgical operations with a large hemorrhage, a crash diet, and severe emotional distress are among the most common causes. Most are self-limiting and will undergo normal reversal.

> A careful patient history with respect to the chronology of events usually reveals the diagnosis and the cause.

In *delayed anagen release*, hair follicles remain in prolonged anagen rather than cycling into telogen. When finally released from anagen, the clinical sign of increased shedding of telogen hair will be found. This type of telogen effluvium underlies postpartum hair loss. During the second half of pregnancy, the percentage of anagen hairs increases from the normal 85–95 %; at this time also the percentage of hairs of large shaft diameter is higher than in nonpregnant women of the same age. After partuition the follicles, in which anagen has been prolonged, rapidly enter catagen and then telogen, with an increased shedding of hair evident after 3–4 months.

> Most women will return to their usual hair growth cycle and pre-pregnancy thickness of hair between 6 and 12 months after birth. In case of persistent postpartum effluvium (>12 months), excessive hair loss may be caused by common conditions, such as female androgenetic alopecia, iron deficiency, or hypothyroidism. Lesser common conditions include persistent hyperprolactinemia (Chiari–Frommel syndrome) and postpartum hypopituitarism (Sheehan syndrome) caused by pituitary necrosis due to blood loss and hypovolemic shock during childbirth.

In *immediate telogen release*, hair follicles normally programmed for release of the club hair after an interval of usually 100 days after the end of anagen are prematurely stimulated to cycle into anagen. There is premature teloptosis. This type of telogen effluvium underlies the shedding of hair upon initiation of therapy with topical minoxidil solution (shedding phase).

Seemingly ironic, upon initiation of treatment with the hair growth-promoting agent minoxidil, patients frequently experience increased shedding of hair. Patients should be prepared and informed that this represents a physiological response to treatment, since minoxidil not only increases the duration of anagen but triggers an immediate telogen release.

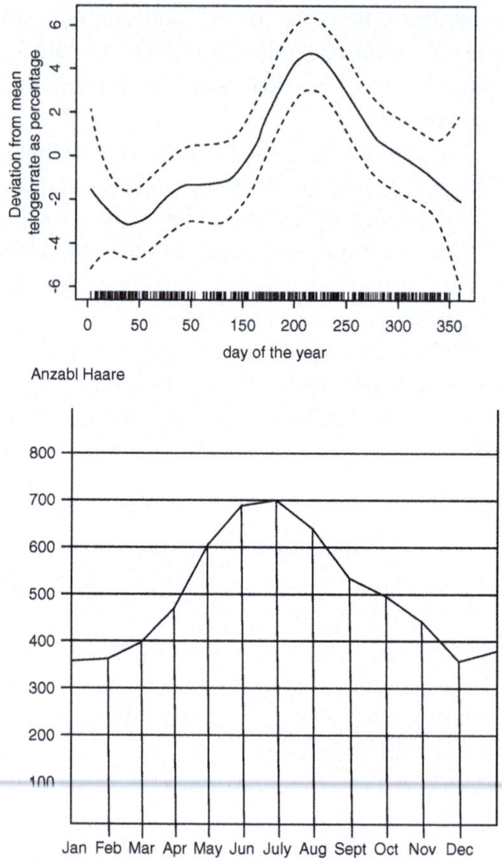

Fig. 4.13 (**a**, **b**) Seasonality of hair growth and shedding. (**a**) Fluctuations in frontal telogen rates ($n=823$) in relation to the day of the year in women complaining of hair loss (From: Kunz et al. 2009) (**b**) Fluctuations of shed hair in a 39-year-old healthy male, counted between 1996 and 2011. The mean counted values were plotted in relation to the month of the year

In *delayed telogen release*, hair follicles remain in prolonged telogen rather than being shed and recycling into anagen. When finally teloptosis sets in, again the clinical sign of increased shedding of club hairs is observed. This process underlies molting in mammals and probably also seasonal shedding of hairs in humans or mild telogen effluvia following travel from low-daylight to high-daylight conditions. The cyclical activities of the hair follicle is the mechanism by which mammals change their coat of hair to meet the exigencies of growth, seasonal changes in the ambient environment, and, perhaps, normal wear and tear. It seems likely that environmental factors, such as the photoperiod, mediate through the optic pathway and the neuroendocrine system coat phenotype and function to photoperiod-dependent environmental changes. Originally, Orentreich reported three women in New York who experienced maximum hair loss in November. Studying a group of 14 men during 18 months, Randall and Ebling showed that the proportion of telogen hair and of hair shedding were maximal in September. Courtois et al. observed ten men, with or without alopecia, for a period of between 8 and 14 years and also demonstrated a maximal proportion of telogen hairs at the end of summer. Some subjects also exhibited a periodicity approximately corresponding to two annual peaks. Ultimately, Kunz et al. published a study of 823 otherwise healthy women with telogen effluvium observed over a period of 6 years and demonstrated the existence of overall annual periodicity in the growth and shedding of hair, manifested by a maximal proportion of telogen hairs in July. A second peak seemed to exist, although less pronounced, in April (Fig. 4.13a). The telogen rate was lowest toward the beginning of February. The fact that human hair follicles, just as those of other mammals, undergo cyclical activity and are influenced by hormones implies that human hair is not unaffected by these phenomena.

From an evolutionary point of view, the maintenance of the low winter level of hair shedding and the postponement of hair fall until the end of summer might, perhaps, are postulated as having a selective advantage with respect to isolation of the head against the cold in winter and protection of the scalp against the midday sun in summer, respectively.

Finally, a 39-year-old long-haired male presented at the Center for Dermatology and to Hair Disease Professor Trüeb with early androgenetic alopecia. He had counted his hairs shed in the course of hair washing every 3 days from the years 1996–2011 and plotted their mean value against the month of the year (Fig. 4.13b). There was a striking congruence with the graphic formerly demonstrated for women by Kunz et al., which proves that men are subject to the same seasonal changes of hair growth and shedding as women.

The difference is that seasonal hair shedding is less noticeable in men, who commonly wear their hair shorter. Moreover, men usually have a lesser sensitivity than women for the condition of their hair.

Finally, the existence of a *short anagen phase* was proposed by Headington in his classification of telogen effluvium. Headington suggested the existence of a mild form of persistent telogen effluvium in association with decreased hair length due to a short anagen phase. The existence of *short anagen hair* as an isolated disorder in otherwise healthy children was later confirmed by Barraud-Klenovsek and Trüeb, who reported two children with a peculiar type of isolated congenital hypotrichosis. Both presented with persistent short, fine hair since birth (Fig. 4.14). Evidence was provided that the short hair observed in these patients was due to a short anagen phase of the hair cycle, with a normal rate of hair growth. Shortening of the anagen phase of the scalp hair cycle leads to a decrease in the maximal hair length and an increase in the number of hairs in telogen, resulting in an increase in hair shedding. Alternatively, Sinclair provided evidence of short anagen hair with a persistent synchronized pattern of scalp hair growth in a 4-year-old boy. One patient had affected family members with an apparently autosomal dominant mode of inheritance. The disorder appears to resolve spontaneously during puberty and adulthood. The syndrome of short anagen hair was

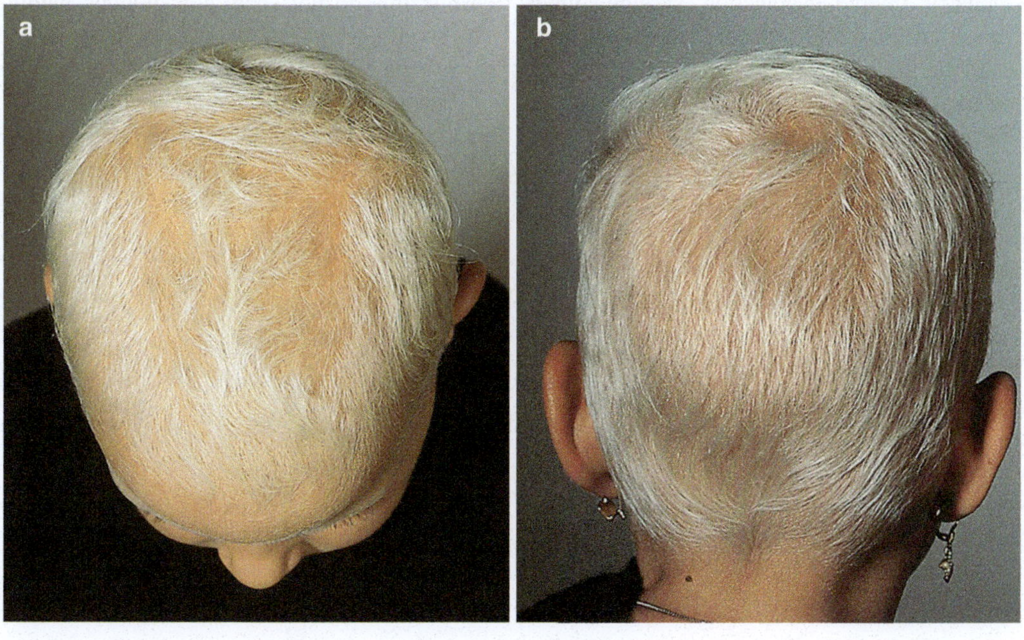

Fig. 4.14 (**a**, **b**) Short anagen hair

subsequently confirmed by Olsen who proposed methods for diagnosing this entity by clinical examination, trichogram, light microscopic examination of the hair shaft, scalp biopsy, and measurement of scalp hair growth rate.

> Short anagen hair appears to be an uncommon though probably underreported condition, whose incidence is poorly documented in the medical literature. The most important differential diagnosis includes short anagen hair in trichodental syndrome, loose anagen hair, hereditary hypotrichosis simplex, and premature androgenetic alopecia. Treatment is not necessary, though one would expect—as in androgenetic alopecia—efficacy of topical minoxidil from reported successful treatment of a short anagen hair nevus.

Chronic telogen effluvium. Diffuse shedding of telogen hairs that persists longer than 6 months either represents a primary disorder and is then a diagnosis of exclusion, or it is secondary to a variety of identifiable systemic disorders, such as iron deficiency, thyroid dysfunction, systemic lupus erythematosus, and syphilis. In comparison, other dietary deficiencies, metabolic diseases, connective tissue disorders, and malignant or chronic infectious diseases are infrequent causes of hair loss in office-based clinical practice. Drugs known to cause hair loss, such as anticoagulants (heparin, warfarin), oral retinoids (acitretin, isotretinoin), interferon, agents with antithyroid action (carbimazole, propylthiouracil, amiodarone), hypolipidemic agents (fibrates), colchicine, antimetabolites (methotrexate, azathioprine, cyclophosphamide), and hormones with pro-androgen action (norethisterone, levonorgestrel, tibolone). Finally, dietary habits should be addressed. Especially in young women, if anorexia nervosa/bulimia is suspected, the aid of a psychiatrist should be sought; in other cases, the informed patient will be happy to abandon any dietary culprit.

> The cause of chronic telogen effluvium may be multifactorial and difficult to establish.

While symptomatic telogen effluvium is triggered by one or several identifiable events, in *primary chronic telogen effluvium*, no specific trigger is evident. It predominantly affects women, while men with short hair tend not to notice increased hair shedding. The presentation of this type of diffuse hair loss tends to be distinctive and was originally described 1959 in detail by Guy and Edmundson as "diffuse cyclic hair loss in women" and revived by Whiting in 1996, who additionally characterized histopathologic features differing the condition from androgenetic alopecia. The typical patient is a vigorous otherwise healthy woman between 30 and 60 with a full, thick head of hair. On examination there are some bitemporal thinning (Fig. 4.15a) and a positive hair pull test equally over the vertex and occiput. There is no widening of the central part, as is common in androgenetic alopecia. Nevertheless, patients are adamant that they previously had more hair and are distressed by the prospect of going bald. Many frequently bring large balls of hair for inspection (Fig. 4.15b) but despite this do not show any obvious balding. The condition tends to run a fluctuating course. It is has been proposed that the disorder may be due to synchronization phenomena of the hair cycle, shortening of the anagen phase, or premature teloptosis.

> On the long run, chronic telogen effluvium appears to be self-limiting, and it is important to reassure patients that this condition represents exaggerated shedding rather than actual hair loss.

In an attempt to find a simple method to evaluate reliably the diagnosis and activity of androgenetic alopecia and telogen effluvium,

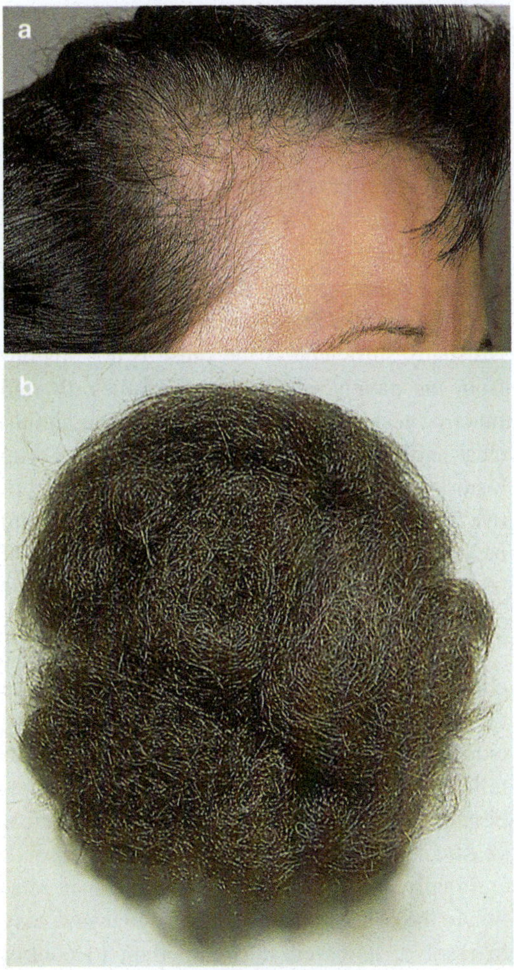

Fig. 4.15 (**a**, **b**) Chronic telogen effluvium: (**a**) Temporal thinning of hair. (**b**) Ball of shed hair

Nevertheless, differential diagnosis of chronic telogen effluvium from androgenetic alopecia is often complicated through considerable overlap. Ultimately, synchronization phenomena of hair cycling, often on a seasonal basis, are more pronounced in androgenetic alopecia, since with a shorter anagen phase there is a tendency to more pronounced synchronization of hair follicles.

More recently, an inflammatory or "autoimmune" type of telogen effluvium has been proposed on the basis of the observation of a high frequency of associated scalp dysesthesia (trichodynia), associated autoimmune phenomena (Hashimoto's thyroiditis), and response to topical corticosteroid treatment.

Up to date, histopathological evidence is lacking for the presence of follicular inflammation in telogen effluvium (as opposed to androgenetic alopecia). In 2002, Sato-Kuwamora et al. suggested naming a peculiar type of inflammatory non-cicatricial alopecia that is characterized by marked female predominance and a uniquely short clinical course *acute diffuse and total alopecia of the female scalp*. It is basically identical with a subtype of alopecia areata presenting with diffuse hair loss as originally proposed in the German literature by Braun-Falco and Zaun 40 years earlier in 1962.

Guarrera et al. adopted the modified wash test, which accomplishes such a task through the assessment of the number of shed hair and the vellus percentage. As in the wash test, 5 days after the last shampoo, the patient is instructed to wash the hair in the sink with its drain covered by a gauze. The hairs entrapped in the gauze are then collected, counted, and divided into ≤3 and ≥5 cm in length. The test demonstrated that in female with androgenetic alopecia the proportion of vellus hairs is significantly higher than in chronic telogen effluvium (58.9 % versus 3.5 %).

Acute diffuse and total alopecia of the female scalp, alopecia areata incognita (yet another synonymous designation proposed by Rebora in 1987), and diffuse alopecia areata all represent the same alopecia areata variant that is characterized by diffuse hair shedding in the absence of the patches otherwise typical for the disease. The condition usually affects women over 40 years of age, who complain of diffuse alopecia and may be misdiagnosed as having telogen effluvium.

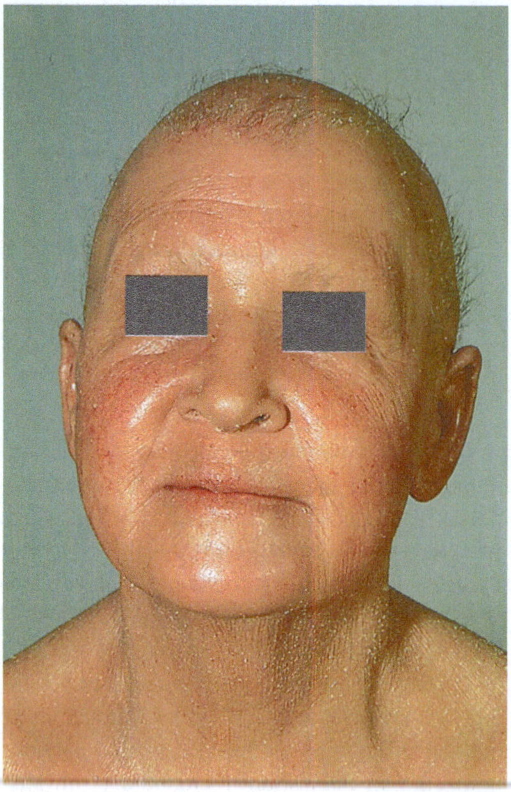

Fig. 4.16 Diffuse inflammatory effluvium due to erythroderma (Sézary syndrome)

The presence of yellow dots and short regrowing miniaturized hairs seen in the terminal hair-bearing scalp by trichoscopy, as well as associated autoimmune phenomena (Hashimoto's thyroiditis and/or circulating antithyroid and anti-parietal cell antibodies), represents important clues to the diagnosis. The diagnosis is usually confirmed by histopathology and/or usually excellent response with complete hair regrowth to a course of systemic corticosteroids.

Ultimately, the designation *inflammatory telogen effluvium* should be reserved for telogen effluvium related to inflammatory conditions of the scalp, such as severe seborrhoeic dermatitis, acute allergic contact dermatitis (usually to PPD in hair coloring agents), erythroderma (of psoriasis or lymphoma: Fig. 4.16), or interface dermatitis from lupus erythematosus or dermatomyositis.

Treatment of telogen effluvium is quite straightforward: Acute telogen effluvium is usually self-limiting (within 6 months by definition), providing that the culprit has been identified and eliminated.

Reassuring patients that they are not going bald and that the telogen effluvium is temporary is usually sufficient. If the cause is not obvious from the patient's history, iron studies, thyroid function tests, syphilis serology, and an antinuclear antibody titer should be performed. A drug history and in women a change in the contraceptive pill or hormone replacement therapy should be inquired about, as these are common causes of telogen effluvium related to female androgenetic alopecia.

Recommendations for treatment of primary chronic telogen effluvium are scanty and include topical or systemic corticosteroids, topical minoxidil, and dietary supplements on the basis of millet extract, pantothenic acid, biotin, their combination, or combinations of L-cystine, medicinal yeast, and pantothenic acid (CYP-complex).

Finally, the issue of overvalued ideas in relation to the condition of the hair is not always easy to resolve; however, it is important to control stress as a complication of hair loss or fear of hair loss. For this purpose, strong psychological support is essential to help limit patient anxiety, and patients need to be educated about the basics of the hair cycle. Information about the hair cycle can be useful to explain how hair loss not related to cycle shortening (as in androgenetic alopecia) generally precedes new regrowth and why considerable patience is required for effective cosmetic recovery.

Most importantly, women with chronic telogen effluvium need to be reassured that it represents exaggerated shedding rather than actual hair loss and that the shed hair is mostly being replaced; therefore, the risk of total baldness is remote.

4.2.4 Alopecia Areata

Novalis (Georg Philipp Friedrich von Hardenberg, poet, author, and philosopher of early German Romanticism, 1772–1801) wrote: "when we dream that we are dreaming, the moment of awaking is at hand." I personally realized the extent of psychological traumatism resulting from the loss of hair in clumps on the occasion of a respective dream during a lecture tour on hair. I dreamt awaking in the morning before my presentation in the hotel room and pulling out hairs in clumps in front of the bathroom mirror when attempting to groom them. In that moment I realized it was alopecia areata but almost simultaneously also that it must be a dream.

Since hair is a power symbol, as the Biblical Samson teaches us in Judges 16, it is customary that hair falling out in dreams is interpreted as loss of power and control. The same type of helpless feeling is experienced in waking life when hair is lost. The hair loss dream is typically a manifestation of a stressful situation. Ultimately, hair dreams represent a situation that is beyond one's control.

Alopecia areata is considered to be of autoimmune origin with an organ-specific, T-cell-mediated assault on the hair follicle at the level of the bulb. The hair bulb is an immune protected site with deficient MHC expression. There is circumstantial evidence suggesting that alopecia areata results from loss of immune privilege with presentation of autoantigens. A peribulbar lymphocytic infiltrate induces hair follicle keratinocytes to undergo apoptosis resulting in inhibition of cell division in the hair matrix. It represents the most frequent cause of dystrophic anagen effluvium, either localized or diffuse, occurring in the otherwise healthy child or adult. It is a common hair loss condition characterized by an acute onset of non-scarring hair loss in usually sharply defined areas. Any hair-bearing area can be affected, but the most noticeable are the scalp, the beard area, and the eyebrows. The characteristic patch of alopecia areata is usually round or oval and is completely bald and smooth. Trichoscopic examination reveals yellow dots, dystrophic hairs (cadaverized hairs, exclamation mark hairs), and/or short regrowing miniaturized hairs.

> The progress of alopecia areata in an individual patient is unpredictable, though a large surface area, a long disease duration, and associated nail abnormalities have been connected with a poorer prognosis.

Some patients lose hair in only a small patch, while others may have more extensive or less frequently diffuse involvement. Alopecia totalis is the loss of all scalp hair; alopecia universalis is the loss of all scalp and body hair.

A recent meta-analysis of published trials on treatment of alopecia areata states that only few treatments have been well evaluated in randomized trials. The authors found no randomized controlled trials on the use of diphenylcyclopropenone (DCP), intralesional corticosteroids, or dithranol, although commonly used in clinical practice. Although topical steroids and minoxidil are widely prescribed and appear to be safe, there is no convincing evidence that they are beneficial in the long term. Most trials have been reported poorly and are so small that any important clinical benefits are inconclusive. Of 17 trials including 6–85 participants with a total of 540 participants assessing a range of interventions that included topical and oral corticosteroids, topical ciclosporin, photodynamic therapy, and topical minoxidil, none showed significant treatment benefit in terms of hair growth when compared with placebo. The authors came to the conclusion that considering the possibility of spontaneous remission, especially for those in the early stages of the disease, the options of not being treated therapeutically or, depending on individual preference, of wearing a wig may be alternative ways of dealing with this condition.

Nonetheless, depending on patient age, surface area, and disease duration, a treatment algorithm can be designed (Fig. 4.17). Any treatment of alopecia areata should fulfill the following criteria:

- Remission rates superior to the spontaneous remission rates of alopecia areata
- Proof of efficacy in half side treatment of alopecia totalis or universalis
- Good safety profile with minimal toxicity

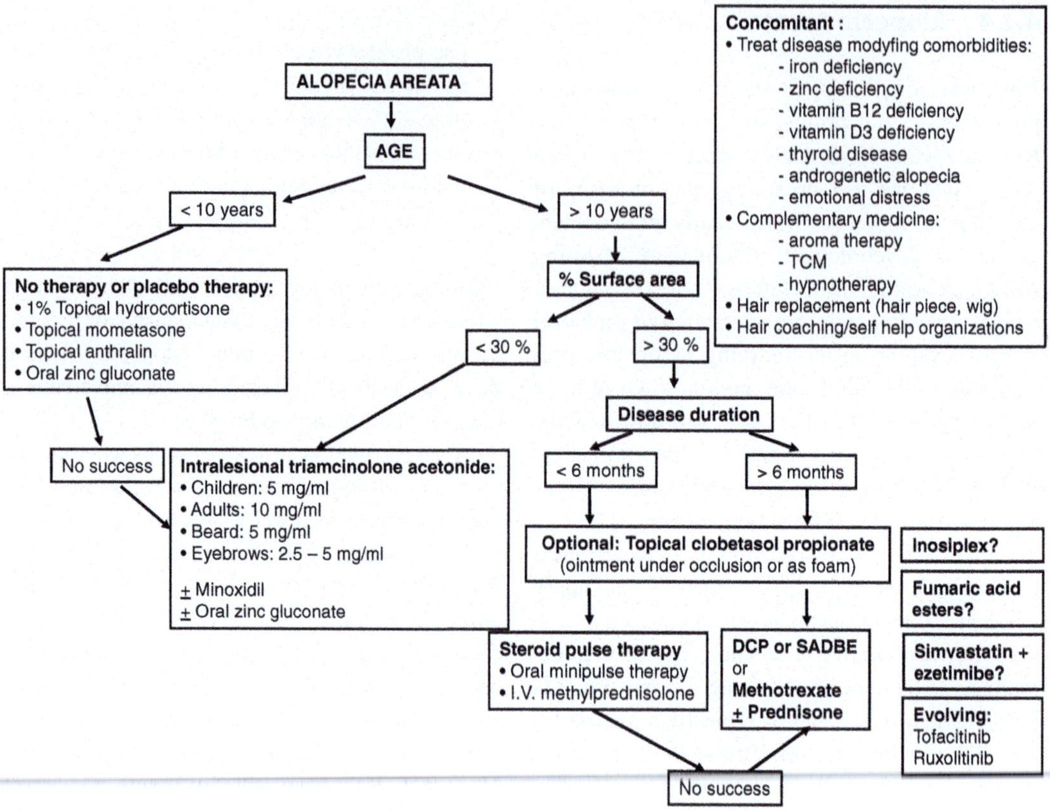

Fig. 4.17 Algorithm for treatment of alopecia areata, depending on patient age, surface area, and disease duration

> The spontaneous remission rates for patchy alopecia areata are one third within 6 months, half within 1 year, and two thirds within 5 years; thereafter, complete remissions are rare. Recurrence rates within 5 years are 80 % and within 20 years 100 %. Total remission rates for alopecia totalis or universalis with a disease duration of 5 years or more are 1 % in children and less than 10 % in adults.

Single patches of alopecia areata are best treated with intralesional triamcinolone acetonide 10 mg/ml by jet injector or insulin syringe on a monthly basis, for an average of three to a maximum of six consecutive treatments (in children 5 mg/ml, for eyebrows 2.5–5 mg/ml, and for beard 5 mg/ml by insulin syringe).

Since patchy alopecia areata is the most prevalent form of the disease and intralesional corticosteroid injections are the most frequently practiced treatment for this condition, Samrao et al. conducted a retrospective cross-sectional case series on 18 patients with patchy alopecia areata treated at 4- to 8-week intervals with intralesional triamcinolone acetonide for at least 20 months to evaluate the effect on bone mineral density (BMD). Patients were evaluated for BMD using dual-energy X-ray absorptiometry (DXA). Follow-up DXA measurements were obtained in those with abnormal findings. Nine out of 18 patients (50 %) had abnormal DXA results. Patients with the following risk factors were more likely to have abnormal BMD: age older than 50 years, body mass index less than 18.5 kg/m^2, lack of weight-bearing exercise, smoking history, postmenopausal status, past stress fracture, family history of osteopenia or osteoporosis, and a cumulative intralesional triamcinolone acetonide dose of greater than 500 mg.

The authors concluded that patients with patchy alopecia areata who receive chronic intralesional triamcinolone acetonide therapy should be counseled on preventive measures for osteoporosis and monitored for effects on BMD.

In an attempt to circumvent side effects related with systemic corticosteroid therapy for widespread disease, pulsed administration of corticosteroids has been proposed in the treatment of alopecia areata: Sharma originally proposed 300 mg oral prednisolone pulses at 4-week intervals, for a minimum of four doses or until cosmetically acceptable hair growth was obtained. 58.3 % of patients with widespread alopecia areata showed cosmetically acceptable hair growth. Response was evident on average after 2–3 months of therapy. In a subsequent study, Sharma and Muralidhar reported efficacy and safety of monthly oral corticosteroid pulse therapy also for treatment of widespread alopecia areata in young patients (up to 18 years of age), including children. Children aged less than 12 years received betamethasone sodium phosphate as soluble equivalent to prednisolone 5 mg/kg body weight every month. Side effects were minimal and included transient giddiness, headache, and epigastric burning.

Subsequently, Kar et al. confirmed in the first placebo-controlled study usefulness of oral prednisolone pulse therapy in alopecia areata.

Agarwal et al. alternatively suggested twice-weekly 5 mg betamethasone oral pulse therapy on two consecutive days per week for a total duration of 12 weeks.

To determine the effectiveness of an intravenous pulse of methylprednisolone, much in the same way as for treatment of other autoimmune diseases, Friedli et al. originally performed an open prospective study of patients with rapid and extensive hair loss for less than 1 year (first occurrence or relapse) with the bald area exceeding 30 % of the scalp. Two hundred and fifty milligram intravenous methylprednisolone was administered twice a day on three consecutive days. A single series of intravenous pulse of methylprednisolone was well tolerated and appeared to be effective in patients with rapidly progressing extensive multifocal alopecia areata, but not those with ophiasic and universal alopecia areata.

Subsequently, Nakajima confirmed the efficacy of intravenous pulse of methylprednisolone in a larger study of 139 patients aged >15 years with alopecia areata. With intravenous pulse corticosteroid therapy (500 mg methylprednisolone on three consecutive days, in three cycles, 4 weeks apart) within 6 months of disease onset, remission rates were 88 % for multilocular alopecia areata with surface area <50 %, 59.4 % with surface area >50 %, and 21.4 % in alopecia totalis/universalis. After 6 months of disease onset, the remission rate was 15.8 %.

Finally, Im et al. studied the outcome in 70 patients with severe alopecia areata treated with intravenous methylprednisolone pulse therapy on three consecutive days. All of patients had rapid and extensive hair loss with the bald area exceeding 50 % of the scalp. Seventy percent of patients showed terminal hair growth, and 41.4 % complete recovery with acceptable cosmetic results.

The prognostic factors that influenced successful outcome of i.v. methylprednisolone pulse therapy of alopecia areata were disease duration before treatment in relation to the type of alopecia areata. A good response was obtained for all types of alopecia areata with a duration of 3 months or less before treatment and for the multifocal type of alopecia areata with a duration of <6 months.

Tosti et al. evaluated topical clobetasol for treatment of widespread and long-standing (severe and refractory) alopecia areata. With

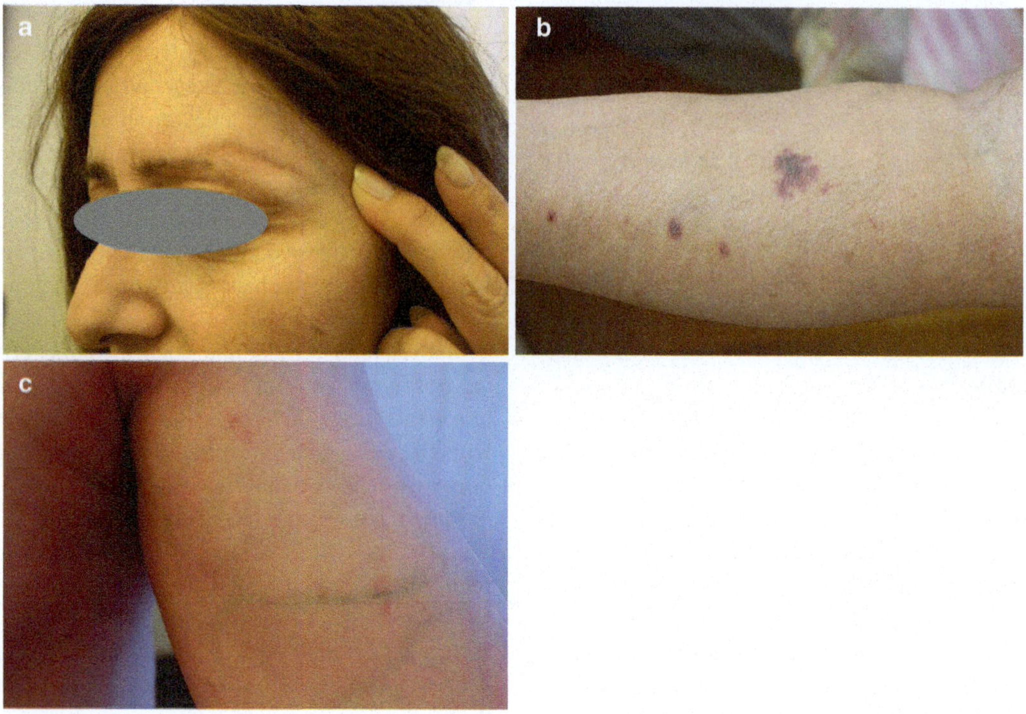

Fig. 4.18 (**a**–**c**) Typical cutaneous adverse effects from corticosteroid treatments: (**a**) subcutaneous atrophy after steroid injection in eyebrow area, (**b**) Bateman's purpura from occlusive clobetasol propionate treatment for alopecia areata in a 76-year-old female patient, (**c**) steroid-induced striae distensae rubrae (stretch marks) of upper arms from uncontrolled use of clobetasol propionate ointment for treatment of alopecia areata in a 38-year-old male patient. The patient also had evidence of adrenal suppression

0.05 % topical clobetasol ointment under occlusion (Saran wrap) on six consecutive nights per week over 6 months, regrowth of hair was achieved in alopecia totalis or universalis in 17.8 %. Negative prognostic features for treatment success were positive family history for alopecia areata, first manifestation of disease before the age of 10 years, and association with atopic disease or autoimmune thyroid disease. Folliculitis and acne were frequent side effects. Despite positive clinical results obtained using clobetasol ointment with occlusive dressing, this approach has a low patient compliance, especially in patients with residual hair. Therefore, in a subsequent study, 0.05 % clobetasol foam was applied twice daily on five consecutive days per week and proved to also be effective, safe, and well tolerated, with good cosmetic acceptance and patient compliance. Folliculitis occurred in a smaller proportion of patients. No significant modifications in cortisol and ACTH blood levels were observed.

In summary, the art of using corticosteroids for treatment of alopecia areata is maximizing efficacy and minimizing toxicity.

Figure 4.18a–c illustrates typical cutaneous adverse effects from the use of intralesional or high-potency topical corticosteroids.

Topical immunotherapy has been used since the 1970s to treat dermatologic conditions understood to result from an altered immunological state, mainly widespread, long-standing alopecia areata and resistant viral warts. Any of three universal contact sensitisers may be used for topical immunotherapy, but diphenylcyclopropenone (D(P)CP) has advantages over dinitrochlorobenzene (DNCB) and squaric acid dibutylester (SADBE). In a retrospective study of 68 patients with severe alopecia areata (>40 % scalp hair loss) treated for at least 5 months with topical DCP, Pericin and Trüeb found an overall response rate of 70.6 % with 30.9 % complete remission and 39.7 % partial remission. Among the investigated prognostic factors for the outcome of DCP therapy, only the extent of alopecia areata at the time of initiation of treatment was found to be of significance. Total remission rates for multilocular alopecia areata were 43.8 %, for subtotal alopecia areata and ophiasis 33.3 %, and for alopecia totalis or universalis 21.4 %, irrespective of disease duration. Subsequent authors confirmed that topical immunotherapy with DCP is effective and usually well tolerated. The extent of hair loss before therapy is the main predictor for therapeutic success. However, DCP therapy is associated with a high relapse rate of which patients should be informed. A long period of therapy is needed and may increase the percentage of responders, especially in alopecia totalis and universalis. Maintenance therapy is recommended to reduce the risk of relapse.

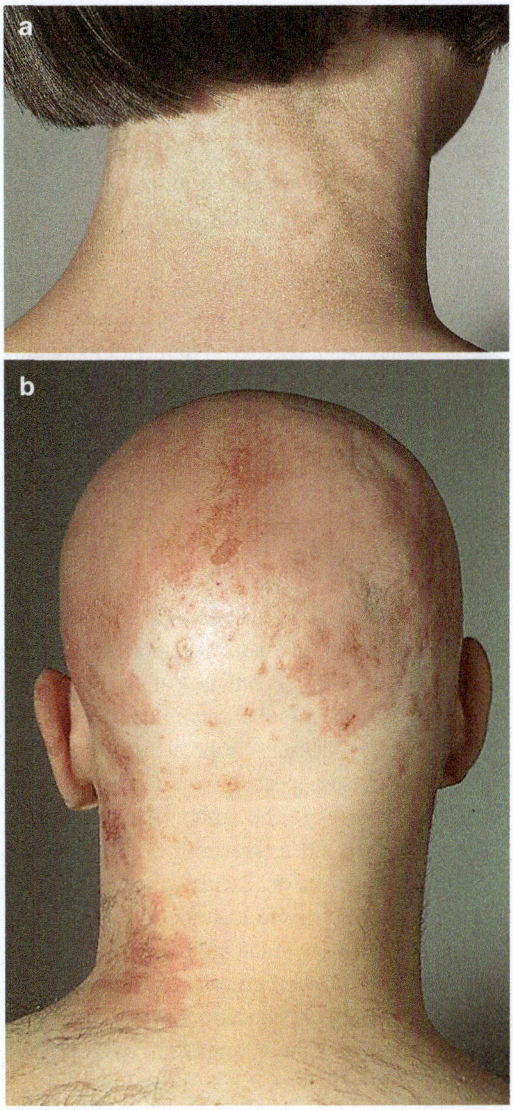

Fig. 4.19 (**a**, **b**) Adverse effects from treatment of alopecia areata with DCP. (**a**) Dyschromia in confetti. (**b**) Erythema multiforme-like eruption

> Ultimately, Tosti et al. found that severity of alopecia areata at time of first consultation is an important prognostic factor, response to topical immunotherapy may be associated with better prognosis, in children the prognosis is worse, and alopecia areata may worsen over time.

Finally, it must be borne in mind that DCP is photosensitive, which is why the substance must be stored in the dark, and the scalp must be protected from light after application of DCP until contact dermatitis is elucidated.

Side effects of DCP therapy include itching, blistering, cervical lymphadenopathy, dyschromia in confetti (Fig. 4.19a), vitiligo, erythema multiforme-like eruption (Fig. 4.19b), exacerbation of (pre-existent) discoid lupus erythematosus, (contact) urticaria, and lentiginous eruption.

> Sensitization of medical, nursing, and pharmacy staff may be avoided by careful handling of the DCP solutions.

Oral fexofenadine, an H1-receptor antagonist, may partially inhibit the itch of contact dermatitis induced by DCP in patients with alopecia areata. Moreover, Inui et al. suggested that oral fexofenadine may enhance the efficacy of contact immunotherapy for extensive alopecia areata in patients with an atopic background (atopic alopecia areata).

Inosine pranobex or Isoprinosine is a combination of inosine, acetamidobenzoic acid, and dimethylaminoisopropanol used as an immunomodulating drug used to treat patients suffering from viral infections such as subacute sclerosing panencephalitis, varicella, and herpes simplex types 1 and 2 and as an adjunct in the treatment of genital warts. Its use for treatment of alopecia areata has been originally reported in the 1980s, with observation of patients with alopecia areata associated with autoantibodies showing response to therapy. Treatment with Isoprinosine produced a clinical response, as judged by total or partial hair growth in 9 of the 14 patients treated. It was striking to observe that seven of the nine responders had autoantibodies prior to treatment. These disappeared or decreased with Isoprinosine therapy. The authors concluded that alopecia areata is a heterogeneous condition subdivided by the presence or absence of autoantibodies, since clinical response to Isoprinosine was mainly obtained in patients with autoantibodies. Subsequent studies failed to confirm efficacy of Isoprinosine in inducing total remission in alopecia areata, either as a monotherapy or in combination with topical immunotherapy with DCP.

Also, treatment of therapy-resistant alopecia areata with fumaric acid esters has been proposed. Fumaric acid or trans-butenedioic acid is the chemical compound with the formula $HO_2CCH{=}CHCO_2H$. This white crystalline compound is one of two isomeric unsaturated dicarboxylic acids, the other being maleic acid. The salts and esters are known as fumarates. Fumarate is also an intermediate in the citric acid cycle used by cells to produce energy in the form of adenosine triphosphate from food. It is formed by the oxidation of succinate by the enzyme succinate dehydrogenase. Fumarate is then converted by the enzyme fumarase to malate. Human skin naturally produces fumaric acid when exposed to sunlight. Dimethylfumarate significantly reduces disability progression in multiple sclerosis and is used for treatment of psoriasis. In patients with relapsing–remitting multiple sclerosis, dimethylfumarate significantly reduced relapse and disability progression in a phase 3 trial. It activates the Nrf2 antioxidant response pathway, the primary cellular defense against the cytotoxic effects of oxidative stress. Fumaric acid ester therapy has also proved to be safe and effective in patients with psoriasis vulgaris. This treatment was introduced nearly 30 years ago but is only now gaining renewed interest among dermatologists. Although the mode of action of fumaric acid esters in the treatment of psoriasis is not fully understood, recent experimental data point toward a skewing of the Th1-dominated T-cell response in psoriasis to a Th2-like pattern and inhibition of proliferation of keratinocytes. More recently, therapy-resistant alopecia areata was treated with fumaric acid esters within the bounds of an open, non-placebo-controlled pilot study for a period of 6 months and a maximum dose of 120 mg dimethylfumarate per day. Six of ten patients took benefit from the therapy with fumaric acid esters, with very good results in three, presenting an almost entire remission. Validation of this therapeutic approach in a placebo-controlled and multicenter study with higher numbers of patients is pending.

Namazani originally proposed the use of statins for treatment of a variety of dermatologic conditions characterized by ingress of activated leukocytes into the skin, including alopecia areata. The 3-hydroxy-3-methylglutaryl coenzyme A (HMG-CoA) reductase inhibitors (statins) atorvastatin, cerivastatin, fluvastatin, pravastatin, lovastatin, and simvastatin are currently used for reducing atherogenesis and cardiovascular morbidity, but there is increasing evidence that they also have immunomodulatory activities. Statins downregulate the expression of adhesion molecules, intercellular adhesion molecule-1 (ICAM-1), monocyte chemotactic protein-1 (MAC-1), and lymphocyte function-associated antigen-1 (LFA-1) on leukocytes and endothelial cells and, through binding to LFA-1, interfere with ICAM-1-LFA-1 interaction, which is crucial for activation of lymphocytes by antigen-presenting cells, ingress of leukocytes into the inflammation sites, and immunologic cytotoxicity. Statins inhibit the inducible expression of major histocompatibility complex class II in several cell types including macrophages and downregulate the expression of T-helper-1 (Th1) chemokine receptors on T-cells, leading further to inhibition of activation of lymphocytes and their infiltration into the inflammation sites. Statins block the induction of inducible nitric oxide synthase and the expression of several pro-inflammatory cytokines such as tumor necrosis factor-alpha and interferon-gamma in macrophages and possess antioxidant effects. These agents inhibit the proliferation of immunocytes and the activation of natural killer cells.

Robins was the first to report hair regrowth following initiation of simvastatin and ezetimibe therapy in a patient with alopecia universalis. Lattouf et al. subsequently reported a case series of 29 alopecia areata patients with 40–70 % scalp involvement who were enrolled for treatment with simvastatin/ezetimibe 40/10 mg daily. Nineteen completed 24 weeks of treatment, and the remaining ten patients were lost to follow-up. Fourteen of nineteen were judged responders. Hair regrowth was evident after 16–24 weeks of treatment. Upon completion of the initial 24 weeks of treatment, the 14 responders were randomized into a group of seven patients who continued treatment for an additional 24 weeks or into a group of seven patients who stopped medication. In the former group, five of seven continued with hair growth or had stable disease, while in the latter group, five of seven patients relapsed. No side effects were observed. Nevertheless, in January 2014 the US Food and Drug Administration released an advice on statin risk reporting that "… they need to be taken with care and knowledge of their side effects." Among them the most common complication is myopathy, ranging from more common clinically benign myalgia to rare and life-threatening rhabdomyolysis. To minimize statin-associated myopathy, clinicians should take into consideration a series of factors that potentially increase this risk: drug–drug interactions, especially with cytochrome P-450 3A4 inhibitors (including grapefruit juice), female gender, advanced age, and comorbidities such as diabetes mellitus, hypothyroidism, and vitamin D deficiency. Moreover, periodic screening of creatine kinase (CK, CPK) levels is recommended. It has been suggested that coenzyme Q10 supplementation (50 mg bid) may reduce statin-related mild to moderate muscular symptoms. A more recent meta-analysis of available randomized controlled trials eventually did not suggest any significant benefit of coenzyme Q10 supplementation in improving statin-induced myopathy.

Finally, Joly proposed the use of methotrexate (MTX) alone or in combination with low doses of oral corticosteroids in the treatment of alopecia areata totalis and universalis with an overall success rate of 64 %. Best results are achieved with subcutaneous MTX in the maximal dosage of 30 mg weekly in combination with 20 mg oral prednisone daily with regrowth of hair beginning within 2–4 months of therapy. Lasting improvement required continuous treatment in most cases. Therefore, drug toxicities are to be carefully weighed out against treatment benefit, and therapeutic drug monitoring following the respective guidelines is strongly recommended.

> Ultimately, potentially disease-modifying comorbidities are to be sought out and simultaneously treated such as deficiencies of iron, zinc, vitamin B12, and vitamin D3, thyroid dysfunction, androgenetic alopecia, and emotional distress.

Since alopecia areata is considered to be an organ-specific autoimmune disease, further laboratory investigation would seem unnecessary or even inappropriate. An increased incidence of other autoimmune diseases, like Hashimoto's thyroiditis and pernicious anemia, is seen among alopecia areata patients, while low serum ferritin, zinc, or vitamin D levels and HIV infection may have an influence on the disease course. Ultimately, the detection of circulating antithyroid or anti-parietal cell autoantibodies may represent markers for autoimmunity in favor of the diagnosis of alopecia areata in an occasional uncertain case.

Ikeda originally classified alopecia areata into four prognostic groups depending on comorbid conditions:

Ikeda type I (no disease associations) accounts for the majority of cases (>80 %), presenting with singular patches of alopecia (alopecia areata vulgaris), usually manifesting between the ages of 20 and 40 years, with duration of the singular patch usually <6 months, disease duration of usually <3 years, and infrequent development to total alopecia (in 10 %).

Ikeda type II (association with atopic disease) accounts for 10 % of cases, presenting with multiple patches of alopecia, reticular alopecia, or ophiasis, often manifesting before the age of 20 years, with sustained duration of patches <1 year, and frequent development to alopecia totalis (in 75 %).

Ikeda type III (prehypertensive type) accounts for <5 % of cases, presenting with the reticular type of alopecia areata, usually in young adults from families with arterial hypertension and development to alopecia totalis in ca. 40 %.

Ikeda type IV (association with autoimmune endocrinopathy) accounts for <5 % of cases, often manifesting after the age of 40 years, with a chronic course, and development to alopecia totalis in 10 %.

Rook later revised the classification, discarding Ikeda type III (prehypertensive type) of alopecia areata.

Kantor et al. studied serum ferritin levels in women with alopecia and found that the mean ferritin levels in patients with alopecia areata were statistically significantly lower than in normals without hair loss, though not in patients with alopecia areata totalis/universalis.

Park et al. evaluated the therapeutic effects of oral zinc supplementation for 12 weeks in alopecia areata patients who had a low serum zinc level. Oral zinc gluconate (50 mg/day) supplementation was given without any other treatment for 12 weeks. The serum zinc level was measured before and after zinc supplementation. Fifteen alopecia areata patients were enrolled in this study. After the therapy, the serum zinc levels increased significantly from 56.9 microg/ to 84.5 microg/dl. Positive therapeutic effects were observed for 9 out of 15 patients (66.7 %). The serum zinc levels of the positive response group increased more than those of the negative response group ($p=0.003$). The authors concluded that zinc supplementation needs to be given to alopecia areata patients who have a low serum zinc level.

Current observations link vitamin D deficiency to many autoimmune diseases. The most frequently reported associations were detected between the relatively high prevalence of multiple sclerosis, diabetes mellitus I, and inflammatory bowel disease in northern regions and the lower exposure to sunlight in these geographic locations. Yilmaz et al. originally reported decreased vitamin D concentrations in patients with alopecia areata. The study, however, was performed in only 42 cases and during summer. At this point, and after originally having reported on a statistical significant seasonality of alopecia areata in adult patients suffering from remitting–relapsing forms, independently from an atopic diathesis and seasonal telogen effluvium, d'Ovidio et al. checked a larger group of 156 patients affected by chronic relapsing/remitting alopecia areata with involvement of more than 25 % of scalp area. The authors confirmed the presence of insufficiency/deficiency of 25-hydroxyvitamin D (25(OH)D) in the patients' group, although the results were not significantly different compared with 148 controls. This was due to the universal tendency to lower values of 25(OH)D also in the "normal" population of central Europe.

Subsequently, Aksu Cerman et al. performed a cross-sectional study on 86 patients with alopecia areata, 44 patients with vitiligo, and 58 healthy controls to evaluate the status of vitamin D and the relationship between vitamin D levels and disease severity in patients with alopecia areata. Serum 25(OH)D levels in patients with alopecia areata were found to be significantly lower than those of the patients with vitiligo and the healthy controls ($p=0.001$ and $p<0.001$, respectively). The prevalence of 25(OH)D deficiency was significantly higher in the patients with alopecia areata (90.7 %) compared with the patients with vitiligo (70.5 %) and the healthy controls (32.8 %) ($p=0.003$ and

$p<0.001$, respectively). Furthermore, a significant inverse correlation was found between disease severity and serum 25(OH)D level in the patients with alopecia areata ($r=-0.409$; $p<0.001$). The authors concluded that patients with alopecia areata present deficient serum 25(OH)D levels that inversely correlate with disease severity. Accordingly, they propose screening alopecia areata patients for vitamin D deficiency for the possibility of vitamin D supplementation.

> The optimal level for 25-hydroxyvitamin D, the most stable and reliable parameter to evaluate vitamin D status, begins at 30 ng/mL even though the level required to maintain optimal immune system homeostasis has not been established yet, although several reports estimate it would be superior to 40 ng/mL (or 100 nmol/mL).

The calculation formulas for saturation and maintenance therapy with vitamin D are the following:

Saturation dose in IU vitamin D

$$= \left(40\ \text{ng/mL} - \text{patient's vitamin D level in ng/mL}\right) \times \frac{\text{patient's body weight in kg}}{70\ \text{kg}} \times \frac{10{,}000\ \text{IU}}{1\ \text{ng/mL}}$$

Maintenance dose in IU vitamin D (per month)

$$= 40\ \text{ng/mL} \times 0.2 \times \frac{\text{patient body weight in kg}}{70\ \text{kg}} \times \frac{10{,}000\ \text{IU}}{1\ \text{ng/mL}}$$

Vitamin D

$1\ \mu g = 40\ \text{IU}$

Vitamin D in blood levels

$1\ \text{ng/mL} = 1\ \mu g/L = 2.5\ \text{nmol/L}$

Vitamin *D* deficiency < 20 ng/mL (< 50 nmol/L)

Vitamin *D* insufficiency 20 – 30 ng/mL (50–75 nmol/L)

Toxic range > 150 ng/mL (> 375 nmol/L)

Corazza et al. originally reported on a possible association between celiac disease and alopecia areata. In a routine clinical practice, the authors initially observed three patients with such an association. In one patient gluten-free diet resulted in complete regrowth of scalp and body hair. A prospective screening program for celiac disease using antigliadin and antiendomysial antibodies was set up in 256 consecutive outpatients with alopecia areata. Three patients that were completely asymptomatic for intestinal diseases were found to be positive and underwent biopsy. Histological analysis was consistent with the diagnosis of celiac disease. The authors concluded that alopecia areata may constitute the only clinical manifestation of celiac disease and that the association between these two conditions is a real one because the observed frequency of association was greater than expected by chance. In subsequent papers, results of gluten-free diet on restoring hair growth in celiac disease-associated alopecia areata have been inconsistent. Finally, in their study of 12 children with alopecia areata, Ertekin et al. found a prevalence of celiac disease of 41.7 %. They detected the prevalence of celiac disease in 1,263 healthy children as 0.87 % in the same city. Therefore, the authors concluded that prevalence of silent celiac disease is very high among children with alopecia areata and suggest that children with alopecia areata should be screened for celiac disease.

In summary, certain laboratory investigations may be indicated to detected associated autoimmune diseases and/or comorbidities that may affect the disease course (Table 4.5).

Alopecia areata may rarely be a presenting symptom of the *autoimmune polyendocrinopathy–candidiasis–ectodermal dystrophy (APECED) syndrome*, the first recognized monogenic autoimmune disease. It is due to a mutation of the autoimmune regulator gene (AIRE) and is clinically characterized by the presence of two of the three following major clinical symptoms: Addison's disease, hypoparathyroidism, and mucocutaneous candidiasis. Additional features may be insulin-dependent diabetes mellitus, chronic atrophic gastritis with pernicious anemia, hypogonadism, alopecia (areata), and vitiligo. Onset is in childhood, candidiasis is usually the

Table 4.5 Proposed comorbidities screening in alopecia areata

Test	Purpose
To detect associated autoimmune disorders	
Antithyroid antibodies	To detect associated thyroid autoimmunity
Anti-parietal cell antibodies	To detect associated parietal cell autoimmunity
Thyroid function tests	To detect associated autoimmune thyroid disease
Vitamin B12 level	To detect associated pernicious anemia
Endomysial antibody IgA, antigliadin antibody IgG and IgA (in children)	To detect celiac disease
To detect potentially disease-modifying comorbidities	
CRP and ferritin level	Iron deficiency
Zinc level	Zinc deficiency
Vitamin D3 level	Vitamin D deficiency
HIV serology	HIV infection/AIDS
To rule out other causes of patchy alopecia	
Antinuclear antibody test	Lupus erythematosus
RPR test (or VDRL and TPPA depending on laboratory)	Syphilis II (alopecia areolaris)

first symptom, and manifestations continue to appear until fifth decade. Böni and Trüeb reported unsuccessful treatment trial of alopecia universalis with DCP in a patient with APECED.

Alopecia areata (universalis) has been reported in association with (acquired) human immunodeficiency virus (HIV) infection, as well as in the setting of immune restoration after highly active antiretroviral therapy (HAART).

Finally, the more recent reports on association of alopecia areata with antitumor necrosis factor-alpha therapy may be fortuitous, since alopecia areata represents a common condition. On the other hand, the observation of alopecia areata during anti-TNF alpha therapy proves the inefficacy of anti-TNF alpha therapy for alopecia areata. Finally, Doyle et al. have demonstrated that anti-TNF alpha therapy-related alopecia may closely mimic alopecia areata but is histologically distinguished by epidermal psoriasiform changes.

Not until the prevalence of alopecia areata in patients treated with anti-TNF alpha agents has been shown to be higher than in the general population can alopecia areata be definitely regarded as a potential side effect of antitumor necrosis factor-alpha therapy.

Most recently, Tauber et al. found no difference in comparison of the effect of TNF blocker withdrawal with TNF blocker maintenance in patients with occurrence of alopecia areata during anti-TNF therapy.

The original report of successful treatment of a case of universal alopecia areata with subcutaneous efalizumab by Kaelin et al. in 2006 could subsequently not been confirmed by a 3- to 6-month placebo-controlled trial with efalizumab in a cohort of 62 patients with moderate-to-severe alopecia areata. In both groups, there was an approximately 8 % response rate for hair regrowth at 12 weeks. Therefore, efalizumab proved not effective in promoting hair regrowth in patients with alopecia areata.

Therefore, single case observations of successful treatment of a condition like alopecia areata where spontaneous remissions may occur need to be confirmed by placebo-controlled trials.

New drug treatment opportunities based on the results of genome-wide association studies that implicate T-cell and natural killer cell activation pathways are paving the way to new approaches in future clinical trials for alopecia areata. Currently, there are ongoing studies with the CTLA4-Ig fusion protein abatacept (blocks co-stimulation of T-cells), anti-IL15Rb monoclonal antibodies (blocks activation of CD8+ T-cells), and the Janus kinase (JAK) 3 inhibitor tofacitinib and JAK 1/3 inhibitor ruxolitinib (block signal transduction at the IL-15 receptor).

Craiglow and King originally reported hair growth in a patient with universal alopecia areata treated with tofacitinib for plaque psoriasis, and Xing et al. subsequently reported successful treatment of three patients with alopecia areata with oral ruxolitinib. The patients achieved near-complete hair regrowth within few months of treatment, suggesting the potential clinical utility of JAK inhibition for treatment of alopecia areata.

Platelet-rich plasma (PRP) is blood plasma that has been enriched with platelets. As a concentrated source of autologous platelets, PRP contains and releases through degranulation several growth factors and cytokines. These include PDGF, TGFβ, FGF, IGF-1 and IGF-2, VEGF, EGF, IL-8, and KGF. PRP has gained popularity among a limited number of dermatologists with a primary commercial interest, though the use and clinical validation of the method for diverse dermatologic conditions is still in the early stages. Results of basic science and preclinical trials have yet to be confirmed in large-scale controlled clinical trials.

A Cochrane review on PRP has been performed in chronic wounds. Even if the conclusion of the respective review were positive, this would have not been surprising, since blood platelets have a physiologic role in wound healing. In contrast, it is more difficult to comprehend the role of platelet-derived growth factors and cytokines for hair growth and treatment of hair growth disorders.

Out of this reason, a stringent evaluation of existing data in favor of PRP for treatment of hair-related disorders is indispensable.

There exists a single, double-blind, placebo- and active-controlled, half-head study to evaluate the effects of PRP on alopecia areata; however, in an era, where a more comprehensive understanding of the immunologic basis of alopecia areata has opened the venue to more targeted treatments of alopecia areata, the proposal of PRP with its poorly defined mode of action rather represents an intellectual step backward.

Alopecia areata has long been recognized to be associated with an increased prevalence of psychiatric disorders, specifically major depression, generalized anxiety disorder, social phobia, and paranoid disorder.

Trüeb and Cavegn reported trichotillomania in connection with alopecia areata and suggested that patients with a mental predisposition may artificially prolong the disfigurement as the hair on the bald patches of alopecia areata regrows, with the aim to maintain gratification of dependency needs, which were being met during alopecia areata.

Some experts therefore advocate combination treatment with antidepressant agents in alopecia areata with comorbid depression. Antidepressants that have been used (with alleged success) include imipramine, paroxetine, and citalopram.

Others suggest that hypnotherapy may enhance the mental well-being of patients with alopecia areata, though no effect on hair regrowth could be shown.

As there is no definite cure for alopecia areata and conventional therapy has its clear limitations, a number of alopecia areata patients resort to complementary and alternative medical remedies and therapies (CAM).

Hay et al. reported a randomized, double-blind, controlled trial of 7 months' duration aromatherapy with follow-up at 3 and 7 months to investigate the efficacy in the treatment of alopecia areata. Eighty-six patients were randomized into two groups. The active group massaged essential oils (thyme, rosemary, lavender, and cedarwood) in a mixture of carrier oils (jojoba and grapeseed) into their scalp daily. The control group used only carrier oils for their massage, also daily. Treatment success was evaluated on sequential photographs. The degree of improvement was measured by two methods: a 6-point scale and computerized analysis of traced areas of alopecia. Nineteen (44 %) of 43 patients in the active group showed improvement compared with 6 (15 %) of 41 patients in the control group ($p=0.008$). The authors concluded that aromatherapy is a safe and effective treatment for alopecia areata.

A more recent review of CAM addressed two pertinent aspects: first, an overview of the published medical literature on CAM used in alopecia areata, and, second, a thorough assessment of the considerations and limitations of the use of CAM for treatment of alopecia areata. A systematic MEDLINE search yielded 13 studies of the clinical use of CAM in the management of alopecia areata, all belonging to one of the five main categories of CAM. Methodological quality was analyzed using objective assessment scores (Wilson and Lawrence scores). No study was of sufficient internal validity to provide robust evidence of the benefit of CAM for treatment of alopecia areata.

Ultimately, the options available for adapting to the disease rather than treating in an effort to cure are to be taken into consideration in selected long-standing widespread cases or recurrent small spot disease.

4.2.5 Chemotherapy-Induced Alopecia

Chemotherapy-induced hair loss is considered a traumatic experience in cancer patient care, since hair loss negatively affects a patient's perception of appearance, body image, and self-esteem. Ultimately, patients feel deprived of their privacy because the hair loss is readily interpreted by the lay public as associated with having cancer.

Chemotherapy-induced hair loss occurs with an estimated overall incidence of 65 %. The incidence and severity of the hair loss are variable and related to the particular chemotherapeutic agent and protocol: multiple classes of anticancer drugs induce alopecia (Table 4.6), with frequencies of chemotherapy-induced hair loss differing for the four major drug classes: more than 80 % for antimicrotubule agents (i.e., paclitaxel), 60–100 % for topoisomerase inhibitors (i.e., doxorubicin), more than 60 % for alkylators (i.e., cyclophosphamide), and 10–50 % for antimetabolites (i.e., 5-fluorouracil plus leucovorin). Combination therapy consisting of two or more agents usually produces greater incidences of more severe hair loss compared with single-agent therapy.

Table 4.6 Cytotoxic agents and hair loss

Cytostatic agents which usually do cause hair loss	
Adriamycin	Docetaxel
Daunorubicin	Paclitaxel
Etoposide	Ifosfamide
Irinotecan	Vindesine
Cyclophosphamide	Vinorelbine
Epirubicin	Topotecan
Cytotoxic agents which sometimes cause hair loss	
Amsacrine	Vincristine
Cytarabine	Vinblastine
Bleomycin	Lomustine
Busulfan	Thiotepa
5-Fluorouracil	Gemcitabine
Melphalan	
Cytotoxic agents which unusually cause hair loss	
Methotrexate	Procarbazine
Carmustine	6-Marcaptopurine
Mitoxantrone	Streptozotocin
Mitomycin C	Fludarabine
Carboplatin	Raltritrexate
Cisplatin	Capecitabine

Chemotherapy-induced hair loss is a consequence of direct toxic insult to the rapidly dividing cells of the hair follicle. It is a major characteristic of the anagen hair follicle that the epithelial compartment undergoes proliferation, with the bulb matrix cells showing the greatest proliferative activity in building up the hair shaft. The abrupt cessation of mitotic activity leads to the weakening of the partially keratinized, proximal portion of the hair shaft, a narrowing, and a subsequent breakage within the hair canal. The consequence is hair shedding that usually begins

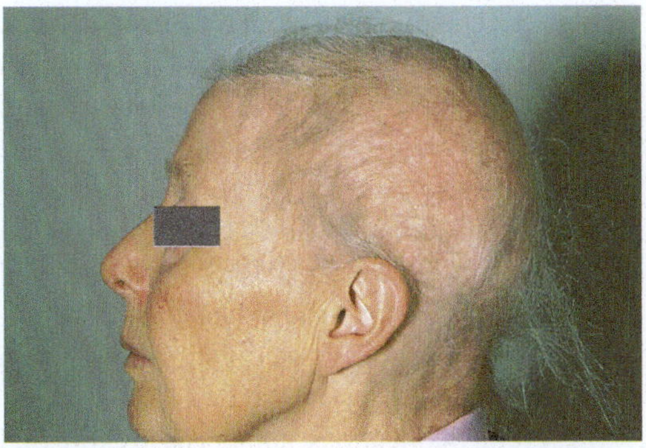

Fig. 4.20 Chemotherapy-induced alopecia (dystrophic anagen effluvium)

at 1–3 weeks after initiation of chemotherapy. Due to its long anagen phase, the scalp is the most common location for hair loss, while other terminal hairs are variably affected depending on the percentage of hairs in anagen. Since normally up to 90 % of scalp hair is in the anagen phase, hair loss is usually copious and the resulting alopecia is quite obvious (Fig. 4.20). Nevertheless, chemotherapy given at high doses for a sufficiently long time and with multiple exposures may also affect the beard, eyebrows, eyelashes, axillary, and pubic hairs.

> While chemotherapy-induced hair loss has traditionally been categorized as acute diffuse hair loss caused by dystrophic anagen effluvium, more recently it has been pointed out that, in fact, chemotherapy-induced hair loss may present with different pathomechanisms and clinical patterns.

Evidence exists that the hair follicle may respond to the same insult capable of stopping mitosis with both shedding patterns, dystrophic anagen effluvium, and telogen effluvium. Accordingly, the hair may fall out very quickly in clumps, or gradually. When mitotic activity is arrested, numerous and interacting factors may influence the shedding pattern. One of these factors is the mitotic activity of the hair follicle at the moment of the insult.

When the hair is in its late anagen phase, in which the mitotic rate is slowing down spontaneously, it simply accelerates its normal path to telogen, while mitotically inactive phases (catagen and telogen) are not affected. Since anagen duration is diminished in androgenetic alopecia, the probability is increased that the antimitotic insult strikes the hair close to the resting phase resulting in telogen effluvium. While synchronization of hair cycles also plays a role, and again in androgenetic alopecia, the hair cycles tend to synchronize due to the diminished duration of anagen, even a minor antimitotic insult may produce marked hair loss.

The hair loss generally is reversible, with hair regrowth typically occurring after a delay of 3–6 months. In some patients, the regrown hair shows changes in color and/or texture. It might be curlier than it was before, or it could be gray until the follicular melanocytes begin functioning again. But the difference is usually temporary.

> However, there is an increasing number of reports of permanent chemotherapy-induced alopecia.

Originally reported in children treated with busulfan and cyclophosphamide after bone marrow transplantation for leukemia, it has been associated with certain risk factors, including chronic graft-*versus*-host reaction, previous exposure to X-ray, and patient age. More recently, reports have accumulated, related specifically to breast cancer chemotherapy with sequential fluorouracil/epirubicin/cyclophosphamide (FEC) and docetaxel.

Miteva et al. studied scalp biopsies from the affected scalp areas of permanent alopecia after systemic chemotherapy. The histology was characterized by a non-scarring pattern with a preserved number of follicular units and lack of fibrosis. The hair count revealed a decreased number of terminal hairs, an increased number of telogen, and miniaturized vellus-like hairs. There was an increased number of fibrous streamers (stelae) in both the reticular dermis and the subcutis, with Arao–Perkins bodies found in the subcutaneous portions of the streamers. The histological findings of permanent alopecia after chemotherapy are similar to those in androgenetic alopecia. It may be speculated that exposure to chemotherapy may lead to an accumulation of DNA damage with defective renewal of hair follicle stem cells, as recently proposed to occur in the aging process of the hair follicle by Nishimura.

A number of preventive measures have been proposed and tried to reduce chemotherapy-induced hair loss. Nevertheless, no treatment exists that can guarantee to prevent chemotherapy-induced hair loss.

> Of the treatments so far investigated, scalp cooling (hypothermia) has been the most widely used and studied.

Of 53 multiple patient studies published between 1973 and 2003 on the results of scalp cooling for the prevention of chemotherapy-induced hair loss, 7 trials were randomized. In six of the seven randomized studies, a significant advantage was observed with scalp cooling. The positive results were most evident when anthracyclines or taxanes were the chemotherapeutic agents.

In the most recent open-label, prospective, non-randomized clinical trial, patients with solid tumors receiving docetaxel in a palliative setting were allocated according to patients' preference to short-term cooling (over 45 min postinfusion) with a Paxman® PSC-2 machine (PAX), with cold cap (CC), or no cooling. The combined endpoint was alopecia World Health Organization (WHO) III or IV, or the necessity to wear a wig. Two hundred thirty-eight patients were included in the trial (128 patients PAX, 71 CC, and 39 no cooling). The number of cycles (median 4) and median docetaxel doses were similar across the three groups (55–60 mg/day on weekly therapy, 135–140 mg/day on 3-weekly therapy). Alopecia occurred with PAX, CC, and no cooling under 3-weekly docetaxel in 23, 27, and 74 % and under weekly docetaxel in 7, 8, and 17 %, respectively. Overall, cooling (PAX and CC combined) reduced risk of alopecia by 78 % (hazard ratio 0.22; 95 % confidence interval 0.12–0.41). CC and PAX prophylaxis led to the same degree of prevention of alopecia. In this first comparison study published to date, both PAX and CC offered efficacious protection against hair loss, in particular when docetaxel was administered in a 3-weekly interval.

In several publications, authors have expressed their concerns about the risk of scalp skin metastases after cooling.

> Therefore, scalp cooling has remained contraindicated for those with hematological malignancies, and its use remains controversial in patients with non-hematological malignancies who undergo curative chemotherapy.

Patients undergoing scalp hypothermia commonly report feeling uncomfortably cold and suffering of headaches.

So far, no approved pharmacological treatment exists for chemotherapy-induced hair loss. Among the agents that so far have been evaluated in cancer patients, the topical hair growth-promoting agent minoxidil was able to shorten the duration, albeit did not prevent chemotherapy-induced hair loss. Minoxidil also failed to induce significant regrowth of hair in busulfan- and cyclophosphamide-induced permanent alopecia.

Advances have been made in the understanding of the pathobiology of chemotherapy-induced hair loss, and several experimental approaches to the development of pharmacologic agents are under evaluation. Because the rapid cell proliferation of hair follicle keratinocytes during anagen renders the hair follicle susceptible to the toxicity of chemotherapy, a strategy to protect against chemotherapy-induced hair loss is arresting the cell cycle to reduce the sensitivity of the follicular epithelium to cell cycle-active antitumor agents. Inhibition of cyclin-dependent kinase 2 (CDK2), a positive regulator of the eukaryotic cell cycle, is believed to represent an approach for prevention of chemotherapy-induced hair loss by arresting the cell cycle. Potent small-molecule inhibitors of CDK2 are currently being developed using structure-based methods. Ultimately, the protection should be selective to the hair follicle, such that the anticancer efficacy of chemotherapy is not hampered. In view of the fact that cancer usually is treated with combinations of chemotherapeutics, an effective treatment of chemotherapy-induced hair loss would likely require agents that are effective for different chemotherapeutics with different action mechanisms. Moreover, variations in patient characteristics must be taken into account, since the pattern of chemotherapy-induced hair loss varies in individual patients.

Since chemotherapy-induced hair loss cannot be reliably prevented, the best way to deal with it is to plan ahead with a focus on making the patient as comfortable as possible with his appearance before, during, and after cancer treatment.

> The major approach to prevent or minimize chemotherapy-induced hair loss remains scalp cooling, while topical minoxidil may speed up hair regrowth.

Even if chemotherapy-induced hair loss cannot be prevented, it can be managed. Anticipating hair loss, coming to terms with the inevitability of hair loss, and taking control are the key steps in coping with chemotherapy-induced hair loss. Recommendations for hair care are summarized in Table 4.7.

Finally, since the estrogen to androgen ratio might be responsible for triggering hair loss in women with genetic susceptibility for androgenetic alopecia, patients following chemotherapy for breast cancer who are under anti-estrogen treatment with tamoxifen or with the aromatase inhibitors letrozole, anastrozole, and formestane may recover some considerable hair with appropriate topical minoxidil therapy.

Table 4.7 Chemotherapy-induced hair loss. Recommendations for hair care

Avoidance of physical or chemical trauma, such as bleaching, coloring, or perming of hair, curling irons, and hot rollers
Gentle hair strategies should be continued throughout chemotherapy, using a satin pillowcase, which is less likely to attract and catch fragile hair, using a soft brush, washing hair only as often as necessary, and using a gentle shampoo
Cutting hair short or shaving hair. Short hair tends to look fuller then long hair, and when the hair is shed, it won't be as noticeable when it is short. Moreover, cutting hair might help to make a better transition to total alopecia. Also, a shaved head may be easier for securing a wig or hairpiece
Appropriate head covering should be planned ahead. Head covering as the hair falls out is a very personal decision. For women in particular, chemotherapy-induced hair loss involves a confrontation with the nature of their disease, while for men it is a normal and inevitable consequence of treatment. Depending on individual preference, temporarily wearing a wig or another head covering until the hair regrows may be the most effective way of dealing with this condition while protecting the scalp from sun and cold exposure at the same time

4.2.6 Adverse Effects of Molecularly Targeted Therapies for Cancer

Molecularly targeted therapy for cancer is a type of medication that blocks the growth of cancer cells by interfering with specific targeted molecules needed for carcinogenesis and tumor growth, rather than by simply interfering with all rapidly dividing cells, as with traditional chemotherapy. Therefore, targeted cancer therapies are expected to be more effective than current treatments while being less harmful to normal cells. Nevertheless, cutaneous adverse effects, including the hair, are among the most frequently observed toxicities, and their intensity can be dose-limiting or lead to discontinuation of therapy. There have been a rapidly emerging number of targeted agents with novel mechanisms of action, and dermatology providers may not be familiar with the full spectrum of associated skin toxicities. In light of the often life-saving nature of targeted therapies for cancer, it is critical that dermatologists recognize the clinical signs and understand the significance of such toxicities in

Table 4.8 Targeted therapies for cancer, hair and scalp toxicities, and recommendations for management

Targeted therapy class	Agents within class	Cancers	Hair and scalp toxicities	Management
Inhibitors of the cellular membrane				
EGFR inhibitors	Cetuximab Panitumumab Erlotinib Gefitinib Lapatinib Canertinib Vandetanib	Colorectal Head and neck Non-small cell lung Breast	Kinking Trichomegaly Upper lip hypertrichosis Alopecia (non-cicatricial and cicatricial) Papulopustular eruption	Non-scarring hair loss: topical minoxidil Hypertrichosis: eyelash trimming Topical eflornithine Scarring hair loss: topical steroids, oral tetracyclines
KIT and BCR-ABL inhibitors	Imatinib Nilotinib Dasatinib	Chronic myelogenous leukemia Gastrointestinal stroma tumor Hypereosinophilic syndrome Dermatofibrosarcoma Systemic mastocytosis AIDS-related Kaposi sarcoma KIT-mutated melanoma	Pigmentary changes	Reversible after treatment is stopped
Multikinase inhibitors	Sorafenib Sunitinib Pazopanib	Multiple	Alopecia Kinking Depigmentation	Topical minoxidil Concealment measures
Inhibitors of intracellular molecular signaling pathway				
RAF inhibitors	Vemurafenib Dabrafenib	BRAFomas Hairy cell leukemia Melanoma Papillary thyroid Serous ovarian Colorectal Prostate	Alopecia Seborrhoeic dermatitis-like eruption	Topical minoxidil Concealment measures Topical imidazoles and steroids
MEK inhibitors	CI-1040 Selumetinib Trametinib	Colorectal Pancreatic Non-small cell lung Hepatocellular Melanoma	Alopecia Trichomegaly Depigmentation	Topical minoxidil Eyelash trimming
mTOR inhibitors	Rapamycin Everolimus Temsirolimus	Multiple	Alopecia Facial hypertrichosis	Topical minoxidil Topical eflornithine
Hedgehog signaling pathway inhibitor	Vismodegib	Basal cell carcinoma	Alopecia	Topical minoxidil Concealment measures

order to provide appropriate counseling of patients and effective clinical management.

Targeted therapies of cancer can be divided into inhibitors of the cellular membrane, such as epidermal growth factor receptor (EGFR) inhibitors, KIT and BCR-ABL inhibitors, and multikinase inhibitors, and inhibitors of intracellular molecular signaling pathways, such as the RAF inhibitors, MEK inhibitors, mTOR inhibitors, and Hedgehog pathway inhibitors (Table 4.8).

EGFR inhibitors are used in the treatment of colorectal, head and neck, non-small cell lung, and breast cancers. Cutaneous adverse events in patients who are taking EGFR inhibitors range in incidence from 50 to 90 %. Well-documented hair changes associated with EGFR inhibitors are transformation of the hair shaft property into curly, fine, and brittle texture, eyelash trichomegaly, upper lip hypertrichosis, and alopecia accompanied by a peculiar diffusely red, atrophic scalp studded with papulopustules, erosions, and crusting. Scarring alopecia may also occur and may represent a severe form of the condition. Associated cutaneous symptoms include papulopustular eruptions, photosensitivity, xerosis, mucositis, and paronychia, onycholysis, and pyogenic granuloma particularly of the great toes.

The severity of EGFR inhibitor-related cutaneous eruptions directly correlates with efficacy of therapy and patient outcomes. Therefore, prophylaxis and early management of cutaneous toxicities may prevent dose reduction or discontinuation of therapy.

Management of hair changes includes topical minoxidil and topical corticosteroids or 1 % topical clindamycin, regular eyelash trimming, and topical eflornithine for upper lip hypertrichosis, and management of cutaneous toxicities includes sunscreen, oral tetracyclines, and low-potency topical corticosteroids.

KIT and BCR-ABL inhibitors are used in the treatment of chronic myelogenous leukemia, gastrointestinal stroma tumors, hypereosinophilic syndrome, dermatofibrosarcoma, systemic mastocytosis, AIDS-related Kaposi sarcoma, and KIT-mutated malignant melanoma. Hansen et al. reported a case of inflammatory non-scarring alopecia associated with nilotinib. Pigmentary changes, which also may include the hair, are consistent with the role of c-kit in the physiology of melanocytes, regulating melanogenesis, proliferation, migration, and survival. Associated skin toxicities are edema, morbilliform eruptions, and new onset or exacerbation of preexisting cutaneous diseases, including lichenoid reactions, psoriasis, pityriasis rosea-like eruption, acute generalized exanthematous pustulosis, DRESS syndrome, Stevens–Johnson syndrome, urticaria, acute neutrophilic dermatosis, photosensitivity, pseudolymphoma, porphyria cutanea tarda, small vessel vasculitis, panniculitis, perforating folliculitis, and erythroderma.

Most adverse effects of KIT and BCR-ABL inhibitors are dose related and reversible after drug discontinuation.

Multikinase inhibitors affect multiple tyrosine kinase systems and therefore result in a vast array of skin- and hair-related adverse effects that overlap with those seen with the more target-specific therapies. Hair changes in texture (kinking) and density (alopecia: Fig. 4.21), and color (depigmentation) may occur, as well as a wide range of skin eruptions. As a general rule, these are reversible after treatment is terminated. Hyperkeratotic hand–foot skin reaction represents a peculiar painful complication of multikinase inhibitor therapy that occurs predominantly over sites of pressure and friction. Patients should be informed of this dose-dependent reaction, and preventive measures

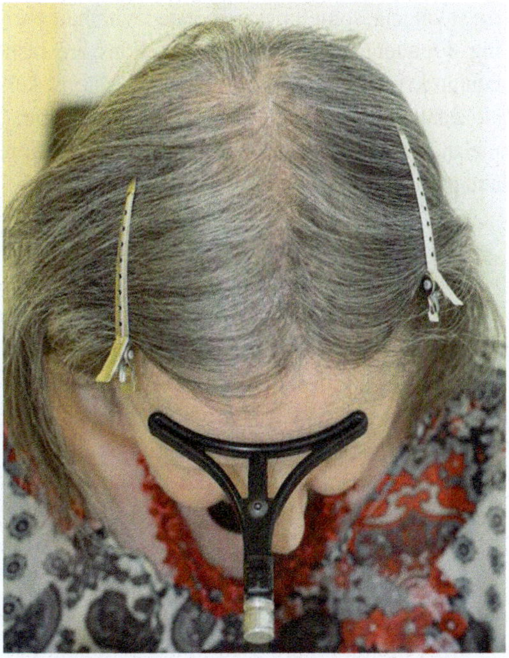

Fig. 4.21 Alopecia from molecularly targeted therapy for cancer (multikinase inhibitor)

should be considered from the onset of treatment, such as pretreatment evaluation with a podiatrist and prescription of orthopedic shoe inserts as needed, along with wide and flexible shoes.

The *RAS-RAF-MEK-ERK or mitogen-activated protein kinase (MAPK) pathway* is one of the most frequently deregulated signaling pathways resulting in increased cellular proliferation in a number of cancers. BRAF, an upstream activator in the MAPK pathway, is one of the most frequently mutated protein kinases found in all human cancers. Malignancies with the highest association with BRAF mutations have been called BRAFomas and include hairy cell leukemia (100 %), melanoma (40–60 %), papillary thyroid carcinoma (ca. 40 %), serous ovarian carcinoma (ca. 30 %), colorectal carcinoma (<10 %), and prostate cancer (<10 %). Of particular interest for dermatologists is that targeted therapies of mutated BRAF have emerged as successful treatments for patients with malignant melanoma, both as monotherapy and in combination with MEK inhibition. Cutaneous adverse effects associated with these agents are frequent and may be dose-limiting. Adverse effects of RAF inhibitors that may affect the scalp are a seborrhoeic dermatitis-like eruption and non-scarring alopecia, sometimes associated with hair curling. Frequent associated skin reactions are rash, benign keratotic squamoproliferative lesions, keratoacanthomas, and squamous cell carcinoma, melanocytic lesions, keratosis pilaris-like reaction, and photosensitivity.

> BRAF inhibition may induce dynamic changes in preexisting nevi or eruptive nevi and development of a second primary melanoma. Data indicate that BRAF blockade in wild-type melanoma cells may in fact accelerate cellular proliferation. Therefore, patients with targeted BRAF inhibitors should undergo frequent monitoring of their melanocytic lesions during therapy.

MEK inhibitors are used in the treatment of a variety of cancers, including colorectal, pancreatic, non-small cell lung, and hepatocellular cancers and malignant melanoma. The side effect profile of MEK inhibitors more closely mirrors that of EGFR inhibitors rather than RAF inhibitors and includes morbilliform and papulopustular eruptions. Hair changes include alopecia, trichomegaly, and hair depigmentation.

> Combination use of MEK and RAF inhibitors improves efficacy of therapy while obviating many of the cutaneous toxicities.

mTOR inhibitors are approved for use in many cancer types, since the PI3K-AKT-mTOR signaling pathway is upregulated in a multitude of malignancies. mTOR inhibitors now in use all preferentially target mTOR complex-1 and therefore share a similar profile of adverse reactions, including stomatitis, inflammatory eruptions, and paronychia. Hair changes that may also be seen with mTOR inhibitors are alopecia and facial hypertrichosis.

The *Hedgehog signaling pathway inhibitor* vismodegib has been successfully developed for the treatment of basal cell carcinoma which has metastasized to other parts of the body, relapsed after surgery, or cannot be treated with surgery or radiation. Nearly all basal cell carcinomas have been shown to contain alterations in the Hedgehog signaling pathway, the most common leading to loss of function of patched homologue 1 (PTCH1). This results in constitutive activation of the smoothened homologue (SMO) with unregulated downstream proliferative activity. Vismodegib is a small-molecule inhibitor of SMO.

> Alopecia is a common cutaneous adverse effect of Hedgehog signaling pathway inhibition, occurring in 51–85 % of patients. Ten to fourteen percent of patients lose >50 % of hair that requires the patient to wear a hairpiece. Non-scarring universal alopecia similar to alopecia universalis may also be seen. Although typically reversible, alopecia is perceived by patients as a significant toxicity of cancer therapy.

With the continued expansion of targeted therapies against cancer, healthcare providers caring for those with cutaneous conditions, including the hair, will become integral partners in the multidisciplinary team approach in modern oncologic care.

4.3 Scarring Alopecias

The scarring alopecias represent a diverse group of disorders that cause permanent destruction of the pilosebaceous unit and irreversible hair loss, characterized by visible loss of follicular ostia and destruction of the hair follicle on histopathologic examination.

> Loss of follicular orifices in an area of alopecia points to an irreversible loss of hair, either due to permanent damage to essential parts of the hair follicle or destruction of the entire hair follicle. Although the scarring alopecias represent the cause of alopecia in a minority of patients, the irreversibility and possible important cosmetic consequences of scarring alopecia demand special diagnostic attention in order to promptly attain a precise diagnosis and specific treatment.

Where there is no obvious physical/chemical injury or acute infectious etiology, clinical differential diagnosis of scarring alopecia is often difficult. The clinical inspection is of limited usefulness in establishing a diagnosis. Overlapping features may blur the distinction between different diseases; moreover, these share the common final pathway of replacement of follicle by fibrous tissue. Finally, there is no characteristic biological marker for most entities.

> Therefore, scarring alopecias pose both a diagnostic and therapeutic challenge to the practitioner. Accurate diagnosis based on a careful patient history, clinical examination, microbiological studies, and scalp biopsy is a prerequisite to therapy.

Diagnostic problems inherent to scalp biopsies are a reluctance of many practitioners in performing them and a lack of familiarity of many pathologists with scalp histopathology. Ultimately, it must be borne in mind that the hair follicle and its derangements are complex and dynamic. A biopsy gives only a momentary snapshot of the underlying pathology.

> Problems related to the treatment of the scarring alopecias include patients' delay, when irreversible scarring has already occurred. Since the causes are mostly unknown, therapy has remained empiric and nonspecific. Published data on recommended therapies have usually low levels of evidence. Ultimately, the goal of therapy is mostly to halt further progression.

4.3.1 Classification

Scarring alopecias may be due to hereditary or developmental defects. Examples of these rare conditions are aplasia cutis congenita, organoid nevi, hereditary epidermolysis bullosa, alopecia ichthyotica, and the follicular keratosis syndromes.

More frequently they are due to acquired, irreparable destruction of critical hair follicle structures (follicular sheath, stem cells, follicular papilla, and their interaction) or of the whole hair follicle. The acquired scarring alopecias are further differentiated into primary and secondary scarring alopecias:

Primary scarring alopecia is due to preferential destruction of the follicle. Well-defined, chronic inflammatory diseases of the scalp amenable to specific therapies are differentiated microscopically from a morphologic point of view on the basis of the pattern of inflammation

Table 4.9 Primary cicatricial alopecias: proposed working classification of NAHRS. Modified

Lymphocytic group
(Classic) lichen planopilaris and variants
Disseminated (Lassueur–Graham Little syndrome)
Patterned
Frontal fibrosing alopecia (Kossard)
Fibrosing alopecia in a pattern distribution (Zinkernagel and Trüeb)
Chronic cutaneous lupus erythematosus
(Classic) pseudopelade of Brocq
Central centrifugal cicatricial alopecia?
Neutrophilic group
Folliculitis decalvans (Quinquaud) and variants
Tufted hair folliculitis (Smith and Sanderson)
Cicatrizing seborrheic eczema (Laymon)
Dissecting cellulitis of the scalp (Perifolliculitis capitis abscedens et suffodiens Hoffman)
Mixed group
Keratosis follicularis spinulosa decalvans (Siemens)/ folliculitis spinulosa decalvans
Folliculitis (acne) keloidalis (nuchae)/dermatitis papillaris capillitii
Folliculitis (acne) necrotica (varioliformis/miliaris)
Erosive pustular dermatosis (of the scalp)
End-stage nonspecific group
Pseudopeladic state (Degos)

and the type of inflammatory cell that predominates (Table 4.9).

Lichen planopilaris is the most common cause of scarring alopecia in the adult. It presents with pruritic central or multifocal alopecic patches with follicular hyperkeratosis and erythema at the hair-bearing margin (Fig. 4.22a). Histopathology reveals a lymphocytic primary scarring alopecia. Non-scalp involvement (mucous membranes, glabrous skin, nails) may be present. The Lassueur–Graham Little (–Piccardi) syndrome is considered a disseminated variant, characterized by the triad of patchy cicatricial alopecia of the scalp, non-cicatricial alopecia of the axilla and groin, and a follicular spinous papule on the body, scalp, or both. With regard to its pathogenesis, lichen planopilaris may be regarded as a T-cell-mediated autoimmune reaction. This autoimmune process triggers apoptosis of the epithelial cells. Several cytokines are involved, including tumor necrosis factor-alpha, interferon-gamma, interleukin-1 alpha, interleukin 6, and interleukin 8. This autoimmune, T-cell-mediated process is thought to be in response to some antigenic change, but a specific antigen has yet not been identified. Harries et al. provide the first evidence that lichen planopilaris may result from an immune privilege collapse of the hair follicle's epithelial stem cell niche. Where a causal or triggering agent is identified, this is termed a lichenoid reaction rather than lichen planus. These may include drug reactions, with the most common inducers including gold salts, beta-blockers, antimalarials, thiazide diuretics, furosemide, spironolactone, metformin, and penicillamine; hepatitis, specifically hepatitis B and hepatitis C infection; and cutaneous graft-*versus*-host disease.

More recently, distinctly patterned forms of lichen planopilaris have been reported, such as Kossard's (postmenopausal) frontal fibrosing alopecia and fibrosing alopecia in a pattern distribution (originally described by Zinkernagel and Trüeb), and the question has arisen to what extent they represent a lichen planus-like reaction on a background of androgenetic alopecia.

Chronic cutaneous or discoid lupus erythematosus presents as symptomatic, erythematous scaly plaques with follicular plugs, telangiectases, atrophy, and depigmentation with time (Fig. 4.22b). In contrast to lichen planopilaris activity tends to be in the center of alopecic patches. Histopathology again reveals a lymphocytic primary scarring alopecia. Among the primary cicatricial alopecias, lupus erythematosus is the only one that may be associated with systemic disease. Patients with only discoid lesions of the scalp uncommonly progress to systemic disease. Nevertheless, patients with systemic disease may also have discoid lesions, including the scalp, though less frequently. Because of the high specificity of the discoid lesion, it has been

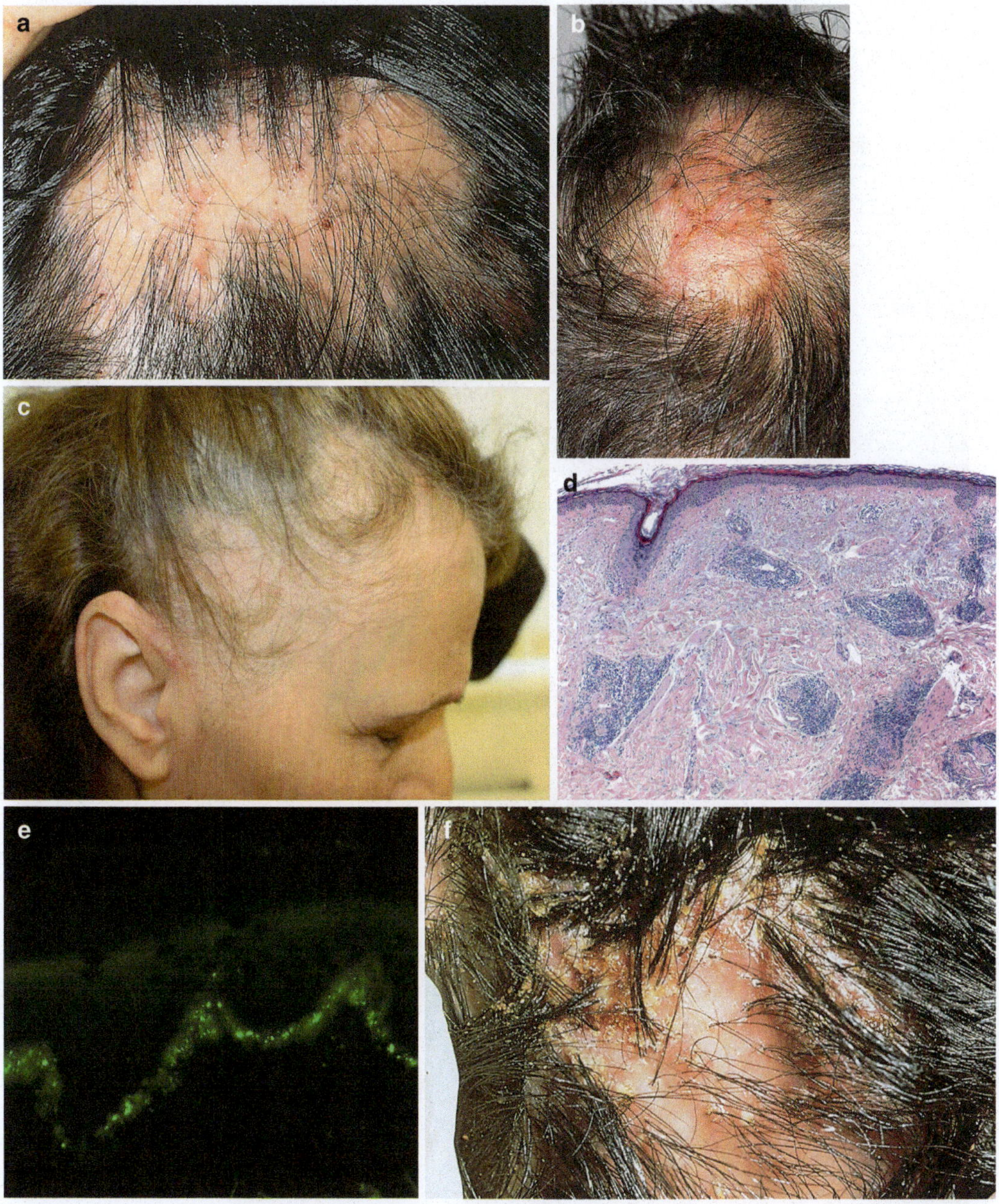

Fig. 4.22 (**a–l**) Scarring alopecia. (**a**) Lichen planopilaris. (**b**) Chronic cutaneous lupus erythematosus. (**c–e**) Histologically verified cutaneous lupus erythematosus presenting as frontal fibrosing alopecia (notice cutaneous lupus erythematosus-typical inflammatory lesion on ear). (**d**) Interface dermatitis (histology) (**e**) immune deposits at the dermo-epidermal junction (direct immunofluorescence). (**f**) Folliculitis decalvans. (**g**) Folliculitis decalvans mimicking laceration injury. (**h**) Pseudopelade Brocq. (**i**) Dissecting cellulitis of scalp. (**j**) Folliculitis keloidalis nuchae. (**k**) Erosive pustular dermatosis of scalp. (**l**) Alopecia parvimaculata Dreuw

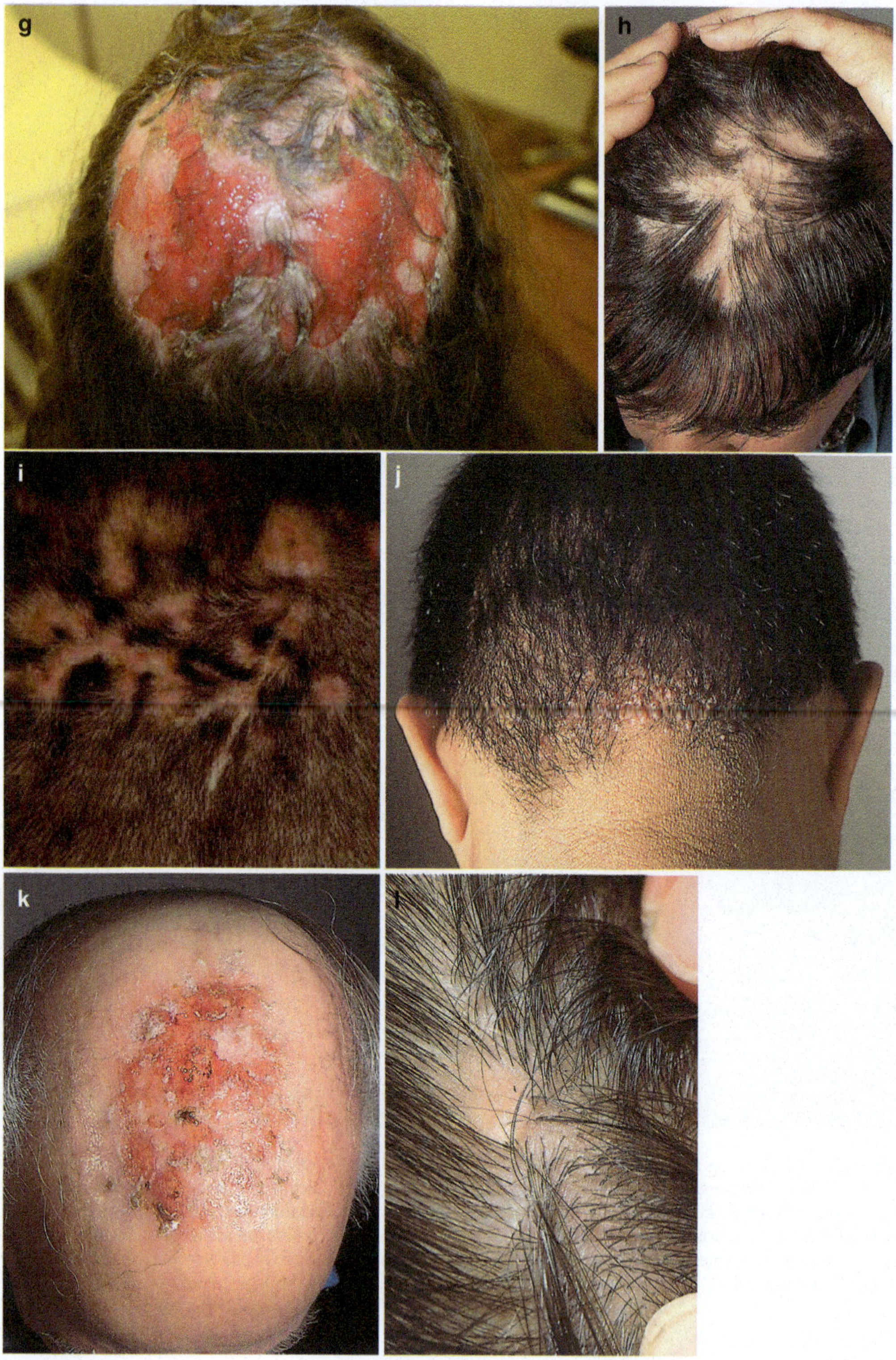

Fig. 4.22 (continued)

Table 4.10 Systemic lupus erythematosus ACR criteria

Criteria	Sensitivity (%)	Specificity (%)
1. *Malar rash* (rash on cheeks)	57	96
2. *Discoid rash* (red, scaly patches on skin that cause scarring)	18	99
3. *Serositis*: pleurisy or pericarditis (pleural is more sensitive; cardiac is more specific)	56	86
4. *Oral ulcers* (includes oral or nasopharyngeal ulcers)	27	96
5. *Arthritis*: nonerosive arthritis of two or more peripheral joints, with tenderness, swelling, or effusion	86	37
6. *Photosensitivity* (exposure to ultraviolet light causes rash, or other symptoms of disease flare up)	43	96
7. *Hematologic disorder*: hemolytic anemia (low red blood cell count) or leukopenia (white blood cell count <4000/μl), lymphopenia (<1500/μl) or thrombocytopenia (<100,000/μl) in the absence of offending drug	59	89
8. *Renal disorder*: more than 0.5 g per day protein in urine or cellular casts seen in urine under a microscope	51	94
9. *Antinuclear antibody test positive*	99	49
10. *Immunologic disorder*: positive anti-Smith, anti-ds DNA, antiphospholipid antibody, and/or false-positive serologic test for syphilis. The presence of anti-ss DNA in 70 % of cases (hypocomplementemia is also seen, due to consumption of C3 and C4 by immune complex-induced inflammation or to congenitally complement deficiency, which may predispose to systemic lupus erythematosus)	85	93
11. *Neurologic disorder*: seizures or psychosis	20	98

included in the American College of Rheumatology (ACR) criteria for the classification of systemic lupus erythematosus (Table 4.10).

For the purpose of identifying patients for clinical studies, a person has systemic lupus erythematosus if any 4 out of 11 symptoms are present simultaneously or serially on two separate occasions.

In addition to the focal and scarring form of alopecia associated with discoid lupus erythematosus, systemic lupus erythematosus patients may experience a diffuse, non-scarring, and transient hair loss associated with exacerbations of their lupus disease process. This diffuse hair loss seen in systemic disease is usually the result of a telogen effluvium. The telogen effluvium is in all probability the result of both severe catabolic effects and elevated levels of circulating proinflammatory cytokines of the lupus disease flare on hair growth cycling.

More recently, discoid lupus erythematosus has been observed to also present as frontal fibrosing alopecia (Fig. 4.22c–e), and it has been discussed to what extent—again—a background of androgenetic alopecia may contribute to this particular clinical presentation of the disease.

> Of patients presenting with discoid lesions, 5–10 % develop clear-cut evidence of systemic disease, with the extent and distribution of the discoid lesions determining the risk: Patients with lesions both above and below the neck (generalized discoid lupus erythematosus) have a higher rate of immunological abnormalities and risk for progression to systemic disease compared to patients with discoid lesions restricted to the head and neck area (localized discoid lupus erythematosus).

Folliculitis decalvans represents a chronic and recurrent pustulofollicular scalp inflammation resulting in scarring alopecia. It usually presents in the central scalp area with exudative crusted areas and grouped follicular pustules at the hair-bearing margin with centrifugal progression (Fig. 4.22f). Very rarely it can present with an extensive ulcerated appearance of the scalp (Fig.4.22g) that has been reported to have been misinterpreted as a laceration of the scalp at the forensic scene. Histopathology reveals a neutrophilic primary scarring alopecia. Invariably pathogenic strains of *S. aureus* can be detected. Only very rarely there may be an association with immune deficiency. A recent study provided evidence of the presence of bacterial biofilms in the infrainfundibular part of human scalp hair follicles to be pathogenic. A biofilm is any group of microorganisms in which cells stick to each other on a surface. These adherent cells are frequently embedded within a self-produced matrix of extracellular polymeric substance. Biofilms form on living or nonliving surfaces and in the case of folliculitis decalvans on the surfaces of the hair shaft. Bacteria living in a biofilm usually have significantly different properties from free-floating bacteria of the same species, as the dense and protected environment of the film allows them to cooperate and interact in various ways. One benefit of this environment is increased resistance to antibiotics, as the dense extracellular matrix and the outer layer of cells protect the interior of the community. Biofilms have been found to be involved in a wide variety of microbial infections in the body, and more recently it has been noted that bacterial biofilms may impair cutaneous wound healing and reduce topical antibacterial efficiency in healing or treating infected skin wounds.

The presence of a bacterial biofilm at the interface of the hair shaft may provide an explanation for the chronicity and high relapse rate of folliculitis decalvans.

Pseudopelade as first described by Brocq in 1888 and redefined by Bergner and Braun-Falco presents with asymptomatic, noninflamed, ivory-white- or flesh-colored, small oval-round, reticulate or large, irregular patches of the central scalp area (Fig. 4.22h). Non-scalp involvement is absent. It is considered a lymphocytic primary scarring alopecia with selective destruction of hair follicles. It is clinically and histologically indistinguishable from end-stage lichen planopilaris, and some suggest that the two entities do not represent distinct diseases, but rather different clinical presentations in a spectrum derived from the same underlying pathogenic mechanism. In an early study, Pierard-Franchimont and Pierard reported massive lymphocyte-mediated apoptosis during the early stage of pseudopelade and suggested that unique aspect is most probably related to the mechanism of apoptosis. Its intensity and extension were more pronounced than in lichen planus and in lupus erythematosus, and the authors suggested that pathogenesis of some cicatricial alopecias could therefore be related to sudden and synchronized cell death of all cells of the epithelial sheaths of the hair follicles without evident relationship with the classical etiologies of inflammatory scar alopecia, i.e., lichen planus and lupus erythematosus.

Ultimately, McElwee et al. explored the degree of similarity between lichen planopilaris and pseudopelade Brocq gene expression patterns and the potential for common and unique gene pathway and gene activity using microarrays. There was limited commonality in the gene expression profiles between the two diseases. Specific genes, such as MMP11, TNFSF13B, and APOL2, were identified with significantly differential expression in association with lichen planopilaris *versus* pseudopelade Brocq. According to the authors, these results suggest that lichen planopilaris and pseudopelade Brocq involve different mechanisms of disease development and should be regarded as biologically distinct cicatricial alopecias with different potential therapeutic targets.

Also using microarray analysis of lichen planopilaris compared to normal scalp biopsies, Karnik et al. identified decreased expression of genes required for lipid metabolism and peroxisome biogenesis. Immunohistochemical analysis showed progressive loss of peroxisomes, proinflammatory lipid accumulation, and infiltration of inflammatory cells followed by destruction of the pilosebaceous unit. The expression of peroxisome proliferator-activated receptor (PPAR) gamma, a transcription factor that regulates these processes, was significantly decreased in lichen planopilaris. The authors proposed that PPAR-gamma-targeted therapy may represent a new strategy in the treatment of lichen planopilaris and subsequently published the first proof of concept with oral pioglitazone.

Two other conditions of primary scarring alopecias predominantly seen in men are dissecting cellulitis of the scalp and folliculitis (or acne) keloidalis nuchae.

Dissecting cellulitis of the scalp also known as perifolliculitis capitis abscedens et suffodiens, or Hoffman's disease, is a rare but well characterized chronic inflammatory disease of the scalp leading to scarring alopecia. Most of those affected are young black males; about 10 % of cases involve white males. Association with acne conglobata was described as early as in 1903. Today, the condition is considered to be part of the follicular occlusion triad, along with acne conglobata and hidradenitis suppurativa (acne inversa), although isolated scalp disease occurs. Deep inflammatory nodules develop on the occipital scalp or vertex and can evolve to extensive confluent boggy plaques with sinus tract formation. Hairs overlying the nodules can be easily plucked, and sinus tracts may discharge purulent material. Ultimately, a multifocal scarring alopecia ensues that is potentially disfiguring (Fig. 4.22i). Histopathology reveals a neutrophilic primary scarring alopecia. Pathogenetically, a defect in follicular keratinization is blamed, leading to poral obstruction and accumulation of sebaceous and keratinous material within dilated pilosebaceous units. Subsequently, follicles burst, and an intense neutrophilic inflammatory reaction with abscess and sinus tract formation follows.

Folliculitis keloidalis nuchae represents yet another form of chronic inflammatory folliculitis. Again, the condition tends to occur preferentially in young black men, although white men may also be affected. It is rarely ever seen in women but has been reported in women of African descent. The disease involves the occipital scalp. Lesions start as firm follicular papules (Fig. 4.22j), a condition that has also been synonymously named *dermatitis papillaris capillitii*. Especially in black men, these may coalesce into larger, keloid-like plaques. Histopathology reveals a mixed cellular primary scarring alopecia.

Yet another peculiar condition, primarily seen on the balding scalp, is *erosive pustular dermatosis of the scalp*. It has also been classified among the mixed group of primary inflammatory alopecia. The condition was originally described by Burton and subsequently delineated by Pye, Peachey, and Burton as a distinctive clinical entity producing chronic extensive pustulation confined to the scalp of elderly individuals and leading to erosion and scarring alopecia (Fig. 4.22k). A high incidence of antecedent local trauma strongly suggests that scalp injury may be important in initiating the dermatosis in a susceptible elderly person with atrophic skin changes of the scalp, particularly due to prolonged exposure of long-standing androgenetic alopecia to UVR. No recognized cause of pustulation is present, and the histology is nonspecific. Response to antibiotics is poor, but the condition is suppressed by potent topical steroids, suggesting a primary inflammatory rather than an infective etiology. The condition has been observed following contusion, laceration, blistering sunburn, shingles, synthetic fiber implantation, craniotomy, and skin grafting of the scalp, as well as following treatment of solar keratoses with 5 % topical fluorouracil cream, cryotherapy and topical tretinoin, and soft X-ray therapy.

> Therefore, one must think of the possibility of erosive pustular dermatosis of the scalp in cases of delayed wound healing following treatment of actinic keratoses on the scalp.

Response to therapy has been variable. Anecdotal reports describe partial response to nimesulide, a phenoxymethane sulfonanilide that inhibits the respiratory burst of human granulocytes, but best responses have been reported to potent topical steroids or topical 0.1 % tacrolimus. Long-term follow-up is advised, since neoplastic change has been reported.

Secondary scarring alopecia results from events outside the follicle, which eventually impinge upon and eradicate the follicle. These include physical or chemical injury, infectious diseases (fungal, bacterial, viral), granulomatous disease (sarcoidosis, necrobiosis lipoidica/ Miescher's granulomatosis disciformis progressiva) or neoplastic processes (primary or metastatic solid tumors, malignant lymphoma), and autoimmune diseases, such as circumscribed scleroderma, cicatricial pemphigoid, and necrotizing temporal arteritis.

Alopecia neoplastica has originally been defined as hair loss secondary to a visceral malignancy that has metastasized to the scalp. More recently, a classification into primary and secondary alopecia neoplastica has been proposed. The clinical presentation may mimic alopecia areata.

> At times, the diagnosis of alopecia neoplastica may antedate the diagnosis of the underlying malignancy. The suspicion must remain high, and a scalp biopsy will reveal the diagnosis.

In a study of 398 patients with malignant tumors of the scalp, basal (41 %) and squamous cell carcinomas (16.6 %) were the most frequent, followed my metastatic tumors to the scalp in 12.8 %, of which lung cancer was the most frequent primary tumor in both male and female patients. Another study of 197 scalp tumors in women identified basal cell carcinoma in 77 % and squamous cell carcinoma in 17 %, in stark contrast to a frequency of 54 % squamous cell carcinoma in men who were in average older.

Primary scalp tumors are infrequently associated with hair loss. Alopecia caused by primary skin neoplasias has been described most frequently in folliculotropic mycosis fungoides.

Secondary alopecia neoplastica seems to predominate in elderly women, in whom breast cancer accounts for over 80 % of primary tumors. Other primary tumors of which scalp metastases presented as neoplasm-related hair loss have been gastric, colon, renal, pancreatic, and prostate carcinoma.

Finally, *pseudopeladic state of Degos* et al. (1954) represents the nonspecific end stage of a variety of at least 60 types of primary or secondary cicatricial alopecias, whereby *pseudopelade of Brocq* (1905) may represent the end stage or a variant of lichen planopilaris, *Sperling's central centrifugal scarring alopecia* (2000) with its predilection for African Americans and close relationship to LoPresti's hot comb alopecia (1968) a USA-specific perspective of Degos' pseudopeladic state due to peculiarities of African American hair grooming habits and hair anatomy, and *alopecia parvimaculata Dreuw* (1911) possibly the pediatric variant of Degos' pseudopeladic state.

Dreuw originally reported an epidemic outbreak of alopecia in schoolboys, in whom hair was lost in very small, irregularly shaped patches (Fig. 4.221). Today, the condition is rather seen sporadically in children and is understood to be of multietiologic origin. Permanent (scarring) alopecia is reported to occur in 10 % of cases and must be differentiated from alopecia areata in this age group.

The relationship of the different groups of scarring alopecia is graphically summarized in Fig. 4.23.

4.3.2 Treatment

Recommended treatment regimens for the most prevalent among the inflammatory scarring alopecias are summarized in Table 4.11.

Since structural changes in the course of scarring alopecia are irreversible, there is a clear need for early intervention. With the expanding technologies for dissecting the immunologic and molecular basis, there is hope for a deeper understanding of the underlying pathogenesis and novel therapeutic interventions. Among these, currently, microarray analysis is used to identify disease-associated gene expression patterns with the aims of further clarification of nosologic classifications and development of targeted therapies of the scarring alopecias.

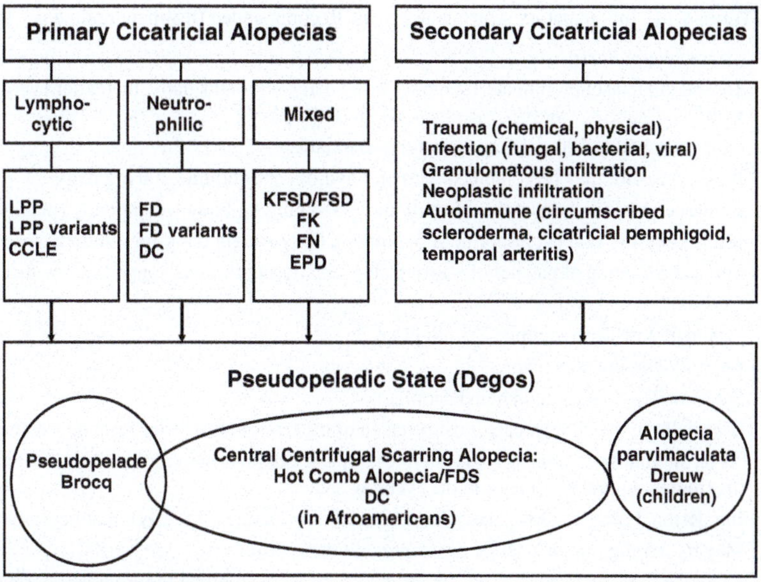

Fig. 4.23 Overview of scarring alopecias. Abbreviations: *LPP* lichen planopilaris, *CCLE* chronic cutaneous lupus erythematosus, *FD* folliculitis decalvans, *DC* dissecting cellulitis, *KFSD* keratosis follicularis spinulosa decalvans, *FSD* folliculitis spinulosa decalvans, *FK* folliculitis keloidalis, *FN* folliculitis necrotica, *EPD* erosive pustular dermatosis

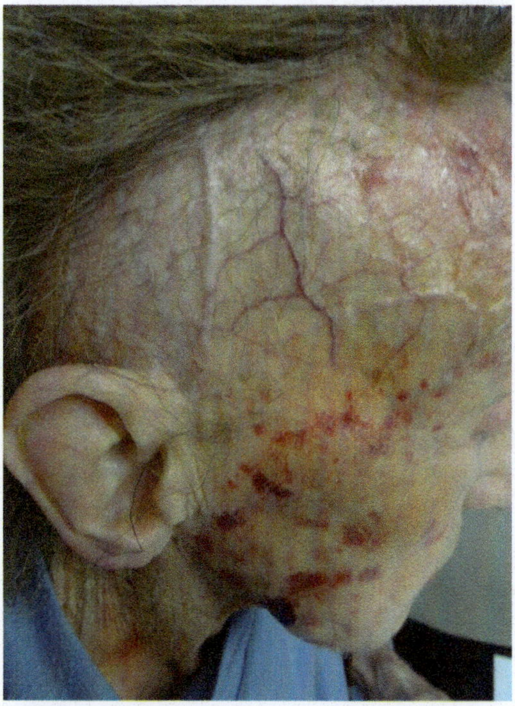

Fig. 4.24 Cutaneous atrophy with Bateman purpura from prolonged and unjudicious use of high-potency topical corticosteroid for treatment of frontal fibrosing alopecia

Where end-stage fibrosis is established, surgical treatment such as reduction plasty, scalp expander technology, and autologous hair transplantation or prosthetic help are taken into consideration.

4.3.3 Graft-*Versus*-Host Disease

Graft-*versus*-host disease (GvHD) is a common complication following allogeneic tissue transplantation and responsible for significant post-therapeutic morbidity, mortality, and decrease in quality of life of affected patients. It is commonly associated with hematopoietic stem cell or bone marrow transplantation, though the term may apply to all forms of tissue grafts. The condition is induced and maintained by immunocompetent cells from the donor tissue (graft) that particularly attack epithelia of fast proliferating tissues of the recipient (host), such as those from the gastrointestinal tract, liver, and the skin. Involvement of the gastrointestinal tract can result in severe intestinal inflammation, with sloughing of the mucosal membrane, severe diarrhea, abdominal pain, nausea, and vomiting, while liver involvement is measured by bilirubin levels.

On the basis of the time of presentation, cutaneous GvHD has traditionally been divided into an acute and chronic disease. Acute GvHD is observed within the first 100 days post-transplant, while chronic GvHD normally occurs after 100

Table 4.11 Inflammatory scarring alopecias. Recommended treatment regimens

Lichen planopilaris
Topical clobetasol propionate 1st month twice daily, 3 months daily, thereafter every second day, in combination with
Oral doxycycline 100–200 mg daily for 3–6 months
If unsuccessful, may be combined with oral hydroxychloroquine 200 mg daily
If unsuccessful, oral mycophenolate mofetil 35–45 mg/kg body weight daily (max. 3 g daily)
If unsuccessful, oral cyclosporine A 3–5 mg/kg body weight daily for 4 months may be combined with
Surgical reduction of patches of scarring alopecia (during immunosuppression with 2.5–5 mg/kg oral cyclosporine A)
Or
Trial with low-dose excimer 308 nm laser
Frontal fibrosing alopecia
Same may be tried as in lichen planopilaris
Especially in the elderly, care must be taken of the risk of corticosteroid-induced cutaneous atrophy (Fig. 4.24)
As an alternative to topical corticosteroids, topical calcineurin inhibitors (pimecrolimus, tacrolimus) may be tried at the frontotemporal hairline or in the eyebrow area
Intralesional triamcinolone acetonide 10 mg/ml is effective for (early) treatment of eyebrows
May try 2.5 mg oral finasteride or 0.5 mg oral dutasteride
Autologous hair transplantation surgery may be effective both at the frontotemporal hairline and for eyebrows
Chronic cutaneous lupus erythematosus
Intralesional triamcinolone acetonide 10 mg/ml every 4 weeks, in combination with
Oral hydroxychloroquine, first 4 weeks 2×200 mg daily and thereafter 200 mg daily
May be combined with 1200 IU vitamin E and 500 mg vitamin C daily (in smokers)
Photoprotection
Folliculitis decalvans
Oral fusidic acid 3×500 mg daily for 3 weeks, in combination with
Oral zinc gluconate 30 mg daily for 6 months
Or
Oral rifampicin 450 mg twice daily in combination with oral flucloxacilline 500 mg four times daily for 2 weeks and thereafter every 3 months for 5 days
Or
Oral rifampicin 300 mg twice daily in combination with oral clindamycin 300 mg twice daily during 10 weeks
Or
Oral levofloxacin 500 mg twice daily for 10 days
Daily antiseptic shampoo treatment with 0.2–2 % chlorhexidine gluconate
Surgical reduction of patches of scarring alopecia (with expander technology as needed) or selective punch excision of hair tufts may be taken into consideration (during oral antibiotic treatment)
Dissecting cellulitis of the scalp
Oral isotretinoin 1 mg/kg body weight daily for at least 6 months, in combination with
Sustained, pathogen-specific, systemic antibiotic (according to antibiogram), and
Oral prednisone, 1 mg/kg body weight with subsequent tapering
Or
Oral dapsone 100–200 mg daily, in combination with
Oral zinc gluconate 30 mg daily, and
Intralesional triamcinolone acetonide 5–10 mg/ml
In severe and refractory cases, large-scale surgical excision in combination with reconstructive surgery
Or
Subcutaneous adalimumab 40 mg every 2 weeks
Folliculitis keloidalis nuchae
Patient should refrain from shaving the nape of the neck

Table 4.11 (continued)

Early lesions may be treated with a combination of cryotherapy and intralesional triamcinolone acetonide 10–40 mg/ml
Daily topical antiseptics or antibiotics, such as povidone–iodine shampoo, shampoo with 0.2–2 % chlorhexidine gluconate, or topical clindamycin solution
During inflammatory phases, oral doxycycline 200 mg daily, or minocycline 100 mg daily, or erythromycin 1–2 g daily
In case of keloid-like plaques may consider CO_2-laser evaporation
Tinea capitis (children)
Systemic antimycotic treatment, in case of endotrich infection with *Trichophyton spp.* with oral terbinafine 6 mg/kg body weight per day for 2–4 weeks, in case of exotrich infection with *Microsporum spp.* with oral itraconazole 5 mg/kg body weight per day for 4–6 weeks, in combination with
Topical antimycotic treatment, either as shampoo (selenium disulfide, ketoconazole, or povidone iodine) or topical antimycotic agent (ciclopiroxolamine, an imidazole, or terbinafine)
May combine oral prednisone 1 mg/kg body weight per day for 1–2 weeks in case of deep inflammatory tinea (Kerion)
Combine with oral antibiotic, preferably an oral macrolide antibiotic, if secondary pathogenic bacterial infection is present
Check for carrier status for sanitation of family members or pets, depending on anthropophilic or zoophilic fungal agent, respectively, detected in mycologic culture

days. This distinction is not arbitrary, since acute and chronic GvHD appear to involve different immune cell subsets, different cytokine profiles, and somewhat different host targets and respond to treatment in different ways.

In acute GVHD, skin involvement is frequent, and the skin is often the initial organ involved. The cutaneous marker of acute GvHD is typically a diffuse maculopapular rash, sometimes in a lacy pattern. Friedman et al. originally reported acute follicular graft-*versus*-host reaction in the form of disseminated follicular papules simulating folliculitis. Histopathologic examination demonstrated features of acute GvHD involving hair follicles, suggesting that follicular epithelium may be an early target of the immunologic injury.

The skin is the most common organ involved in chronic GvHD. Patients may have pruritus, rash, pain, dyspigmentation, and fibrotic or sclerodermatous changes. While the cutaneous, mucosal, and nail manifestations of chronic GvHD are well recognized, involvement of the hair follicle has so far found lesser attention.

Miyazaki et al. reported the first case of chronic GvHD with follicular involvement. The indicator case developed pruritic follicular red papules over the trunk and extremities 8 months after undergoing an allogeneic bone marrow transplant for aplastic anemia. A biopsy specimen revealed histological exocytosis of lymphocytes into the hair follicles and basal cell vacuolization of the follicular epithelium. Analysis of T-lymphocyte subpopulations in the dermis revealed a predominance of CD4-positive cells.

Chronic GvHD of the scalp may present (personal observation) with perifollicular erythema, follicular keratosis, and obliterations of follicular orifices of the central scalp region reminiscent of fibrosing alopecia in a pattern distribution, underscoring the role of autoantigen-driven cytotoxic CD4+ T-cells, possibly on a background of androgenetic alopecia, for the pathogenesis of the clinical syndrome. There may be associated mucosal (usually lichen planus-like), skin (lichenoid, or scleroderma-like), and/or nail involvement (longitudinal ridging, longitudinal erythronychia, pterygium, or onychoatrophy in order of frequency).

Systemic corticosteroids are the standard of care in GvHD, while methotrexate, ciclosporin, and tacrolimus are commonly used for GvHD prophylaxis. However, high-dose immunosuppression raises the risk both of infections and of tumor relapse. Therefore, it is desirable to taper off the post-transplant high-level immunosuppression to lower levels, at which point the appearance of mild GVHD may be welcome, especially in HLA mismatched patients, as it is associated with a graft-*versus*-tumor effect. Treatment options for supportive therapy in cutaneous GvHD include topical therapies, such as corticosteroids, calcineurin inhibitors, and phototherapy. GvHD of the scalp presenting as fibrosing alopecia in a pattern distribution may be successfully treated with a topical compound of 5 % minoxidil and 0.2 % triamcinolone acetonide solution (personal observation).

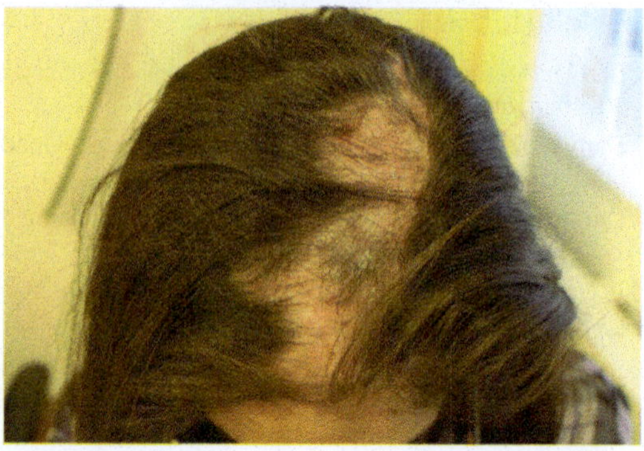

Fig. 4.25 Anti-TNF alpha therapy-induced psoriasis-like dermatitis of scalp with diffuse alopecia

4.3.4 Antitumor Necrosis Factor-Alpha Therapy-Induced Alopecia

Tumor necrosis factor (TNF) alpha inhibitors (infliximab, etanercept, adalimumab) are increasingly being used for the treatment of a variety of autoimmune diseases, such as rheumatoid arthritis, ankylosing spondylitis, Crohn's disease, and plaque psoriasis. During these treatments, adverse effects involving the hair and scalp have been reported.

> The most consistent among the anti-TNF alpha therapy-induced adverse effects affecting the condition of the scalp has been a psoriasis-like dermatitis with diffuse alopecia and the risk of irreversible, scarring hair loss (Fig. 4.25).

Cullen et al. reported on 30 subjects who developed a psoriatic rash while receiving anti-TNF therapy for inflammatory bowel disease and reviewed the data from another 120 published cases of anti-TNF-induced psoriasis in inflammatory bowel disease. They found anti-TNF-induced psoriasis in inflammatory bowel disease to be more common in women (70 %). The most common distributions were palmoplantar (43 %) and scalp (42 %). Follow-up in 148 cases showed that 41 % responded to topical therapy and were able to continue anti-TNF therapy, while 43 % required definitive withdrawal of anti-TNF therapy due to the rash. A second anti-TNF was tried in 27 cases with recurrence or persistence of the rash in 14 (52 %).

Joyau et al. have pointed out that psoriasis occurring during anti-TNF therapy is de novo psoriasis and not an aggravation of a preexisting psoriasis. To this day, several hypotheses have been proposed to explain the underlying immunologic mechanisms. It appears to be a class effect.

Finally, Puig et al. reported on a 47-year-old woman who developed incapacitating palmoplantar pustulosis, a psoriasis vulgaris flare, and severe scalp and nail involvement after 5 months of treatment with adalimumab for psoriatic arthritis. Several treatments, including topical corticosteroids, photochemotherapy, ciclosporin, acitretin, and etanercept 50 mg twice a day for 1 month, were ineffective or not tolerated. Treatment with ustekinumab 45 mg provided complete resolution of skin lesions with acceptable therapeutic control of the arthritis.

4.4 Red Scalp

Red scalp was originally described by Thestrup-Pedersen and Hjorth in 1987 and subsequently commented on by Moschella in 1992, who stated on the difficult problem of "diffuse red scalp disease which can also be itchy and burning. .... It is non responsive to any therapy including potent

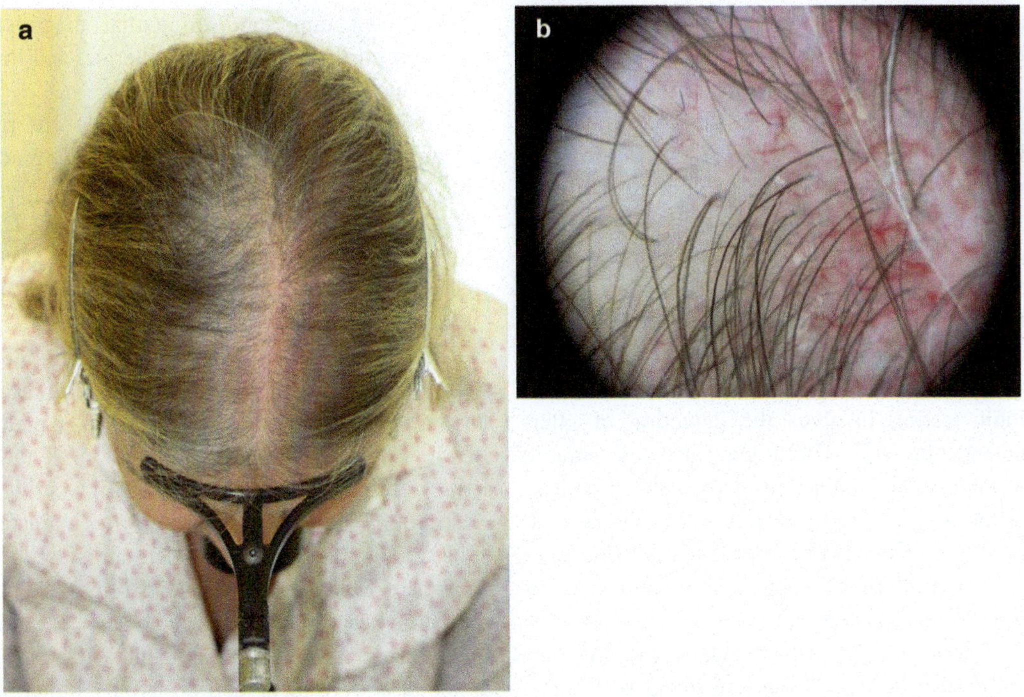

Fig. 4.26 (**a**, **b**) Red scalp: (**a**) in a peculiar half-and-half pattern, (**b**) dermoscopic finding of telangiectatic erythema

topical steroids or anti-seborrhoeic therapy" (Fig. 4.26). Patients frequently report aggravation in the sun or report repeated episodes of sunburn of the scalp.

Grimalt et al. presented their findings in 18 patients with "red scalp syndrome" at the 2000 Annual Meeting of the European Hair Research Society: The majority were middle-aged females consulting for hair loss. The scalp redness was associated with androgenetic alopecia in 13 out of 18 patients, and three of ten biopsies performed were compatible with a cicatricial alopecia (not otherwise specified). Some patients reported associated discomfort of the scalp.

> Today, by definition red scalp is a condition of persistent redness of the scalp, not explained by a specific dermatologic disease of the scalp, with or without sensation of itching or burning, that is refractory to topical corticosteroids and antiseborrheic agents and shows aggravation in the sun.

The most prevalent speculations with respect to the pathogenesis of scalp discomfort with the dermoscopic finding of scalp telangiectasia in the absence of a specific dermatologic disease are perifollicular inflammation and/or increased expression of neuropeptide substance P in the vicinity of affected hair follicles.

In some cases, there exists some relationship to atopy and atopic disease and in others to rosacea and rosacea-like dermatosis of the scalp.

4.4.1 Atopic Dermatitis of the Head and Neck Type

Atopic dermatitis, also known as atopic eczema, is a common, chronic, relapsing, inflammatory skin disorder that may affect the scalp in a significant manner. In infantile eczema, much of the body may be affected, while the typical scalp manifestation is cradle cap. As the children get older, the flector aspects of the extremities are most commonly affected. In adults, the hands and feet are often affected, and a subset of patients suffer of head and neck dermatitis.

The pathogenesis of atopic dermatitis is complex and involves genetics, environmental factors, disrupted permeability of the skin, and immunologic mechanisms.

The diagnosis is based primarily on the clinical presentation, while skin prick tests, serologic testing, and the atopy patch tests may serve as diagnostic tools. Skin prick tests involve the identification of immediate-type allergic reactions (within 15 min), and serologic testing involves the detection of allergen-specific IgE. The atopy patch test aims at reproducing delayed-type allergic skin reactions (after 24–72 h) to immediate-type allergens, in an effort to determine whether a specific IgE-mediated allergen is causing the symptoms of the eczematous skin reaction.

The subset of patients with head and neck dermatitis may have a reaction to resident *Malassezia* flora fueling their condition. This reaction is likely related to both humoral- and cell-mediated immunity. Even in the absence of differences in *Malassezia* spp. colonization, patients with head and neck atopic dermatitis are more likely to have positive skin prick test results and *Malassezia*-specific IgE compared to healthy control subjects and to patients with atopy without head and neck dermatitis. However, no clear relationship with atopy patch testing has been found.

> Clinically, *Malassezia* allergy may be suspected in patients with atopic disease and (1) eczema involving the head and neck region, (2) exacerbations during adolescence or early adulthood, (3) lesions recalcitrant to conventional therapy.

There is literature to suggest that these patients may benefit from a 1- to 2-month course of daily oral itraconazole followed by long-term weekly treatment in combination with regular use of ketoconazole shampoo.

The most important differential diagnoses include seborrhoeic dermatitis, allergic, and irritant contact dermatitis.

Seborrhoeic dermatitis represents a chronic recurrent condition characterized by scaling and poorly defined erythematous patches with a predilection for areas rich in sebaceous glands. The scalp is almost invariably affected, and other areas of skin involved (in order of frequency) are the face, chest, and intertriginous areas. The cause of seborrhoeic dermatitis is again understood to involve fungi of the genus *Malassezia*. The inflammatory process is believed to be mediated by fungal metabolites, specifically free fatty acids released from sebaceous triglycerides. Accordingly, antifungal agents are the mainstay of treatment of seborrhoeic dermatitis, with a number of well-performed studies proving superiority of ketoconazole and ciclopirox olamine shampoo over placebo for treatment. With respect to the use of topical corticosteroids either as lotion, cream, or foam, there is a consensus that they are useful in the short term, mainly to control erythema and itching, but no data are available regarding the question whether the combination of topical antifungal agents with topical corticosteroid results in a greater benefit than single-agent therapy.

A typically successful therapy for seborrhoeic dermatitis of the scalp would be using a 2 % ketoconazole or a 1.5 % ciclopirox olamine shampoo every other day during the first 2 weeks and thereafter twice weekly, depending on severity, either as monotherapy or in the more severe cases in combination with systemic itraconazole 200 mg daily during the first 7 days of treatment (and thereafter 200 mg every second week) and topical clobetasol propionate 0.05 % foam as needed.

Allergic contact dermatitis represents the manifestation of an allergic response of the skin caused by contact with a substance the individual is sensitized to. In contrast to irritant contact dermatitis, allergic contact dermatitis represents a hypersensitivity reaction that is atypical within the general population.

Allergic reactions to cosmetics are usually overestimated by consumers. Less than 10 % of the population report an intolerance reaction to a cosmetic product, of those 1 % is caused by a contact allergen that is identified with patch testing.

Common contact allergens in cosmetics include (in order of frequency) fragrances, hair dyes (*p*-phenylenediamine or PPD and *p*-toluenediamine or PTD), and preservatives (formaldehyde, parabens, quaternium-15, imidazolinylurea, DMDM hydantoin, and bronopol). In cases where an allergic contact dermatitis is suspected, respective patch testing is recommended.

The ratings "paraben-free," "silicone-free," and "sulfate-free" are rather in the interest of marketing purposes than consumer protection.

Contact sensitivity to parabens is generally overestimated. Paraben-sensitive persons, who react to parabens on patch testing and develop a dermatitis when paraben-containing products are used on compromised skin, may continue to use paraben-containing product on areas of intact skin, without adverse reaction. This phenomenon has been termed the "paraben paradox" by Fisher in 1973. Originally, Fisher included in the definition of "paraben paradox" also the fact that paraben-containing personal products, which are the cause of an allergic contact dermatitis, often produce false-negative patch test reactions when applied to the skin of the back. The explanation for this phenomenon is again that the patch testing is being performed on intact skin.

More frequently, complaints of scalp discomfort related to the use of a hair cosmetic agent is due to irritant contact dermatitis. Typical contact irritants are sodium lauryl sulfate and cocamidopropyl betaine.

4.4.2 Rosacea-Like Dermatosis of the Scalp

An interesting analogy of red scalp exists to rosacea, where patients with the telangiectatic variant of rosacea report stinging sensation to the topical application of 5 % lactic acid on the cheeks more frequently than patients with the papulopustular type of rosacea or normal controls.

In a published series of 403 patients complaining of hair loss examined for trichodynia, Willimann and Trüeb found the dermatoscopic finding of scalp telangiectasia to strongly correlate with the presence of trichodynia. On the one hand, these findings suggest a connection between sensory or subjective irritation and cutaneous vascular reactivity. On the other hand, dilated and tortuous vessels are typically found in photodamaged skin.

Oberholzer et al. reported on patients with red scalp disease with clinical and histopathologic findings consistent with rosacea and response to oral tetracycline therapy. On the basis of the observation of clinical and histopathologic features of rosacea and response to oral tetracycline therapy, patients complaining of red scalp accompanied with scalp discomfort were suggested to suffer of a rosacea-like dermatosis of the scalp. Careful examination of the affected scalp, including dermoscopy, invariably reveals erythema, telangiectasia, follicular papules, and pustules. Histology demonstrates ectatic venules and a usually sparse perivascular infiltrate, in the case of papules a more pleomorphic perifollicular infiltration with granuloma formation, including neutrophils. Intrafollicular collections of neutrophils are found when pustules are observed.

Rosacea is a chronic inflammatory disorder usually affecting the central parts of the face with flushing, persistent erythema, and telangiectasia, in combination with episodes of swelling, papules, and pustules. It typically presents either as erythematotelangiectatic rosacea or as the papulopustular type with a predilection for the centrofacial area. Eye involvement (ocular rosacea) is common and well appreciated.

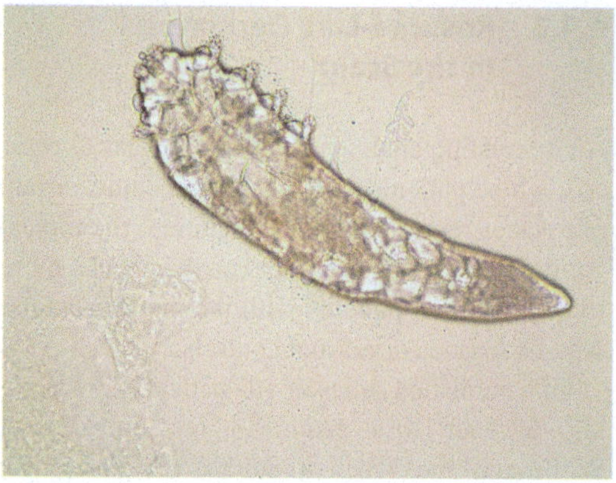

Fig. 4.27 *Demodex* mite extracted from an inflammatory follicular lesion in scalp demodicosis (light microscopy)

Other extrafacial locations of rosacea may be involved more frequently than appreciated because of failure to search, in particular, rosacea affecting the upper forehead and scalp.

Demodex infestation of the scalp has previously been put forward as a possible etiologic factor in some cases of scalp rosacea. However, demodex mites are common commensals of the pilosebaceous unit (Fig. 4.27). Moreover, there is no consensus to what degree demodex mites are causative of skin pathology and how they might contribute to disease in humans. Nevertheless, *Demodex folliculorum* and *D. brevis* have been identified and implied to play a role in pustular folliculitis of the face, papulopustular scalp eruptions, perioral dermatitis, and blepharitis. In general, the clinical presentations of demodicidosis have been classified into three main groups: "pityriasis folliculorum," "rosacea-like demodicidosis," and "granulomatous rosacea-like demodicidosis gravis."

Methods used for diagnostic purposes include cyanoacrylic adhesives, comedone extractor, cellophane tape preparations, skin scraping, punch biopsy, and standardized surface skin biopsy.

Therapy includes oral metronidazole (250 mg bid for 30 days), 5 % topical permethrin cream bid, and 0.02 % miconazole shampoo on a regular basis.

4.4.3 Scalp Burnout

Burnout syndrome is defined as a condition of emotional exhaustion with reduced capacity. It is understood to represent a development lign that starts with enthusiastic idealism leading through frustrating experiences to disillusionment, psychosomatic disorders, depression, and aggressivity.

Just as the burnout syndrome is not recognized to represent a true medical condition by the scientific community, but is rather defined as a coping problem in ICD-10, we encounter individuals in daily clinical practice with an analogous patient's career with regard to the condition of the scalp, which represents rather a question of problem solving than a specific dermatologic condition.

Management begins with protection of the scalp from further noxious environmental, medical, or cosmetic exposures and acting toward its appeasement and restoration while regaining the confidence of the patient.

The first step consists in adapting the frequency of hair washing to condition of the hair and scalp. Persons with greasy hair (seborrhea) should shampoo their hair often, sometimes even daily, whereas persons with dry hair (sebostasis) should shampoo less often. A mild shampoo must be selected, avoiding ingredients with irritation potential or containing frequent contact allergens. Of particular interest are herbal special care ingredients with anti-irritant activity from traditional phytomedicine, such as chamomile (*Matricaria chamomilla*), heartseed (*Cardiospermum halicacabum*), peony (*Paeonia lactiflora*), and Virginian witch hazel (*Hamamelis virginiana:* Fig. 4.28).

When Europeans originally encountered Native Americans, the American Indian tribes dwelling in the Northeastern regions utilized about 275 plants for medicinal purpose. The native North American Virginian witch hazel *H. virginiana* was among the most important of those plants and was used for treatment of superficial skin wounds and inflammatory skin

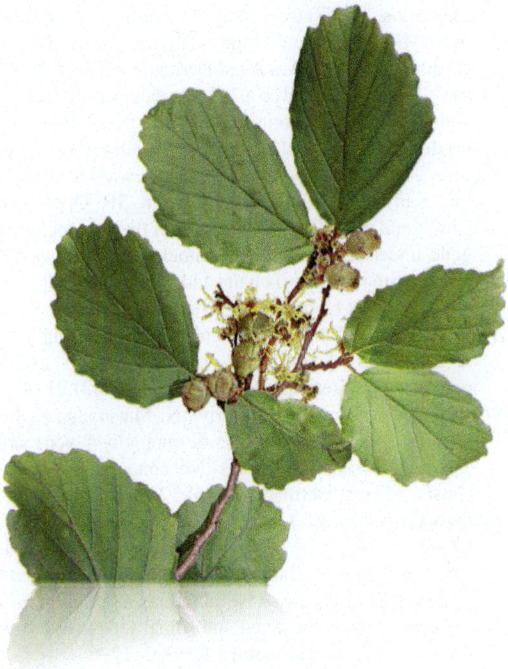

Fig. 4.28 North American Virginian witch hazel (*Hamamelis virginiana*)

conditions. The Native Americans produced witch hazel extract by boiling the stems of the shrub and producing a decoction, which was used to treat inflammatory conditions. Early Puritan settlers in New England adopted this remedy from the natives. A missionary, Dr. Charles Hawes, eventually learned of the preparation's therapeutic properties and further determined that the product of the plant's twigs was even more efficacious. Hawes' process was further refined by Thomas Newton Dickinson, Sr., who is credited with starting the commercial production of witch hazel extract in 1866 and establishing its wide use. From the middle of the nineteenth century onward, Hamamelis finally became a constituent of the official American and European medicine. The leaves (*Hamamelidis folium*) as well as the bark (*Hamamelidis cortex*) of the plant are used. The main constituents of the extract include tannin, gallic acid, catechins, proanthocyanidins, flavonoids (kaempferol, quercetin), essential oils (carvacrol, eugenol, hexenol), choline, and saponins. It is a strong antioxidant and astringent, which makes it useful as a natural remedy also for acne, psoriasis, eczema, aftershave applications, ingrown nails, and cracked or blistered skin and for treating insect bites.

> In shampoo form, witch hazel (*Hamamelis virginiana*) is particularly useful in the treatment of the red scalp syndrome and in preventing or soothing scalp irritation resulting from sustained use of ethanolic topical minoxidil solutions.

Originally, an observational study was carried out at the Department of Dermatology, University Hospital of Zurich, over a period of 6 months, from October 2009 to March 2010, during which a *Hamamelis* product (Erol® Energy shampoo and tonic) was dispensed to patients complaining of scalp irritation, with or without clinical signs of inflammation. Many patients had previously used various medicinal shampoos, mainly against seborrhea and dandruff, as well as topical corticosteroids without success. After a period of application of 4 weeks, the majority of patients reported an improvement of subjective manifestations of irritation and rated the tolerance of both products as good to excellent. Overall, the majority of the patients were satisfied with the products. Since then, in the period between August 2010 and December 2013, Erol® Energy shampoo has been applied successfully in 1,373 patients (1,233 women and 140 men) at the Center for Dermatology and Hair Disease Professor Trüeb to treat irritable scalp conditions or as concomitant treatment to minoxidil therapy for androgenetic alopecia. During this period, 369 (26.9 %) have received Erol® shampoo more than once. Experience shows that 2 and 5 % topical minoxidil in an alcohol base for treatment of androgenetic alopecia may lead to irritation of the scalp, which has a negative impact on patient compliance. The complaints of patients and the redness of the scalp are often misinterpreted as seborrhoeic dermatitis and treated with anti-dandruff shampoos and alcohol-based topical corticosteroids (scalp applications) that only aggravate the problem through additional irritation. An alternative is to compound the minoxidil into a topical solution of *Hamamelis* distillate.

Further Reading

Congenital Atrichia and Hypotrichosis

Ahmad W, Faiyaz ul Haque M, Brancolini V, Tsou HC, ul Haque S, Lam H, Aita VM, Owen J, deBlaquiere M, Frank J, Cserhalmi-Friedman PB, Leask A, McGrath JA, Peacocke M, Ahmad M, Ott J, Christiano AM (1998) Alopecia universalis associated with a mutation in the human hairless gene. Science 279: 720–724

Baumer A, Belli S, Trüeb RM, Schinzel A (2000) An autosomal dominant form of hereditary hypotrichosis simplex maps to 18p11.32-p11.23 in an Italian family. Eur J Hum Genet 8:443–448

Bolling MC, Jonkman MF (2009) Skin and heart: une liaison dangereuse. Exp Dermatol 18(8):658–668

Böni R, Böni RH, Tsambaos D, Spycher MA, Trüeb RM (1995a) Trichorhinophalangeal syndrome. Dermatology 190(2):152–155

Breslau-Siderius EJ, Lavrijsen APM, Otten FWA, van der Schroeff JG, Swart JGN (1991) The Rapp-Hodgkin syndrome. Am J Med Genet 38:107–110

Clements SE, Techanukul T, Holden ST, Mellerio JE, Dorkins H, Escande F, McGrath JA (2010) Rapp-Hodgkin and Hay-Wells ectodermal dysplasia syndromes represent a variable spectrum of the same genetic disorder. Br J Dermatol 163(3):624–629

Fosko SW, Stenn KS, Bolognia JL (1992) Ectodermal dysplasias associated with clefting: significance of scalp dermatitis. J Am Acad Dermatol 27: 249–256

Freire-Maia N, Pinheiro M (1984) Ectodermal dysplasias: a clinical and genetic study. Lidd, New York

Henn W, Zlotogorski A, Lam H, Martinez-Mir A, Zaun H, Christiano AM (2002) Atrichia with papular lesions resulting from compound heterozygous mutations in the hairless gene: a lesson for differential diagnosis of alopecia universalis. J Am Acad Dermatol 47: 519–523

Hillmer AM, Kruse R, Betz RC, Schumacher J, Heyn U, Propping P, Nothen MM, Cichon S (2001) Variant 1859G-A (arg620 to gln) of the 'hairless' gene: absence of association with papular atrichia or androgenetic alopecia. (Letter). Am J Hum Genet 69: 235–237

Just M, Ribera M, Fuente MJ, Bielsa I, Ferrándiz C (1998) Hereditary hypotrichosis simplex. Dermatology 196(3):339–342

Podjasek JO, Hand JL (2011) Marie-Unna hereditary hypotrichosis: case report and review of the literature. Pediatr Dermatol 28(2):202–204

Protonotarios N, Tsatsopoulou A (2004) Naxos disease and Carvajal syndrome: cardiocutaneous disorders that highlight the pathogenesis and broaden the spectrum of arrhythmogenic right ventricular cardiomyopathy. Cardiovasc Pathol 13(4):185–194

Protonotarios N, Tsatsopoulou A, Fontaine G (2001) Naxos disease: keratoderma, scalp modifications, and cardiomyopathy. J Am Acad Dermatol 44(2):309–311

Richards KA, Mancini AJ (2002) Three members of a family with pili torti and sensorineural hearing loss: the Bjornstad syndrome. J Am Acad Dermatol 46(2):301–303

Schaffer JV, Bazzi H, Vitebsky A, Witkiewicz A, Kovich OI, Kamino H, Shapiro LS, Amin SP, Orlow SJ, Christiano AM (2006) Mutations in the desmoglein 4 gene underlie localized autosomal recessive hypotrichosis with monilethrix hairs and congenital scalp erosions. J Invest Dermatol 126(6):1286–1289

Selvaag E (2000) Pili torti and sensorineural hearing loss. A follow-up of Bjørnstad's original patients and a review of the literature. Eur J Dermatol 10(2):91–97

Shimomura Y, Sakamoto F, Kariya N, Matsunaga K, Ito M (2006) Mutations in the desmoglein 4 gene are associated with monilethrix-like congenital hypotrichosis. J Invest Dermatol 126(6):1281–1285

Zlotogorski A, Marek D, Horev L, Abu A, Ben-Amitai D, Gerad L, Ingber A, Frydman M, Reznik-Wolf H, Vardy DA, Pras E (2006) An autosomal recessive form of monilethrix is caused by mutations in DSG4: clinical overlap with localized autosomal recessive hypotrichosis. J Invest Dermatol 126:1292–1296

Challenges in Non-scarring Alopecia: Androgenetic Alopecia

Abdel Fattah NS, Darwish YW (2011) Androgenetic alopecia and insulin resistance: are they truly associated? Int J Dermatol 50:417–422

Acibucu F, Kayatas M, Candan F (2010) The association of insulin resistance and metabolic syndrome in early androgenetic alopecia. Singapore Med J 51:931–936

Amory JK, Wang C, Swerdloff RS et al (2007) The effect of 5alpha-reductase inhibition with dutasteride and finasteride on semen parameters and serum hormones in healthy men. J Clin Endocrinol Metab 92:1659–1665

Arias-Santiago S, Gutierrez-Salmeron MT, Buendia-Eisman A et al (2010a) Hypertension and aldosterone levels in women with early-onset androgenetic alopecia. Br J Dermatol 162:786–789

Arias-Santiago S, Gutierrez-Salmeron MT, Buendia-Eisman A et al (2010b) Lipid levels in women with androgenetic alopecia. Int J Dermatol 49:1340–1342

Arias-Santiago S, Gutierrez-Salmeron MT, Buendia-Eisman A et al (2010c) A comparative study of dyslipidaemia in men and woman with androgenic alopecia. Acta Derm Venereol 90:485–487

Arias-Santiago S, Gutierrez-Salmeron MT, Buendia-Eisman A et al (2011) Sex hormone-binding globulin and risk of hyperglycemia in patients with androgenetic alopecia. J Am Acad Dermatol 65:48–53

Arias-Santiago S, Gutiérrez-Salmerón MT, Castellote-Caballero L, Buendía-Eisman A, Naranjo-Sintes R

(2010d) Androgenetic alopecia and cardiovascular risk factors in men and women: a comparative study. J Am Acad Dermatol 63(3):420–429
Armenores P, Shirato K, Reid C, Sidhu S (2010) Frontal fibrosing alopecia associated with generalized hair loss. Australas J Dermatol 51:183–185
Bahta AW, Farjo N, Farjo B, Philpott M (2008) Premature senescence of balding dermal papilla cells in vitro is associated with p16(INK4a) expression. J Invest Dermatol 128(5):1088–1094
Bangha E, Elsner P, Kistler GS (1996) Suppression of UV-induced erythema by topical treatment with melatonin (N-acetyl-5-methoxytryptamine). Arch Dermatol Res 288:522–526
Birch MP, Messenger JF, Messenger AG (2001a) Hair density, hair diameter and the prevalence of female pattern hair loss. Br J Dermatol 144:297–304
Blume-Peytavi U, Blumeyer A, Tosti A, Finner A, Marmol V, Trakatelli M, Reygagne P, Messenger A, European Consensus Group (2001) S1 guideline for diagnostic evaluation in androgenetic alopecia in men, women and adolescents. Br J Dermatol 164:5–15
Blume-Peytavi U, Kunte C, Krisp A, Garcia Bartels N, Ellwanger U, Hoffmann R (2007) Comparison of the efficacy and safety of topical minoxidil and topical alfatradiol in the treatment of androgenetic alopecia in women. J Dtsch Dermatol Ges 5:391–395
Blumeyer A, Tosti A, Messenger A et al (2011) Evidence-based (S3) guideline for the treatment of androgenetic alopecia in women and in men. J Dtsch Dermatol Ges 9(Suppl 6):S1–S57
Buzney E, Sheu J, Buzney C, Reynolds RV (2014) Polycystic ovary syndrome: a review for dermatologists: part II. Treatment. J Am Acad Dermatol 71(5):859–873
Camacho F, Moreno JC, Garcia-Hernández MJ (1996) Telogen alopecia from UV rays. Arch Dermatol 132:1398–1399
Chew AL, Bashir SJ, Wain EM, Fenton DA, Stefanato CM (2010) Expanding the spectrum of frontal fibrosing alopecia: a unifying concept. J Am Acad Dermatol 63:653–660
Choi JW, Na SY, Park KC, Youn SW, Huh CH (2012) Relation between treatment efficacy and cumulative dose of 3% topical minoxidil in male pattern baldness. J Am Acad Dermatol 66(1):e10–e12
Cotton SG, Nixon JM, Carpenter RG et al (1972) Factors discriminating men with coronary heart disease from healthy controls. Br Heart J 34:458–464
Dardour JC, Pugash E, Aziza R (1988) The one-stage preauricular flap for male pattern baldness: long-term results and risk factors. Plast Reconstr Surg 81:907–912
Davis MG, Thomas JH, van de Velde S, Boissy Y, Dawson TL Jr, Iveson R, Sutton K (2011) A novel cosmetic approach to treat thinning hair. Br J Dermatol 165(Suppl 3):24–30
de Lacharrière O, Deloche C, Misciali C et al (2001) Hair diameter diversity: a clinical sign reflecting the follicle miniaturization. Arch Dermatol 137(5):641–646
De Villez RL, Jacobs JP, Szpunar CA, Warner ML (1994) Androgenetic alopecia in the female. Treatment with 2% topical minoxidil solution. Arch Dermatol 3:303–307
Dogramaci AC, Balci DD, Balci A et al (2009) Is androgenetic alopecia a risk for atherosclerosis? J Eur Acad Dermatol Venereol 23:673–677
Donati A, Molina L, Doche I et al (2011) Facial papules in frontal fibrosing alopecia: evidence of vellus follicle involvement. Arch Dermatol 147(12):1424–1427
Drake LA, Dinehart SM, Farmer ER et al (1996) Guidelines of care for androgenetic alopecia. American Academy of Dermatology. J Am Acad Dermatol 35:465–469
Drake L, Hordinsky M, Fiedler V et al (1999) The effects of finasteride on scalp skin and serum androgen levels in men with androgenetic alopecia. J Am Acad Dermatol 41:550–554
Duskova M, Hill M, Starka L (2010) Changes of metabolic profile in men treated for androgenetic alopecia with 1 mg finasteride. Endocr Regul 44:3–8
Eun HC, Kwon OS, Yeon JH et al (2010) Efficacy, safety, and tolerability of dutasteride 0.5 mg once daily in male patients with male pattern hair loss: a randomized, double-blind, placebo-controlled, phase III study. J Am Acad Dermatol 63:252–258
Finasteride Male Pattern Hair Loss Study Group (2002) Long-term (5-year) multinational experience with finasteride 1 mg in the treatment of men with androgenetic alopecia. Eur J Dermatol 12:38–49
Galliker NA, Trüeb RM (2012) Value of trichoscopy versus trichogram for diagnosis of female androgenetic alopecia. Int J Trichology 4:19–22
Georgala S, Befon A, Maniatopoulou E, Georgala C (2007) Topical use of minoxidil in children and systemic side effects. Dermatology 214:101–102
Goren A, Castano JA, McCoy J, Bermudez F, Lotti T (2014) Novel enzymatic assay predicts minoxidil response in the treatment of androgenetic alopecia. Dermatol Ther 27(3):171–173
Goren A, Shapiro J, Roberts J, McCoy J, Desai N, Zarrab Z, Pietrzak A, Lotti T (2015) Clinical utility and validity of minoxidil response testing in androgenetic alopecia. Dermatol Ther 28(1):13–16
Gubelin Harcha W, Barboza Martínez J, Tsai TF, Katsuoka K, Kawashima M, Tsuboi R, Barnes A, Ferron-Brady G, Chetty D (2014) A randomized, active- and placebo-controlled study of the efficacy and safety of different doses of dutasteride versus placebo and finasteride in the treatment of male subjects with androgenetic alopecia. J Am Acad Dermatol 70(3):489–498
Haley NJ, Hoffmann D (1985) Analysis for nicotine and cotinine in hair to determine cigarette smoker status. Clin Chem 31:1598–1600
Hayakawa K, Shimizu T, Ohba Y et al (1992) Intrapair differences of physical aging and longevity in identical twins. Acta Genet Med Gemellol (Roma) 141:177–185
Hamilton JB (1951) Patterned loss of hair in men; types and incidence. Ann N Y Acad Sci 53:708–728
Hirsso P, Rajala U, Hiltunen L, Jokelainen J, Keinänen-Kiukaanniemi S, Näyhä S (2007) Obesity and low-

grade inflammation among young Finnish men with early-onset alopecia. Dermatology 214(2):125–129
Housman E, Reynolds RV (2014) Polycystic ovary syndrome: a review for dermatologists: part I. Diagnosis and manifestations. J Am Acad Dermatol 71(5):847
Iorizzo M, Vincenzi C, Voudouris S et al (2006) Finasteride treatment of female pattern hair loss. Arch Dermatol 142(3):298–302
Iyengar B (1998) The hair follicle: a specialized UV receptor in the human skin? Biol Signals Recept 7:188–194
Jaworsky C, Kligman AM, Murphy GF (1992) Characterisation of inflammatory infiltrates in male pattern alopecia: implication for pathogenesis. Br J Dermatol 127:239–246
Jung JY, Yeon JH, Choi JW, Kwon SH, Kim BJ, Youn SW, Park KC, Huh CH (2014) Effect of dutasteride 0.5 mg/d in men with androgenetic alopecia recalcitrant to finasteride. Int J Dermatol 53(11):1351–1357
Kaufman KD, Olsen EA, Whiting D et al (1998) Finasteride in the treatment of men with androgenetic alopecia. Finasteride Male Pattern Hair Loss Study Group. J Am Acad Dermatol 39:578–589
Kaufman KD, Rotonda J, Shah AK et al (2008) Long-term treatment with finasteride 1 mg decreases the likelihood of developing further visible hair loss in men with androgenetic alopecia (male pattern hair loss). Eur J Dermatol 18:400–406
Kawashima M, Hayashi N, Igarashi A et al (2004) Finasteride in the treatment of Japanese men with male pattern hair loss. Eur J Dermatol 14:247–254
Kossard S (1994a) Postmenopausal frontal fibrosing alopecia: scarring alopecia in a pattern distribution. Arch Dermatol 130:770–774
Kossard S, Lee MS, Wilkinson B (1997) Postmenopausal frontal fibrosing alopecia: a frontal variant of lichen planopilaris. J Am Acad Dermatol 36:59–66
Lesko SM, Rosenberg L, Shapiro S (1993) A case-control study of baldness in relation to myocardial infarction in men. JAMA 269:998–1003
Leyden J, Dunlap F, Miller B et al (1999) Finasteride in the treatment of men with frontal male pattern hair loss. J Am Acad Dermatol 40:930–937
Li M, Marubayashi A, Nakaya Y, Fukui K, Arase S (2001) Minoxidil-induced hair growth is mediated by adenosine in cultured dermal papilla cells: possible involvement of sulfonylurea receptor 2B as a target of minoxidil. J Invest Dermatol 117:1594–1600
Liu CS, Kao SH, Wei YH (1997) Smoking-associated mitochondrial DNA mutations in human hair follicles. Environ Mol Mutagen 30:47–55
Ludwig E (1977) Classification of the types of androgenetic alopecia (common baldness) occurring in the female sex. Br J Dermatol 97:247–254
Mahé YF, Michelet JF, Billoni N et al (2000) Androgenetic alopecia and microinflammation. Int J Dermatol 39:576–584
Moltz L (1988) Hormonale Diagnostik der sogenannten androgenetischen Alopezie der Frau. Geburtshilfe Frauenheilk 48:203–214
Mosley JG, Gibbs CC (1996a) Premature grey hair and hair loss among smokers: a new opportunity for health education? BMJ 313:1616
Mumcuoglu C, Ekmekci TR, Ucak S (2011) The investigation of insulin resistance and metabolic syndrome in male patients with early-onset androgenetic alopecia. Eur J Dermatol 21:79–82
Naito A, Midorikawa T, Yoshino T, Ohdera M (2008) Lipid peroxides induce early onset of catagen phase in murine hair cycles.Int J Mol Med 22:725–729.
Norwood OT (1975) Male pattern baldness: classification and incidence. South Med J 68:1359–1365
Olsen EA (2005) Female pattern hair loss and its relationship to permanent/cicatricial alopecia: a new perspective. J Investig Dermatol Symp Proc 10:217–221
Olsen EA, Hordinsky M, Whiting D et al (2006) The importance of dual 5alpha-reductase inhibition in the treatment of male pattern hair loss: results of a randomized placebo-controlled study of dutasteride versus finasteride. J Am Acad Dermatol 55:1014–1023
Olsen EA, Weiner MS, Amara IA et al (1990) Five-year follow-up of men with androgenetic alopecia treated with topical minoxidil. J Am Acad Dermatol 22:643–646
Olsen EA, Weiner MS, Delong ER et al (1985) Topical minoxidil in early male pattern baldness. J Am Acad Dermatol 13:185–192
Olsen EA, DeLong ER, Weiner MS (1987) Long-term follow-up of men with male pattern baldness treated with topical minoxidil. J Am Acad Dermatol 16:688–695
Olsen EA, Dunlap FE, Funicella T et al (2002) A randomized clinical trial of 5% topical minoxidil versus 2% topical minoxidil and placebo in the treatment of androgenetic alopecia in men. J Am Acad Dermatol 47:377–385
Olsen EA, Messenger AG, Shapiro J et al (2005) Evaluation and treatment of male and female pattern hair loss. J Am Acad Dermatol 52:301–311
Olszewska M, Rudnicka L (2005) Effective treatment of female androgenic alopecia with dutasteride. J Drugs Dermatol 4(5):637–640
Orfanos CE, Hertel H (1988) Disorder of hair growth in hyperprolactinemia. Z Hautkr 63:23–26
Osawa Y, Tochigi B, Tochigi M et al (1990) Aromatase inhibitors in cigarette smoke, tobacco leaves and other plants. J Enzyme Inhib 4:187–200
Piérard-Franchimont C, Uhoda I, Saint-Léger D, Piérard GE (2002) Androgenetic alopecia and stress-induced premature senescence by cumulative ultraviolet light exposure. Exogenous Dermatol 1:203–206
Price VH (1999) Treatment of hair loss. N Engl J Med 341:964–973
Price VH, Menefee E, Sanchez M et al (2006) Changes in hair weight in men with androgenetic alopecia after treatment with finasteride (1 mg daily): three- and 4-year results. J Am Acad Dermatol 55:71–74
Rakowska A, Slowinska M, Kowalska-Oledzka E, Olszewska M, Rudnicka L (2009) Dermoscopy in female androgenic alopecia: method standardization and diagnostic criteria. Int J Trichology 1(2):123–130

Roberts J, Desai N, McCoy J, Goren A (2014) Sulfotransferase activity in plucked hair follicles predicts response to topical minoxidil in the treatment of female androgenetic alopecia. Dermatol Ther 27: 252–254
Rushton DH, Ramsay ID, James KC et al (1990) Biochemical and trichological characterization of diffuse alopecia in women. Br J Dermatol 123:187–197
Schmidt JB, Lindmaer A, Spona J (1991) Hyperprolactinemia and hypophyseal hypothyroidism as cofactors in hirsutism and androgen-induced alopecia in women. Hautarzt 42:168–172
Severi G, Sinclair R, Hopper JL et al (2003) Androgenetic alopecia in men aged 40–69 years: prevalence and risk factors. Br J Dermatol 149:1207–1213
Starka L, Duskova M, Cermakova I et al (2005) Premature androgenic alopecia and insulin resistance. Male equivalent of polycystic ovary syndrome? Endocr Regul 39(4):127–131
Stough D (2007) Dutasteride improves male pattern hair loss in a randomized study in identical twins. J Cosmet Dermatol 6:9–13
Su L-S, Chen TH-H (2007) Association of androgenetic alopecia with smoking and its prevalence among Asian men. Arch Dermatol 143:1401–1406
Su LH, Chen LS, Lin SC et al (2013) Association of androgenetic alopecia with mortality from diabetes mellitus and heart disease. JAMA Dermatol 149:601–606
Tosti A (2007) Dermoscopy of hair and scalp disorders with clinical and pathological correlations. Informa Healthcare, Hampshire
Tosti A, Iorizzo M, Piraccini BM (2005) Androgenetic alopecia in children: report of 20 cases. Br J Dermatol 152:556–559
Trüeb RM (1993) Female pattern baldness in men. J Am Acad Dermatol 29:782–783
Trüeb RM (2003a) Association between smoking and hair loss: another opportunity for health education against smoking? Dermatology 206:189–191
Trüeb RM (2003b) Is androgenetic alopecia a photoaggravated dermatosis? Dermatology 207:343–348
Tsuboi R, Itami S, Inui S et al (2012) Guidelines for the management of androgenetic alopecia. J Dermatol 39:113–120
van Bon BW, Gilissen C, Grange DK et al (2012) Cantú syndrome is caused by mutations in ABCC9. Am J Hum Genet 90(6):1094–1101
Van Neste D, Fuh V, Sanchez-Pedreno P et al (2000) Finasteride increases anagen hair in men with androgenetic alopecia. Br J Dermatol 143:804–810
Venning VA, Dawber RP (1988) Patterned androgenic alopecia in women. J Am Acad Dermatol 18: 1073–1077
Weitz JL, Crowley KA, Landman SL et al (1987) Increased neutrophil elastase activity in cigarette smokers. Ann Intern Med 107:680–682
Whiting DA (1993) Diagnostic and predictive value of horizontal sections of scalp biopsy specimens in male pattern androgenetic alopecia. J Am Acad Dermatol 128:755–763
Whiting DA, Waldstreicher J, Sanchez M et al (1999) Measuring reversal of hair miniaturization in androgenetic alopecia by follicular counts in horizontal sections of serial scalp biopsies: results of finasteride 1 mg treatment of men and postmenopausal women. J Investig Dermatol Symp Proc 4:282–284
Yang CC, Hsieh FN, Lin LY, Hsu CK, Sheu HM, Chen W (2014) Higher body mass index is associated with greater severity of alopecia in men with male-pattern androgenetic alopecia in Taiwan: a cross-sectional study. J Am Acad Dermatol 70(2):297–302
Yi SM, Son SW, Lee KG et al (2012) Gender-specific association of androgenetic alopecia with metabolic syndrome in a middle-aged Korean population. Br J Dermatol 167:306–313
Yin L, Morita A, Tsuji T (2000) Alterations of extracellular matrix induced by tobacco smoke extract. Arch Dermatol Res 292:188–194
Zinkernagel MS, Trüeb RM (2000a) Fibrosing alopecia in a pattern distribution. Patterned lichen planopilaris or androgenetic alopecia with a lichenoid tissue reaction pattern? Arch Dermatol 136:205–211

Challenges in Non-scarring Alopecia: Aging Hair

Arafah BM (2001) Increased need for thyroxine in women with hypothyroidism during estrogen therapy. N Engl J Med 344(23):1743–1749
Arck PC, Overall R, Spatz K et al (2006) Towards a "free radical theory of graying": melanocyte apoptosis in the aging human hair follicle is an indicator of oxidative stress induced tissue damage. FASEB J 20:1567–1569
Billoni N, Buan B, Gautier B, Gaillard O, Mahé YF, Bernard BA (2000) Thyroid hormone receptor beta1 is expressed in the human hair follicle. Br J Dermatol 142:645–652
Birch MP, Messenger JF, Messenger AG (2001b) Hair density, hair diameter and the prevalence of female pattern hair loss. Br J Dermatol 144:297–304
Brenner S, Matz H (1999) Improvement in androgenetic alopecia in 53-76-year-old men using oral finasteride. Int J Dermatol 38:92–930
Carmina E, Lobo RA (2003) Treatment of hyperandrogenic alopecia in women. Fertil Steril 79:91–95
Castro RF, Azzalis LA, Feder D et al (2012) Safety and efficacy analysis of liposomal insulin-like growth factor-1 in a fluid gel formulation for hair-loss treatment in a hamster model. Clin Exp Dermatol 37(8):909–912
Chang IM (2001) Anti-aging and health-promoting constituents derived from traditional oriental herbal remedies: information retrieval using the TradiMed 2000 DB. Ann N Y Acad Sci 928:281–286
Chein E (1998) Age reversal, from hormones to telomeres. WorldLink Medical Publishing
Comaisch S (1985) The thyroid and hair growth. Semin Dermatol 4:4–8

Commo S, Gaillard O, Bernard BA (2004) Human hair greying is linked to a specific depletion of hair follicle melanocytes affecting both the bulb and the outer root sheath. Br J Dermatol 150:435–443

Courtois M, Loussouarn G, Hourseau C, Grollier JF (1995) Aging and hair cycles. Br J Dermatol 132:86–93

Eichmüller S, van der Veen C, Mill I et al (1998) Clusters of perifollicular macrophages in normal murine skin: physiological degeneration of selected hair follicles by programmed organ deletion. J Histochem Cytochem 46:361–370

Giesen M, Gruedl S, Holtkoetter O et al (2011) Ageing processes influence keratin and KAP expression in human hair follicles. Exp Dermatol 20(9):759–761

Giesen M, Welss T, zur Wiesche ES et al (2009) Coenzyme Q10 has anti-aging effects on human hair. Int J Cosmet Sci 31:154–155

Gnann LA, Castro RF, Azzalis LA et al (2013) Hematological and hepatic effects of vascular epidermal growth factor (VEGF) used to stimulate hair growth in an animal model. BMC Dermatol 13:15

Harley CB, Futcher AB, Greider CW (1990) Telomeres shorten during ageing of human fibroblasts. Nature 345(6274):458–460

Hollfelder B, Blankenburg G, Wolfram LJ, Höcker H (1995) Chemical and physical properties of pigmented and non-pigmented hair ('grey hair'). Int J Cosmet Sci 17:87–89

Horsley V, Aliprantis AO, Polak L et al (2008) NFATc1 balances quiescence and proliferation of skin stem cells. Cell 132(2):299–310

Jeon SY, Pi LQ, Lee WS (2008) Comparison of hair shaft damage after UVA and UVB irradiation. J Cosmet Sci 59:151–156

Kao SH, Liu CS, Wang SY, Wei YH (1997) Ageing-associated large-scale deletions of mitochondrial DNA in human hair follicles. Biochem Mol Biol Int 42(2):285–298

Keene S, Goren A (2011) Therapeutic hotline. Genetic variations in the androgen receptor gene and finasteride response in women with androgenetic alopecia mediated by epigenetics. Dermatol Ther 24(2): 296–300

Keyes BE, Segal JP, Heller E et al (2013) Nfatc1 orchestrates aging in hair follicle stem cells. Proc Natl Acad Sci U S A 110(51):E4950–E4959

Kim NW, Piatyszek MA, Prowse K (1994) Specific association of human telomerase activity with immortal cells and cancer. Science 266(5193):2011–2015

Kligman AM (1988) The comparative histopathology of male-pattern baldness and senescent baldness. Clin Dermatol 16:108–118

Lee S, Tanglertsampan C, Tanchotikul M, Worapunpong N (2014) Minoxidil 2% lotion for eyebrow enhancement: a randomized, double-blind, placebo-controlled, spilt-face comparative study. J Dermatol 41(2): 149–152

Li JJ, Mitchell LH, Dow RL (2010) Thyroid receptor agonists for the treatment of androgenetic alopecia. Bioorg Med Chem Lett 20(1):306–308

Liu CS, Chen HW, Lii CK, Tsai CS, Kuo CL, Wei YH (2002) Alterations of plasma antioxidants and mitochondrial DNA mutation in hair follicles of smokers. Environ Mol Mutagen 40(3):168–174

Lurie R, Ben-Amitai D, Laron Z (2004) Laron syndrome (primary growth hormone insensitivity): a unique model to explore the effect of insulin-like growth factor 1 deficiency on human hair. Dermatology 208: 314–318

Macieira-Coelho A (2003) Biology of aging. Progress in molecular and subcellular biology. Springer, Heidelberg, pp 50–52

Mosley JG, Gibbs CC (1996b) Premature grey hair and hair loss among smokers: a new opportunity for health education? BMJ 313:1616

Nagl W (1995) Different growth rates of pigmented and white hair in the beard: differentiation vs. proliferation? Br J Dermatol 132:94–97

Nakauchi Y, Kumon Y, Yamasaki H et al (1995) Scalp hair loss caused by octreotide in a patient with acromegaly: a case report. Endocr J 42(3):385–389

Nagase S, Kajiura Y, Mamada A, Abe H, Shibuichi S, Satoh N, Itou T, Shinohara Y, Amemiya Y (2009) Changes in structure and geometric properties of human hair by aging. J Cosmet Sci 60(6):637–648

Nagase S, Tsuchiya M, Matsui T, Shibuichi S, Tsujimura H, Masukawa Y, Satoh N, Itou T, Koike K, Tsujii K (2008) Characterization of curved hair of Japanese women with reference to internal structures and amino acid composition. J Cosmet Sci 59(4):317–332

Nishimura EK, Granter SR, Fisher DE (2005) Mechanisms of hair graying: incomplete melanocyte stem cell maintenance in the niche. Science 307:720–724

Nishimura EK, Jordan SA, Oshima H et al (2002) Dominant role of the niche in melanocyte stem-cell fate determination. Nature 416:854–860

Nogueira AC, Dicelio LE, Joekes I (2006) About photodamage of human hair. Photochem Photobiol Sci 5:165–169

Olszewska M, Warszawik O, Rakowska A et al (2010) Methods of hair loss evaluation in patients with endocrine disorders. Endokrynol Pol 61(4):406–411

Otsuka H, Nemoto T (1988) Study on Japanese hair. Koshokashi 12:192–197

Panchaprateep R, Asawanonda P (2014) Insulin-like growth factor-1: roles in androgenetic alopecia. Exp Dermatol 23(3):216–218

Paradi M, Shahee O, Shaza D et al (2007) Comparison of senescent and androgenetic alopecia using microarray analysis. In: Fifth international hair research societies meeting, Abstract O-10-3, Vancouver

Price VH, Roberts JL, Hordinsky M et al (2000) Lack of efficacy of finasteride in postmenopausal women with androgenetic alopecia. J Am Acad Dermatol 43: 768–776

Price V, Sawaya M, Headington J, Kibarian M (2001) Histology and hormonal activity in senescent thinning in males (abstract 266). J Invest Dermatol 117:434

Robbins C, Mirmirani P, Messenger AG, Birch MP, Youngquist RS, Tamura M, Filloon T, Luo F, Dawson

TLJ (2012) What women want – quantifying the perception of hair amount: an analysis of hair diameter and density changes with age in caucasian women. Br J Dermatol 167:324–332
Rudolph KL, Chang S, Lee HW et al (1999) Longevity, stress response, and cancer in aging telomerase-deficient mice. Cell 96(5):701–712
Rundegren J (2004) Pattern alopecia: what clinical features determine the response to topical minoxidil treatment? IHRS 2004 abstract B2.4. JDDG 2:500
Santos Nogueira AC, Joekes I (2004) Hair color changes and protein damage caused by ultraviolet radiation. J Photochem Photobiol B 74:109–117
Schallreuter KU, Wood JM, Pittelkow MR et al (1994) Regulation of melanin biosynthesis in the human epidermis by tetrahydrobiopterin. Science 263:1444–1446
Schell H, Kiesewetter F, Seidel C, von Hintzenstern J (1991) Cell cycle kinetics of human anagen scalp hair bulbs in thyroid disorders determined by DNA flow cytometry. Dermatologica 182:23–26
Schindler AE (2003) Thyroid function and postmenopause. Gynecol Endocrinol 17(1):79–85
Shum KW, Cullen DR, Messenger AG (2002) Hair loss in women with hyperandrogenism: four cases responding to finasteride. J Am Acad Dermatol 47:733–739
Spencer JD, Gibbons NC, Böhm M, Schallreuter KU (2008) The Ca_{2+} – binding capacity of epidermal furin is disrupted by H_2O_2-mediated oxidation in vitiligo. Endocrinology 149:163–1645
Spencer JD, Gibbons NC, Rokos H et al (2007) Oxidative stress via hydrogen peroxide affects propriomelanocortin peptides directly in the epidermis of patients with vitiligo. J Invest Dermatol 127:411–420
Tang L, Bernardo O, Bolduc C et al (2003) The expression of insulin-like growth factor 1 in follicular dermal papillae correlates with therapeutic efficacy of finasteride in androgenetic alopecia. J Am Acad Dermatol 49(2):229–233
Thai KE, Sinclair RD (2002) Finasteride for female androgenetic alopecia. Br J Dermatol 147:812–813
Tobin DJ (2008) Biology of hair follicle pigmentation. In: Blume-Peytavi U, Tosti A, Whiting DA, Trüeb R (eds) Hair growth and disorders. Springer, Berlin/Heidelberg, p 51 ff
Tobin DJ, Paus R (2001) Graying: gerontobiology of the hair follicle pigmentary unit. Exp Gerontol 36:29–54
Trüeb RM (2005) Aging of hair. J Cosmet Dermatol 4(2):60–67
Trüeb RM (2006a) Anti-aging. Von der Antike zur Moderne. Steinkopff, Darmstadt
Trüeb RM (2006b) Pharmacologic interventions in aging hair. Clin Interv Aging 1(2):121–129
Trüeb RM (2009a) Oxidative stress in ageing of hair. Int J Trichology 1(1):6–14
Trüeb RM, Swiss Trichology Study Group (2004) Finasteride treatment of patterned hair loss in normoandrogenic postmenopausal women. Dermatology 209:202–207
van Neste D (2004) Thickness, medullation and growth rate of female scalp hair are subject to significant variation according to pigmentation of scalp location during aging. Eur J Dermatol 14:28–32
van Neste D, Tobin DJ (2004) Hair cycle and hair pigmentation: dynamic interactions and changes associated with aging. Micron 35:193–200
Whiting DA, Olsen EA, Savin R et al (2003) Efficacy and tolerability of finasteride 1 mg in men aged 41 to 60 years with male pattern hair loss. Eur J Dermatol 13:150–160
Wood JM, Decker H, Hartmann H et al (2009) Senile hair graying: H_2O_2-mediated oxidative stress affects human hair color by blunting methionine sulfoxide repair. FASEB J 23:2065–2075
Yamada S, Fukuhara N, Nishioka H et al (2013) Scalp hair loss after transsphenoidal adenomectomy in patients with acromegaly. Clin Endocrinol (Oxf) 79(3):386–393

Challenges in Non-scarring Alopecia: Telogen Effluvium

Ahrens J (1994) Systemische Behandlung des diffusen Haarausfalls. Therapiewoche Schweiz 10:551–554
Antaya RJ, Sideridou E, Olsen EA (2005) Short anagen syndrome. J Am Acad Dermatol 53(2 Suppl 1):S130–S134
Barraud-Klenovsek MM, Trüeb RM (2000) Congenital hypotrichosis due to short anagen. Br J Dermatol 143:612–617
Braun-Falco O, Zaun H (1962) Über die Beteiligung des gesamten Capillitiums bei Alopecia areata. Hautarzt 13:342–348
Budde J, Tronnier H, Rahlfs VW, Frei-Kleiner S (1993) Systemische Therapie von diffusem Effluvium und Haarstrukturschäden. Hautarzt 44:380–384
Chartier MB, Hoss DMM, Grant-Kels JM (2002) Approach to the adult female patient with diffuse nonscarring alopecia. J Am Acad Dermatol 47:809–818
Courtois M, Loussouarn G, Hourseau S, Grollier JF (1996) Periodicity in the growth and shedding of hair. Br J Dermatol 134:47–54
Dupré A, Lassère J, Christol B et al (1977) Traitement des alopécies diffuses chroniques par le panthénol et la D.biotine injectables. Rev Med Toulouse 13:675–677
Floersheim GL (1992) Prüfung der Wirkung von Biotin auf Haarausfall und Haarqualität. Z Hautkr 67:246–255
Guarrera M, Rebora A (1996) Anagen hairs may fail to replace telogen hairs in early androgenic female alopecia. Dermatology 192:28–31
Guarrera M, Rebora A (2005) Kenogen in female androgenetic alopecia. A longitudinal study. Dermatology 210:18–20
Guy WB, Edmundson WF (1960) Diffuse cyclic hair loss in women. Arch Dermatol 81:205–227
Headington JT (1993) Telogen effluvium. New concepts and review. Arch Dermatol 129:356–363
Inui S, Nakajima T, Itami S (2008) Significance of dermoscopy in acute diffuse and total alopecia of the female scalp: review of twenty cases. Dermatology 217:333–336

Kligman AM (1961) Pathologic dynamics of human hair loss, I: telogen effluvium. Arch Dermatol 83:175–198
Kunz M, Seifert B, Trüeb RM (2009) Seasonality of hair shedding in healthy women complaining of hair loss. Dermatology 219:105–110
Lengg N, Heidecker B, Seifert B, Trüeb RM (2007) Dietary supplement increases anagen hair rate in women with telogen effluvium: results of a double-blind placebo-controlled trial. Therapy 4:59–65
Lew BL, Shin MK, Sim WY (2009) Acute diffuse and total alopecia: a new subtype of alopecia areata with a favorable prognosis. J Am Acad Dermatol 60:85–93
Loussouarn G, El Rawadi C, Pineau I, Jouanique C, Hamidou Z, Michelin C, Reygange P. Stemoxydine and hair kenogen phase in androgenetic alopecia (poster). In: Sixteenth annual meeting of the European Hair Research Society, Barcelona, 21–23 June 2012
Orentreich N (1969) Scalp replacement in man. In: Montagna W, Bobson RL (eds) Advances in biology of skin, vol IX, Hair growth. Pergamon, Oxford, pp 99–108
Paus R (1996) Control of the hair cycle and hair diseases as cycling disorders. Curr Opin Dermatol 3:248–258
Paus R, Cotsarelis G (1999) The biology of hair follicles. N Engl J Med 341:491–497
Petri H, Perchalla P, Tronnier H (1990) Die Wirksamkeit einer medikamentösen Therapie bei Haarstrukturschäden und diffusen Effluvien – vergleichende Doppelblindstudie. Schweiz Rundsch Med Prax 79:1457–1462
Piérard-Franchimont C, Piérard GE (2001) Teloptosis, a turning point in hair shedding biorhythms. Dermatology 203:115–117
Randall VA, Ebling FJG (1991) Seasonal changes in human hair growth. Br J Dermatol 124:146–151
Rathman-Josserand M, Genty G, Lecardonnel J, Chabane S, Cousson A, François Michelet J, Bernard BA (2013) Human hair follicle stem/progenitor cells express hypoxia markers. J Invest Dermatol 133:2094–2097
Rebora A (1987) Alopecia areata incognita: a hypothesis. Dermatologica 174:214–218
Rebora A (1997) Telogen effluvium. Dermatology 195: 209–212
Rebora A (2014) Telogen effluvium revisited. G Ital Dermatol Venereol 149(1):47–54
Rebora A, Guarrera M (2002) Kenogen. A new phase of the hair cycle? Dermatology 205:108–110
Rebora A, Guarrera M (2004) Teloptosis and kenogen: two new concepts in human trichology. Arch Dermatol 140:619–620
Sato-Kawamura M, Aiba S, Tagami H (2002) Acute diffuse and total alopecia of the female scalp. A new subtype of diffuse alopecia areata that has a favorable prognosis. Dermatology 205:367–373
Sinclair R (1999) Diffuse hair loss. Int J Dermatol 38(Suppl 1):8–18
Stenn K (2005) Exogen is an active, separately controlled phase of the hair growth cycle. J Am Acad Dermatol 52:374–375
Stroud JP (1987) Diagnosis and management of the hair loss patient. Cutis 40:272–276
Thai KE, Sinclair RD (2003) Short anagen hair with persistent synchronized pattern of scalp hair growth. J Am Acad Dermatol 49:949–951
Tosti A, Misciali C, Piraccini BM et al (1994) Drug-induced hair loss and hair growth. Incidence, management and avoidance. Drug Saf 10:310–317
Trüeb RM (2000) Idiopathic chronic telogen effluvium in women. Hautarzt 51:899–905
Trüeb RM (2010) Systematic approach to hair loss in women. J Dtsch Dermatol Ges 8:284–298
Whiting DA (1996) Chronic telogen effluvium: increased scalp hair shedding in middle-aged women. J Am Acad Dermatol 35:899–906
York J, Nicholson T, Minors P, Duncan DF (1998) Stressful life events and loss of hair among adult women, a case-control study. Psychol Rep 82:1044–1046

Challenges in Non-scarring Alopecia: Alopecia Areata

Abedini H, Farshi S, Mirabzadeh A, Keshavarz S (2014) Antidepressant effects of citalopram on treatment of alopecia areata in patients with major depressive disorder. J Dermatolog Treat 25(2):153–155
Abell E, Munro DD (1973) Intralesional treatment of alopecia areata with triamcinolone acetonide by jet injector. Br J Dermatol 88:55–59
Agarwal A, Nath J, Barua KN (2006) Twice weekly 5 mg betamethasone oral pulse therapy in the treatment of alopecia areata. J Eur Acad Dermatol Venereol 20(10):1375–1376
Aksu Cerman A, Sarikaya Solak S, Kivanc Altunay I (2014) Vitamin D deficiency in alopecia areata. Br J Dermatol 170(6):1299–1304
Ali A, Martin JM (2010) Hair growth in patients alopecia areata totalis after treatment with simvastatin and ezetimibe. J Drugs Dermatol 9(1):62–64
Banach M, Serban C, Sahebkar A et al (2015) Effects of coenzyme Q10 on statin-induced myopathy: a meta-analysis of randomized controlled trials. Mayo Clin Proc 90(1):24–34
Bardella MT, Marino R, Barbareschi M et al (2000) Alopecia areata and coeliac disease: no effect of a gluten-free diet on hair growth. Dermatology 200(2):108–110
Berth-Jones J, Hutchinson PE (1991) Treatment of alopecia totalis with a combination of inosine pranobex and diphencyprone compared to each treatment alone. Clin Exp Dermatol 16(3):172–175
Bondavalli P, Quadri G, Parodi A, Rebora A (1998) Failure of gluten-free diet in celiac disease-associated alopecia areata. Acta Derm Venereol 78(4):319
Böni R, Trüeb RM, Wüthrich B (1995b) Alopecia areata in a patient with candidiasis-endocrinopathy syndrome: unsuccessful treatment trial with diphenylcyclopropenone. Dermatology 191(1):68–71
Buckley DA, du Vivier AW (1999) Topical immunotherapy in dermatology. Int J Clin Pract 53(2):130–137

Chartaux E, Joly P (2010) Long-term follow-up of the efficacy of methotrexate alone or in combination with low doses of oral corticosteroids in the treatment of alopecia areata totalis or universalis. Ann Dermatol Venereol 137(8–9):507–513

Chaves Y, Duarte G, Ben-Said B, Tebib J, Berard F, Nicolas JF (2008) Alopecia areata universalis during treatment of rheumatoid arthritis with anti-TNF-alpha antibody (adalimumab). Dermatology 217:380

Cipriani R, Perini GI, Rampinelli S (2001) Paroxetine in alopecia areata. Int J Dermatol 40:600–601

Corazza GR, Andreani ML, Venturo N et al (1995) Celiac disease and alopecia areata: report of a new association. Gastroenterology 109(4):1333–1337

Craiglow BG, King BA (2014) Killing two birds with one stone: oral tofacitinib reverses alopecia areata universalis in a patient with plaque psoriasis. J Invest Dermatol 134(12):2988–2990

Delamere FM, Sladden MM, Dobbins HM, Leonardi-Bee J (2008) Interventions for alopecia areata. Cochrane Database Syst Rev (2):CD004413

Divito SJ, Kupper TS (2014) Inhibiting Janus kinases to treat alopecia areata. Nat Med 20(9):989–990

d'Ovidio R, d'Ovidio FD (1995) Recidive stagionali dell'alopecia areata. G Ital Dermatol Venereol 295: 130–134

d'Ovidio R, Vessio M, d'Ovidio FD (2013) Reduced level of 25-hydroxyvitamin D in chronic/relapsing alopecia areata. Dermatoendocrinol 5(2):271–273

Doyle LA, Sperling LC, Baksh S, Lackey J, Thomas B, Vleugels RA, Qureshi AA, Velazquez EF (2011) Psoriatic alopecia/alopecia areata-like reactions secondary to anti-tumor necrosis factor-α therapy: a novel cause of noncicatricial alopecia. Am J Dermatopathol 33:161–166

El-Zawahry BM, Bassiouny DA, Khella A, Zaki N (2010) Five-year experience in the treatment of alopecia areata with DPC. J Eur Acad Dermatol Venereol 24(3):264–269

Ettefagh L, Nedorost S, Mirmirani P (2004) Alopecia areata in a patient using infliximab: new insights into the role of tumor necrosis factor on human hair follicles. Arch Dermatol 140:1012

Ertekin V, Tosun MS, Erdem T (2014) Screening of celiac disease in children with alopecia areata. Indian J Dermatol 59(3):317

Fabre C, Dereure O (2008) Worsening alopecia areata and de novo occurrence of multiple halo nevi in a patient receiving infliximab. Dermatology 216:185–186

Falto-Aizpurua L, Choudhary S, Tosti A (2014) Emerging treatments in alopecia. Expert Opin Emerg Drugs 19(4):545–556

Fessatou S, Kostaki M, Karpathios T (2003) Coeliac disease and alopecia areata in childhood. J Paediatr Child Health 39(2):152–154

Francomano M, Seidenari S (2002) Urticaria after topical immunotherapy with diphenylcyclopropenone. Contact Dermatitis 47(5):310–311

Friedli A, Labarthe MP, Engelhardt E, Feldmann R, Salomon D, Saurat JH (1998) Pulse methylprednisolone therapy for severe alopecia areata: an open prospective study of 45 patients. J Am Acad Dermatol 39:597–602

Garcia Bartels N, Lee HH, Worm M, Burmester GR, Sterry W, Blume-Peytavi U (2006) Development of alopecia areata universalis in a patient receiving adalimumab. Arch Dermatol 142:1654–1655

García-Hernández MJ, Ruiz-Doblado S, Rodriguez-Pichardo A, Camacho F (1999) Alopecia areata, stress and psychiatric disorders: a review. J Dermatol 26(10):625–632

Georgala S, Katoulis AC, Befon A, Georgala K, Stavropoulos PG (2006) Inosiplex for treatment of alopecia areata: a randomized placebo-controlled study. Acta Derm Venereol 86(5):422–424

Hay IC, Jamieson M, Ormerod AD (1998) Randomized trial of aromatherapy. Successful treatment for alopecia areata. Arch Dermatol 134(11):1349–1352

Hernández MV, Nogués S, Ruiz-Esquide V, Alsina M, Cañete JD, Sanmartí R (2009) Development of alopecia areata after biological therapy with TNF-alpha blockers: description of a case and review of the literature. Clin Exp Rheumatol 27:892–893

Hordinsky MK (2011) Treatment of alopecia areata: "what is new on the horizon?". Dermatol Ther 24: 364–368

Ikeda T (1965) A new classification of alopecia areata. Dermatologica 131(6):421–445

Im M, Lee SS, Lee Y et al (2011) Prognostic factors in methylprednisolone pulse therapy for alopecia areata. J Dermatol 38(8):767–772

Inui S, Nakajima T, Toda N, Itami S (2009) Fexofenadine hydrochloride enhances the efficacy of contact immunotherapy for extensive alopecia areata: retrospective analysis of 121 cases. J Dermatol 36(6):323–327

Joly P (2006) The use of methotrexate alone or in combination with low doses of oral corticosteroids in the treatment of alopecia totalis or universalis. J Am Acad Dermatol 55:632–636

Kaelin U, Hassan AS, Braathen LR, Yawalkar N (2006) Treatment of alopecia areata partim universalis with efalizumab. J Am Acad Dermatol 55(3): 529–532

Kantor J, Kessler LJ, Brooks DG, Cotsarelis G (2003) Decreased serum ferritin is associated with alopecia in women. J Invest Dermatol 121(5):985–988

Kar BR, Handa S, Dogra S, Kumar B (2005) Placebo-controlled oral pulse prednisolone therapy in alopecia areata. J Am Acad Dermatol 52(2):287–290

Katagiri K, Arakawa S, Hatano Y, Fujiwara S (2006) Fexofenadine, an H1-receptor antagonist, partially but rapidly inhibits the itch of contact dermatitis induced by diphenylcyclopropenone in patients with alopecia areata. J Dermatol 33(2):75–79

Kirshen C, Kanigsberg N (2009) Alopecia areata following adalimumab. J Cutan Med Surg 13:48–50

Koo JY, Shellow WV, Hallman CP, Edwards JE (1994) Alopecia areata and increased prevalence of psychiatric disorders. Int J Dermatol 33(12): 849–850

Lattouf C, Jimenez JJ, Tosti A et al (2015) Treatment of alopecia areata with simvastatin/ezetimibe. J Am Acad Dermatol 72(2):359–361

Lowy M, Ledoux-Corbusier M, Achten G, Wybran J (1985) Clinical and immunologic response to Isoprinosine in alopecia areata and alopecia universalis: association with autoantibodies. J Am Acad Dermatol 12:78–84

Magni P, Macchi C, Morlotti B, Sirtori CR, Ruscica M (2015) Risk identification and possible countermeasures for muscle adverse effects during statin therapy. Eur J Intern Med 26:82–88. doi:10.1016/j.ejim.2015.01.002, pii: S0953-6205(15)00003-5

Martinez-Zapata MJ, Martí-Carvajal AJ, Solà I, Expósito JA, Bolíbar I, Rodríguez L, Garcia J (2012) Autologous platelet-rich plasma for treating chronic wounds. Cochrane Database Syst Rev 10:CD006899

Mrowietz U, Christophers E, Altmeyer P (1999) Treatment of severe psoriasis with fumaric acid esters: scientific background and guidelines for therapeutic use. The German Fumaric Acid Ester Consensus Conference. Br J Dermatol 141(3):424–429

Nakajima T, Inui S, Itami S (2007) Pulse corticosteroid therapy for alopecia areata: study of 139 patients. Dermatology 215:320–324

Namazi MR (2004) Statins: novel additions to the dermatologic arsenal? Exp Dermatol 13(6):337–339

Naveh Y, Rosenthal E, Ben-Arieh Y, Etzioni A (1999) Celiac disease-associated alopecia in childhood. J Pediatr 134(3):362–364

Ohlmeier MC, Traupe H, Luger TA, Böhm M (2012) Topical immunotherapy with diphenylcyclopropenone of patients with alopecia areata–a large retrospective study on 142 patients with a self-controlled design. J Eur Acad Dermatol Venereol 26(4):503–507

Pan Y, Rao NA (2009) Alopecia areata during etanercept therapy. Ocul Immunol Inflamm 17:127–129

Park H, Kim CW, Kim SS, Park CW (2009) The therapeutic effect and the changed serum zinc level after zinc supplementation in alopecia areata patients who had a low serum zinc level. Ann Dermatol 21:142–146

Pelivani N, Hassan AS, Braathen LR, Hunger RE, Yawalkar N (2008) Alopecia areata universalis elicited during treatment with adalimumab. Dermatology 216:320–323

Pericin M, Trüeb RM (1998) Topical immunotherapy of severe alopecia areata with diphenylcyclopropenone: evaluation of 68 cases. Dermatology 196:418–421

Perini G, Zara M, Cipriani R et al (1994) Imipramine in alopecia areata. A double-blind, placebo-controlled study. Psychother Psychosom 61:195–198

Perret CM, Steijlen PM, Zaun H, Happle R (1990) Erythema multiforme-like eruptions: a rare side effect of topical immunotherapy with diphenylcyclopropenone. Dermatologica 180(1):5–7

Petukhova L, Duvic M, Hordinsky M, Norris D, Price V, Shimomura Y, Kim H, Singh P, Lee A, Chen WV, Meyer KC, Paus R, Jahoda CA, Amos CI, Gregersen PK, Christiano AM (2010) Genome-wide association study in alopecia areata implicates both innate and adaptive immunity. Nature 466:113–117

Pires MC, Martins JM, Montealegre F, Gatti FR (2010) Vitiligo after diphencyprone for alopecia areata. Dermatol Res Pract 2010:17

Price VH, Hordinsky MK, Olsen EA et al (2008) Subcutaneous efalizumab is not effective in the treatment of alopecia areata. J Am Acad Dermatol 58:395–402

Ricciardi A, Ruberto A, García-Hernández MJ et al (2006) Alopecia areata with comorbid depression: early resolution with combined paroxetine-triamcinolone treatment. J Eur Acad Dermatol Venereol 20:1000–1001

Robins DN (2007) Case reports: alopecia universalis: hair growth following initiation of simvastatin and ezetimibe therapy. J Drugs Dermatol 6(9):946–947

Rook AJ (1977) Common baldness and alopecia areata. In: Rook AJ (ed) Recent advances in dermatology. Blackwell, Oxford, pp 236–238

Samrao A, Fu JM, Harris ST, Price VH (2013) Bone mineral density in patients with alopecia areata treated with long-term intralesional corticosteroids. J Drugs Dermatol 12(2):e36–e40

Sereti I, Sarlis NJ, Arioglu E, Turner ML, Mican JM (2001) Alopecia universalis and Graves' disease in the setting of immune restoration after highly active antiretroviral therapy. AIDS 15:138–140

Shimaoka Y, Hatamochi A, Hamasaki Y, Suzuki H, Ikeda H, Yamazaki S (2008) Discoid lupus erythematosus exacerbated by contact dermatitis caused by use of squaric acid dibutylester for topical immunotherapy in a patient with alopecia areata. J Dermatol 35(3):151–153

Sharma VK (1996) Pulsed administration of corticosteroids in the treatment of alopecia areata. Int J Dermatol 35(2):133–136

Sharma VK, Muralidhar S (1998) Treatment of widespread alopecia areata in young patients with monthly oral corticosteroid pulse. Pediatr Dermatol 15(4):313–317

Smith A, Trüeb RM, Theiler M et al (2015) Methylprednisolone pulse therapy for severe childhood alopecia areata. Ped Dermatol Apr 15 [Epub ahead of print]

Sotiriadis D, Patsatsi A, Lazaridou E, Kastanis A, Vakirlis E, Chrysomallis F (2007) Topical immunotherapy with diphenylcyclopropenone in the treatment of chronic extensive alopecia areata. Clin Exp Dermatol 32(1):48–51

Stewart MI, Smoller BR (1993) Alopecia universalis in an HIV-positive patient: possible insight into pathogenesis. J Cutan Pathol 20(2):180–183

Tauber M, Buche S, Reygagne P et al (2014) Alopecia areata occurring during anti-TNF therapy: a national multicenter prospective study. J Am Acad Dermatol 70:1146–1148

Tosti A, Bellavista S, Iorizzo M (2006a) Alopecia areata: a long term follow-up study of 191 patients. J Am Acad Dermatol 55(3):438–441

Tosti A, Iorizzo M, Botta GL, Milani M (2006b) Efficacy and safety of a new clobetasol propionate 0.05% foam in alopecia areata: a randomized, double-blind placebo-controlled trial. J Eur Acad Dermatol Venereol 20:1243–1247

Tosti A, Piraccini BM, Misciali C, Vincenzi C (2003a) Lentiginous eruption due to topical immunotherapy. Arch Dermatol 139(4):544–545

Tosti A, Piraccini BM, Pazzaglia M, Vincenzi C (2003b) Clobetasol propionate 0.05% under occlusion in the treatment of alopecia totalis/universalis. J Am Acad Dermatol 49:96–98

Trink A, Sorbellini E, Bezzola P, Rodella L, Rezzani R, Ramot Y, Rinaldi F (2013) A randomized, double-blind, placebo- and active-controlled, half-head study to evaluate the effects of platelet-rich plasma on alopecia areata. Br J Dermatol 169(3):690–694

Trost LB, Bergfeld WF, Calogeras E (2006) The diagnosis and treatment of iron deficiency and its potential relationship to hair loss. J Am Acad Dermatol 54: 824–844

Trüeb RM, Cavegn B (1996) Trichotillomania in connection with alopecia areata. Cutis 58:67–70

van den Biggelaar FJ, Smolders J, Jansen JF (2010) Complementary and alternative medicine in alopecia areata. Am J Clin Dermatol 11(1):11–20

van der Steen P, Happle R (1992) 'Dyschromia in confetti' as a side effect of topical immunotherapy with diphenylcyclopropenone. Arch Dermatol 128(4):518–520

Venten I, Hess N, Hirschmüller A, Altmeyer P, Brockmeyer N (2006) Treatment of therapy-resistant alopecia areata with fumaric acid esters. Eur J Med Res 11(7):300–305

Viola F, Barbato M, Formisano M et al (1999) Reappearance of alopecia areata in a coeliac patient during an unintentional challenge with gluten. Minerva Gastroenterol Dietol 45(4):283–285

von Helden R (2014) Gesund in sieben Tagen. Erfolge mit der Vitamin-D-Therapie. Hygeia-Verlag, Dresden, p 78ff

Waldmann TA (2013) The biology of IL-15: implications for cancer therapy and the treatment of autoimmune disorders. J Investig Dermatol Symp Proc 16:S28–S30

Willemsen R, Vanderlinden J, Deconinck A, Roseeuw D (2006) Hypnotherapeutic management of alopecia areata. J Am Acad Dermatol 55:233–237

Willemsen R, Haentjens P, Roseeuw D, Vanderlinden J (2010) Hypnosis in refractory alopecia areata significantly improves depression, anxiety, and life quality but not hair regrowth. J Am Acad Dermatol 62:517–518

Willemsen R, Haentjens P, Roseeuw D, Vanderlinden J (2011) Hypnosis and alopecia areata: long-term beneficial effects on psychological well-being. Acta Derm Venereol 91:35–39

Xing L, Dai Z, Jabbari A et al (2014) Alopecia areata is driven by cytotoxic T lymphocytes and is reversed by JAK inhibition. Nat Med 20(9):1043–1049

Yilmaz N, Serarslan G, Gokce C (2012) Vitamin D concentration are decreased in patients with alopecia areata. Vitam Trace Elem 1:105–109

Zampetti M, Filippetti R (2008) Alopecia areata and celiac disease. G Ital Dermatol Venereol 143(2): 168

Challenges in Non-scarring Alopecia: Chemotherapy-Induced Alopecia

Baker B, Wilson C, Davis A et al (1991) Busulphan/cyclophosphamide conditioning for bone marrow transplantation may lead to failure of hair regrowth. Bone Marrow Transplant 7:43–47

Betticher DC, Delmore G, Breitenstein U, Anchisi S, Zimmerli-Schwab B, Müller A, von Moos R, Hügli-Dayer AM, Schefer H, Bodenmann S, Bühler V, Trüeb RM (2013) Efficacy and tolerability of two scalp cooling systems for the prevention of alopecia associated with docetaxel treatment. Support Care Cancer 21(9):2565–2573

Grevelman EG, Breed WPM (2005) Prevention of chemotherapy-induced hair loss by scalp cooling. Ann Oncol 16:352–358

Kluger N, Jacot W, Frouin E, Rigau V, Poujol S, Dereure O, Guillot B, Romieu G, Bessis D (2012) Permanent scalp alopecia related to breast cancer chemotherapy by sequential fluorouracil/epirubicin/cyclophosphamide (FEC) and docetaxel: a prospective study of 20 patients. Ann Oncol 23(11):2879–2884

Miteva M, Misciali C, Fanti PA, Vincenzi C, Romanelli P, Tosti A (2011) Permanent alopecia after systemic chemotherapy: a clinicopathological study of 10 cases. Am J Dermatopathol 33(4):345–350

McGarvey EL, Baum LD, Pinkerton RC et al (2001) Psychological sequelae and alopecia among women with cancer. Cancer Pract 9:283–289

Mundstedt K, Manthey N, Sachsse S et al (1997) Changes in self-concept and body image during alopecia induced cancer chemotherapy. Support Care Cancer 5:139–143

Rosman S (2004) Cancer and stigma: experience of patients with chemotherapy-induced alopecia. Patient Educ Couns 52:333–339

Tran D, Sinclair RD, Schwarer AP et al (2000) Permanent alopecia following chemotherapy and bone marrow transplantation. Australas J Dermatol 41:106–108

Trüeb RM (2009b) Chemotherapy-induced alopecia. Semin Cutan Med Surg 28:11–14

Trüeb RM (2007) Chemotherapy-induced anagen effluvium: diffuse or patterned? Dermatology 215:1–2

Vowels M, Chan LL, Giri N et al (1993) Factors affecting hair regrowth after bone marrow transplantation. Bone Marrow Transplant 12:347–350

Wang J, Lu Z, Au JLS (2006) Protection against chemotherapy-induced alopecia. Pharm Res 23: 2505–2514

Challenges in Non-scarring Alopecia: Adverse Effects of Molecularly Targeted Therapies for Cancer

Donovan JC, Ghazarian DM, Shaw JC (2008) Scarring alopecia associated with use of the epidermal growth factor receptor inhibitor gefitinib. Arch Dermatol 144:1524–1525

Graves JE, Jones BF, Lind AC, Heffernan MP (2006) Nonscarring inflammatory alopecia associated with the epidermal growth factor receptor inhibitor gefitinib. J Am Acad Dermatol 55:349–353

Hansen T, Little AJ, Miller JJ, Ioffreda MD (2013) A case of inflammatory nonscarring alopecia associated with the tyrosine kinase inhibitor nilotinib. JAMA Dermatol 149:330–332

Hepper DM, Wu P, Anadkat MJ (2011) Scarring alopecia associated with the epidermal growth factor receptor inhibitor erlotinib. J Am Acad Dermatol 64:996–998

Lacouture ME, Schadendorf D, Chu CY, Uttenreuther-Fischer M, Stammberger U, O'Brien D, Hauschild A (2013) Dermatologic adverse events associated with afatinib: an oral ErbB family blocker. Expert Rev Anticancer Ther 13:721–728

Macdonald JB, Macdonald B, Golitz LE, LoRusso P, Sekulic A (2015a) Cutaneous adverse effects of targeted therapies: part I: inhibitors of the cellular membrane. J Am Acad Dermatol 72(2):203–218

Macdonald JB, Macdonald B, Golitz LE, LoRusso P, Sekulic A (2015b) Cutaneous adverse effects of targeted therapies: part II: inhibitors of intracellular molecular signaling pathways. J Am Acad Dermatol 72(2):221–236

Nakamura-Wakatsuki T, Yamamoto T (2012) Purpuric drug eruption and alopecia induced by erlotinib. Dermatol Online J 18:16

Pongpudpunth M, Demierre MF, Goldberg LJ (2009) A case report of inflammatory nonscarring alopecia associated with the epidermal growth factor receptor inhibitor erlotinib. J Cutan Pathol 36:1303–1307

Toda N, Fujimoto N, Kato T, Fujii N, Nakanishi G, Nagao T, Tanaka T (2012) Erosive pustular dermatosis of the scalp-like eruption due to gefitinib: case report and review of the literature of alopecia associated with EGFR inhibitors. Dermatology 225:18–21

Wu CY, Chen GS, Lan CC (2008) Erosive pustular dermatosis of the scalp after gefitinib and radiotherapy for brain metastases secondary to lung cancer. Clin Exp Dermatol 33:106–107

Yang BH, Bang CY, Byun JW, Han SH, Song HJ, In SG, Shin JH, Choi GS (2011) A case of cicatricial alopecia associated with erlotinib. Ann Dermatol 23(Suppl 3):S350–S353

Scarring Alopecias: Classification

Bergner T, Braun-Falco O (1991) Pseudopelade of Brocq. J Am Acad Dermatol 25:865–866

Burton JL, Peachey RDG, Pye RJ (1988) Erosive pustular dermatosis of the scalp – a definition. Br J Dermatol 119:411

Chicarilli ZN (1987) Follicular occlusion triad: hidradenitis suppurativa, acne conglobata, and dissecting cellulitis of the scalp. Ann Plast Surg 18:230–237

Chiu CS, Lin CY, Kuo TT, Kuan YZ, Chen MJ, Ho HC, Yang LC, Chen CH, Shih IH, Hong HS, Chuang YH (2007) Malignant cutaneous tumors of the scalp: a study of demographic characteristics and histologic distributions of 398 Taiwanese patients. J Am Acad Dermatol 56:448–452

Cohen PR (2009) Primary alopecia neoplastica versus secondary alopecia neoplastica: a new classification for neoplasm-associated scalp hair loss. J Cutan Pathol 36:917–918

Degos R, Rabut R, Duperrat B, Leclerq R (1954) Pseudopeladic state; comments on one hundred cases of circumscribed cicatricial alopecia, apparently primary, of pseudopelade type. Ann Dermatol Syphiligr (Paris) 81(1):5–26

Dreuw H (1910) Klinische Beobachtungen bei 101 haarkranken Schulknaben. Monatsh prakt Dermatol 51:103–118

Elston DM, McCollough ML, Angeloni VL (1995) Vertical and transverse sections of alopecia biopsy specimens. Combining the two to maximize diagnostic yield. J Am Acad Dermatol 32:454–457

Gaffney DC, Sinclair RD, Yong-Gee S (2013) Discoid lupus alopecia complicated by frontal fibrosing alopecia on a background of androgenetic alopecia. Br J Dermatol 169(1):217–218

Gathers RC, Lim HW (2009) Central centrifugal cicatricial alopecia: past, present, and future. J Am Acad Dermatol 60(4):660–668

Grattan CEH, Peachu RD, Boon A (1988) Evidence for a role of local trauma in the pathogenesis of erosive pustular dermatosis of the scalp. Clin Exp Dermatol 13:7–10

Harries MJ, Meyer K, Chaudhry I et al (2013) Lichen planopilaris is characterized by immune privilege collapse of the hair follicle's epithelial stem cell niche. J Pathol 231(2):236–247

Harries MJ, Trueb RM, Tosti A et al (2009) How not to get scar(r)ed: pointers to the correct diagnosis in patients with suspected primary cicatricial alopecia. Br J Dermatol 160:482–501

Headington JT (1996) Cicatricial alopecia. Dermatol Clin 14:773–782

Höfer W (1964) Sporadisches Auftreten von Alopecia parvimaculata. Dermatol Wschr 149:381–386

James C, Langlois NE (2013) Folliculitis decalvans: a rare scarring alopecia misinterpreted as a laceration of the scalp at the scene. Forensic Sci Med Pathol 9(4):594–595

Karnik P, Tekeste Z, McCormick TS, Gilliam AC, Price VH, Cooper KD, Mirmirani P (2009) Hair follicle

stem cell-specific PPARgamma deletion causes scarring alopecia. J Invest Dermatol 129(5):1243–1245
Katz TM, Silapunt S, Goldberg LH, Jih MH, Kimyai-Asadi A (2005) Analysis of 197 female scalp tumors treated with Mohs micrographic surgery. J Am Acad Dermatol 52:291–294
Kossard S (1994b) Postmenopausal frontal fibrosing alopecia: scarring alopecia in a pattern distribution. Arch Dermatol 130:770–774
Laffitte E, Panizzon RG, Saurat JH (2004) Delayed wound healing on the scalp following treatment of actinic keratoses: erosive pustular dermatosis of the scalp. Dermatol Surg 30:1610
Laymon CW (1947) The cicatricial alopecias: historical and clinical review, and histologic investigation. J Invest Dermatol 8:99–122
Ljubojevic S, Pasic A, Lipozencic J, Skerlev M (2005) Perifolliculitis capitis abscedens etsuffodiens. J Eur Acad Dermatol Venereol 19:719–721
LoPresti P, Papa CM, Kligman AM (1968) Hot comb alopecia. Arch Dermatol 98(3):234–238
Lovell CR, Harmann RM, Bradfield JW (1980) Cutaneous carcinoma arising in erosive pustular dermatosis of the scalp. Br J Dermatol 102:325–328
Matard B, Meylheuc T, Briandet R, Casin I, Assouly P, Cavelier-balloy B, Reygagne P (2012) First evidence of bacterial biofilms in the anaerobe part of scalp hair follicles: a pilot comparative study in folliculitis decalvans. J Eur Acad Dermatol Venereol 27:853–860
Nayar M, Schomberg K, Dawber RPR, Millard PR (1993) A clinicopathological study of scarring alopecia. Br J Dermatol 128:533–536
Ogunbiyi A, George A (2005) Acne keloidalis in females: case report and review of literature. J Natl Med Assoc 97(5):736–738
Olsen EA, Bergfeld WF, Cotsarelis G et al (2003) Summary of North American Hair Research Society (NAHRS)-sponsored Workshop on Cicatricial Alopecia, Duke University Medical Center, February 10 and 11, 2001. J Am Acad Dermatol 48:103–110
Petronić-Rosić V, Krunić A, Mijusković M, Vesić S (1999) Tufted hair folliculitis: a pattern of scarring alopecia? J Am Acad Dermatol 41(1):112–114
Pierard-Franchimont C, Pierard GE (1986) Massive lymphocyte-mediated apoptosis during the early stage of pseudopelade. Dermatologica 172(5):254–257
Price V, Mirmirani P (2011) Cicatricial alopecia. An approach to diagnosis and management. Springer, New York/Dordrecht/Heidelberg/London
Pye RJ, Peachey RDG, Burton JL (1979) Erosive pustular dermatosis of the scalp. Br J Dermatol 100: 559–566
Richmond HM, Duvic M, Macfarlane DF (2010) Primary and metastatic malignant tumors of the scalp: an update. Am J Clin Dermatol 11:233–246
Ross EK, Tan E, Shapiro J (2005) Update on primary cicatricial alopecias. J Am Acad Dermatol 53:1–37
Smith NP, Sanderson KV (1978) Tufted hair folliculitis of the scalp. J R Soc Med 71:606–608
Solomon AR (1994) The transversely sectioned scalp biopsy specimen: the technique and a algorithm for ist use in the diagnosis of alopecia. Adv Dermatol 9:127–157
Sperling LC (2001) Scarring alopecia and the dermatopathologist. J Cutan Pathol 28:333–342
Sperling LC, Homoky C, Pratt L, Sau P (2000a) Acne keloidalis is a form of primary scarring alopecia. Arch Dermatol 136(4):479–484
Sperling LC, Sau P (1992) The follicular degeneration syndrome in black patients. 'Hot comb alopecia' revisited and revised. Arch Dermatol 128(1):68–74
Sperling LC, Solomon AR, Whiting DA (2000b) A new look at scarring alopecia. Arch Dermatol 136:235–242
Templeton SF, Solomon AR (1994) Scarring alopecia: a classification based on microscopic criteria. J Cutan Pathol 21:97–109
Trachsler S, Trüeb RM (2005) Value of direct immunofluorescence for differential diagnosis of cicatricial alopecia. Dermatology 211:98–102
Trüeb RM, Krasovec M (1999) Erosive pustular dermatosis of the scalp following radiation therapy for solar keratoses. Br J Dermatol 141:763–765
Yu M, Bell RH, Ross EK, Lo BK, Isaac-Renton M, Martinka M, Haegert A, Shapiro J, McElwee KJ (2010) Lichen planopilaris and pseudopelade of Brocq involve distinct disease associated gene expression patterns by microarray. J Dermatol Sci 57(1):27–36
Zinkernagel MS, Trüeb RM (2000b) Fibrosing alopecia in a pattern distribution. Patterned lichen planopilaris or androgenetic alopecia with a lichenoid tissue reaction pattern? Arch Dermatol 136:205–211

Scarring Alopecias: Treatment

Abeck D, Korting HC, Braun-Falco O (1992) Folliculitis decalvans. Long-lasting response to combined therapy with fusidic acid and zinc. Acta Derm Venereol 72(2):143–145
Callender VD, Lawson CN, Onwudiwe OC (2014) Hair transplantation in the surgical treatment of central centrifugal cicatricial alopecia. Dermatol Surg 40(10):1125–1131
Cho BK, Sah D, Chwalek J, Roseborough I, Ochoa B, Chiang C, Price VH (2010) Efficacy and safety of mycophenolate mofetil for lichen planopilaris. J Am Acad Dermatol 62(3):393–397
Donovan JC, Samrao A, Ruben BS, Price VH (2010) Eyebrow regrowth in patients with frontal fibrosing alopecia treated with intralesional triamcinolone acetonide. Br J Dermatol 163:1142–1144
Kakourou T, Uksal U, European Society for Pediatric Dermatology (2010) Guidelines for the management of tinea capitis in children. Pediatr Dermatol 27(3):226–228

Kantor GR, Ratz JL, Wheeland R (1986) Treatment of acne keloidalis nuchae with carbon dioxide laser. J Am Acad Dermatol 14:263–267
Laffitte E, Kaya G, Piguet V, Saurat JH (2003) Erosive pustular dermatosis of the scalp: treatment with topical tacrolimus. Arch Dermatol 139:712–714
Mirmirani P, Karnik P (2009) Lichen planopilaris treated with a peroxisome proliferator-activated receptor gamma agonist. Arch Dermatol 145(12): 1363–1366
Navarini AA, Kolios AG, Prinz-Vavricka BM et al (2011) Low-dose excimer 308-nm laser for treatment of lichen planopilaris. Arch Dermatol 147:1325–1326
Navarini AA, Trüeb RM (2010) 3 cases of dissecting cellulitis of the scalp treated with adalimumab: control of inflammation within residual structural disease. Arch Dermatol 146(5):517–520
Powell JJ, Dawber RP, Gatter K (1999) Folliculitis decalvans including tufted folliculitis: clinical, histological and therapeutic findings. Br J Dermatol 140(2): 328–333
Trüeb RM, Pericin M, Hafner J, Burg G (1997) Tufted hair folliculitis. Hautarzt 48(4):266–269

Scarring Alopecias: Grat-Versus-Host Disease

Friedman KJ, LeBoit PE, Farmer ER (1988) Acute follicular graft-vs-host reaction. A distinct clinicopathologic presentation. Arch Dermatol 124(5):688–691
Häusermann P, Walter RB, Halter J, Biedermann BC, Tichelli A, Itin P, Gratwohl A (2008) Cutaneous graft-versus-host disease: a guide for the dermatologist. Dermatology 216:287–304
Marks C, Stadler M, Häusermann P, Wolff D, Buchholz S, Stary G, Lee S, Lawitschka A, Bertz H (2011) German-Austrian-Swiss Consensus Conference on clinical practice in chronic graft-versus-host disease (GVHD): guidance for supportive therapy of chronic cutaneous and musculoskeletal GVHD. Br J Dermatol 165(1):18–29
Miyazaki K, Higaki S, Maruyama T, Takahashi S, Morohashi M, Ito K (1993) Chronic graft-versus-host disease with follicular involvement. J Dermatol 20(4):242–246

Scarring Alopecias: Anti-tumor Necrosis Factor Alpha Therapy-Induced Alopecia

Cullen G, Kroshinsky D, Cheifetz AS, Korzenik JR (2011) Psoriasis associated with anti-tumour necrosis factor therapy in inflammatory bowel disease: a new series and a review of 120 cases from the literature. Aliment Pharmacol Ther 34(11–12):1318–1327
El Shabrawi-Caelen L, La Placa M, Vincenzi C, Haidn T, Muellegger R, Tosti A (2010) Adalimumab-induced psoriasis of the scalp with diffuse alopecia: a severe potentially irreversible cutaneous side effect of TNF-alpha blockers. Inflamm Bowel Dis 16:182–183
Ettler J, Wetter DA, Pittelkow MR (2012) Pityriasis amiantacea: a distinctive presentation of psoriasis associated with tumour necrosis factor-α inhibitor therapy. Clin Exp Dermatol 37:639–641
Joyau C, Veyrac G, Dixneuf V, Jolliet P (2012) Anti-tumour necrosis factor alpha therapy and increased risk of de novo psoriasis: is it really a paradoxical side effect? Clin Exp Rheumatol 30:700–706
Nakagomi D, Harada K, Yagasaki A, Kawamura T, Shibagaki N, Shimada S (2009) Psoriasiform eruption associated with alopecia areata during infliximab therapy. Clin Exp Dermatol 34:923–924
Osório F, Magro F, Lisboa C, Lopes S, Macedo G, Bettencourt H, Azevedo F, Magina S (2012) Anti-TNF-alpha induced psoriasiform eruptions with severe scalp involvement and alopecia: report of five cases and review of the literature. Dermatology 225:163–167
Papadavid E, Gazi S, Dalamaga M, Stavrianeas N, Ntelis V (2008) Palmoplantar and scalp psoriasis occurring during anti-tumour necrosis factor-alpha therapy: a case series of four patients and guidelines for management. J Eur Acad Dermatol Venereol 22(3): 380–382
Puig L, Morales-Múnera CE, López-Ferrer A, Geli C (2012) Ustekinumab treatment of TNF antagonist-induced paradoxical psoriasis flare in a patient with psoriatic arthritis: case report and review. Dermatology 225(1):14–17

Red Scalp

Grimalt R, Lacueva L, Hasmann G, Ferrando J (2000) Red scalp syndrome. Annual meeting of the European Hair Research Society (EHRS), Abstract F11, p 22
Moschella SL (1994) Written personal communication. August 14, 1992. In: Bernhard JD (ed) Itch: mechanisms and management of pruritus. McGraw-Hill, New York, p 51
Thestrup-Pedersen K, Hjorth N (1987) Rod skalp. En ikke tidligere beskrevet harbundssygdom? Ugeskr Laeger 149:2141–2142

Red Scalp: Atopic Dermatitis of the Head and Neck Type

Bayrou O, Pecquet C, Flahault A, Artigou C, Abuaf N, Leynadier F (2005) Head and neck atopic dermatitis and malassezia-furfur-specific IgE antibodies. Dermatology 211(2):107–113
Broberg A, Faergemann J (1995) Topical antimycotic treatment of atopic dermatitis in the head/neck area: a

double-blind randomized study. Acta Derm Venereol 75:46–49
Brodská P, Panzner P, Pizinger K, Schmid-Grendelmeier P (2014) IgE-mediated sensitization to malassezia in atopic dermatitis: more common in male patients and in head and neck type. Dermatitis 25(3):120–126
Clemmensen S, Hjorth N (1983) Treatment of dermatitis of the head and neck with ketoconazole in patients with type 1 sensitivity to Pityrosporum ovale. Semin Dermatol 2:26–29
Darabi K, Hostetler SG, Bechtel MA, Zirwas M (2009) The role of Malassezia in atopic dermatitis affecting the head and neck of adults. J Am Acad Dermatol 60(1):125–136
Devos SA, van der Valk PG (2000) The relevance of skin prick tests for Pityrosporum ovale in patients with head and neck dermatitis. Allergy 55(11):1056–1058
Ikezawa Z, Kondo M, Okajima M, Nishimura Y, Kono M (2001) Clinical usefulness of oral itraconazole, an antimycotic drug, for refractory atopic dermatitis. Eur J Dermatol 14:400–406
Kim TY, Jang IG, Park YM, Kim HO, Kim CW (1999) Head and neck dermatitis: the role of Malassezia furfur, topical steroid use and environmental factors in its causation. Clin Exp Dermatol 24(3):226–231
Mayser P, Kupfer J, Nemetz D, Schäfer U, Nilles M, Hort W, Gieler U (2006) Treatment of head and neck dermatitis with ciclopiroxolamine cream–results of a double-blind, placebo-controlled study. Skin Pharmacol Physiol 19(3):153–158
Schmid-Grendelmeier P, Scheynius A, Cramer R (2006) The role of sensitization to Malassezia sympodialis in atopic eczema. Chem Immunol Allergy 91:98–109
Svejgaard El, Larsen PØ, Deleuran M, Ternowitz T, Roed-Petersen J, Nilsson J (2004) Treatment of head and neck dermatitis comparing itraconazole 200 mg and 400 mg daily for 1 week with placebo. J Eur Acad Dermatol Venereol 18(4):445–449
Waersted A, Hjorth N (1985) Pityrosporum orbiculare–a pathogenic factor in atopic dermatitis of the face, scalp and neck? Acta Derm Venereol Suppl (Stockh) 114:146–148

Red Scalp: Rosacea-Like Dermatosis of the Scalp

Ayres S Jr (1987) Extrafacial rosacea is rare but does exist. J Am Acad Dermatol 16:391–392
Baima B, Sticherling M (2002) Demodicidosis revisited. Acta Derm Venereol 82:3–6
Dupont C (1986) How common is extrafacial rosacea? J Am Acad Dermatol 14:839
Gajewska M (1975) Rosacea of common male baldness. Br J Dermatol 93:63–66
Karaman U, Celik T, Calik S, Sener S, Aydin NE, Daldal UN (2008) Demodex spp. in hairy skin biopsy specimens. Turkiye Parazitol Derg 32:343–345
Lonne-Rahm SB, Fischer T, Berg M (1999) Stinging and rosacea. Acta Derm Venereol 79(6):460–461
Marks R, Jones EW (1969) Disseminated rosacea. Br J Dermatol 81:16–28
Miskjian HG (1951) Demodicidosis (demodex infestation of the scalp). AMA Arch Derm Syphilol 63:282–283
Oberholzer PA, Nobbe S, Kolm I et al (2009) Red scalp disease–a rosacea-like dermatosis of the scalp? Successful therapy with oral tetracycline. Dermatology 219:179–181
Pereira TM, Vieira AP, Basto AS (2008) Rosacea with extensive extrafacial lesions. Int J Dermatol 47:52–55
Sabater-Marco V, Escutia-Muñoz B, Botella-Estrada R (2015) Eosinophilic follicular reaction induced by Demodex folliculorum mite: a different disease from eosinophilic folliculitis. Clin Exp Dermatol 40:413–415. doi:10.1111/ced.12566
Wilkin J, Dahl M, Detmar M et al (2002) Standard classification of rosacea: report of the national rosacea society expert committee on the classification and staging of rosacea. J Am Acad Dermatol 46:584–587
Wilkin JK (1980) Epigastric rosacea. Arch Dermatol 116:584
Wong CS, Kirby B (2004) Demodicidosis in scalp rosacea? Clin Exp Dermatol 29:318–319

Red Scalp: Scalp Burnout

Trüeb RM (2014) North American Virginian witch hazel (Hamamelis virginiana)-based scalp care and protection for sensitive scalp, red scalp, and scalp burn-out. Int J Trichology 6(3):100–103
World Health Organization (2015) ICD-10: international classification of diseases. World Health Organization, Geneva
Willimann B, Trüeb RM (2002) Hair pain (trichodynia): frequency and relationship to hair loss and patient gender. Dermatology 205(4):374–377

Psychopathological Disorders

5

The educated among the physicians make an effort into an understanding of the mind.

Aristotle (384–322 BC), Nicomachean Ethics

It is a common experience among dermatologists that a significant number of their patients have psychological overlays to their chief complaints. This particularly holds true for complaints related to conditions of the hair and scalp. The exact incidence in any particular dermatologic practice most likely depends on the dermatologist's interest; however, even for those dermatologists who are not specially interested in the psychological aspects of dermatologic disease, some patients have such overt psychopathologic conditions, such as trichotillomania, factitial dermatitis, or delusions of parasitosis, that even the least psychologically minded dermatologist feels obliged somehow to address the psychological issues. Ideally, this would be accomplished simply through referral of the patient to a mental health professional. In reality, the majority of psychodermatologic patients are reluctant to be referred to a psychiatrist. Many lack the insight regarding the psychological contribution to their dermatologic complaints; others fear the social stigmatization of coming under the care of a psychiatrist.

The dermatologist is often the physician designated by the patient to handle their chief complaint, even if the main disorder is a psychological one. Therefore, it is essential for dermatologists dealing with such patients to expand their clinical acumen and therapeutic armamentarium to effectively handle the psychodermatologic cases in their practice. To accomplish this goal, the following steps are required:

1. *Learn to classify and diagnose psychodermatologic disorders*. Because so many different types of conditions lie in between the fields of dermatology and psychiatry, it is paramount to have classification systems that will help clinicians understand what they are dealing with. There are two ways to classify psychocutaneous cases: first, by the category of the dermatologic presentation, e.g., neurotic excoriation, and, second, by the nature of the underlying psychopathologic condition, e.g., depressive disorder, generalized anxiety disorder, or obsessive–compulsive disorder.

R.M. Trüeb, *The Difficult Hair Loss Patient: Guide to Successful Management of Alopecia and Related Conditions*, DOI 10.1007/978-3-319-19701-2_5

2. *Become familiar with the various therapeutic options available*, both nonpharmacologic and psychopharmacologic.
3. *Recognize the limits of what can be accomplished in a dermatologic practice*: Typically, a dermatologist does not have the time, training, or inclination necessary to administer most nonpharmacologic approaches. If a dermatologist seriously considers the challenge of treating these patients with psychopharmacologic agents, the selection of appropriate agents is dictated by the nature of the underlying psychopathologies that need to be treated. In order to prescribe effectively and safely for these patients, the dermatologist must have a basic understanding of the pharmacology of psychotropic agents.
4. *Optimize working relationships with psychiatrists*, since dermatologists and psychiatrists tend to have different perspectives when analyzing a clinical situation, different styles of communication, and different approaches to management.

5.1 Classification

Most psychocutaneous conditions of the hair and scalp can be grouped into the following four categories:

Psychophysiological disorders, in which the scalp disorder is exacerbated by emotional factors, e.g., hyperhidrosis, atopic dermatitis, psoriasis, and seborrheic dermatitis of the scalp

Primary psychiatric disorders, in which there is no real skin condition, but all symptoms are either self-induced or delusional, e.g., trichotillomania, neurotic excoriations, factitial dermatitis, delusion of parasitosis, or psychogenic pseudoeffluvium

Cutaneous sensory disorders, in which the patient has various abnormal sensations of the scalp with no primary dermatologic lesions and no diagnosable internal medical condition responsible for the sensations

Secondary psychiatric disorders, in which patients develop emotional problems as a result of hair loss, usually as a consequence of disfigurement

5.2 Psychophysiological Disorders

Psychophysiological disorders is the term used for psychocutaneous cases in which specific dermatologic skin disorders, such as psoriasis and eczema, are exacerbated by emotional stress in a significant proportion of patients. Examples affecting the scalp include hyperhidrosis, atopic dermatitis, psoriasis, and seborrheic dermatitis. In each of these conditions, one comes across two types of patients: those who experience a close chronologic association between stressful experiences and exacerbation of their dermatologic condition and those for whom the emotional state seems not to influence the natural course of their disease. These two groups are referred to as "stress responders" and "non-stress responders," respectively. The relative proportion of stress responders versus non-stress responders varies among the different psychophysiological conditions.

A study involving a large number of subjects from the Harvard health-care system in Boston, Massachusetts, determined the proportion with emotional trigger to be 100 % in patients with hyperhidrosis, 70 % in those with atopic dermatitis, 62 % with psoriasis, and 41 % with seborrheic dermatitis.

This category also includes the *psychosomatic disorders* – the physical symptomatic representation of unsolved emotional conflicts. For classification, we may consider the different levels of psychosomatic disorder:

The *first level* is physiological and includes bodily sensations in response to emotional shifts, great or small. In health these bodily sensations make little or no impact on consciousness.

At the *second level*, the person becomes more or less constantly aware of the somatic sensations, which are of purely functional nature at this time point, attempts to analyze them, and becomes anxious that they might signify some serious organic disease.

The *third level* is the important one, at which internal somatic medicine and psychiatry meet. The organs and parts of the body have enormous elasticity and rebound, but if the underlying emotional distress is too prolonged, they supposedly lose their elasticity, no longer being able to cope, and finally protest in terms of the psychosomatic organ lesion or organ pathology.

It has long been recognized that psychosomatic factors play a role in dermatologic disease. It has been hypothesized that an organ system is vulnerable to psychosomatic ailments when several etiologic factors are operable. These factors include emotional factors mediated by the central nervous system; intrapsychic processes such as self-concept, identity, and eroticism; specific correlations between the emotional drive and the target organ, i.e., social values and standards linked with the organ system; and a constitutional vulnerability of the target organ.

5.2.1 Folliculitis Necrotica

Folliculitis necrotica is a peculiar dermatosis of the scalp that preferentially affects adult males, with chronic symptoms that wax and wane over time. Traditionally, the condition has been nosologically classified among the primary scarring alopecias. There is circumstantial evidence to also classify it among the psychophysiological disorders.

The disorder is characterized by minute and usually intensely pruritic follicular erythematous papules and pustules of the scalp that may become sore and crusted due to repeated scratching. The lesions may concentrate along the frontal hairline but can appear anywhere on the scalp, varying in number from just a few to numerous lesions covering the scalp (Fig. 5.1). The disease has been classified into *acne necrotica miliaris* and *acne necrotica varioliformis*. The former affects the superficial portion of the hair follicle, allowing for hair regrowth after successful treatment. Miliaris refers to a millet, a term for a small seed. The latter represents deeper lesions that progress to scabs that leave smallpox-like (varioliform) scars in their wake. Focal permanent alopecia may occur where the scalp has been scarred.

> Patients with folliculitis necrotica tend to be middle-aged executives, with lesions often triggered by stress. Many have jobs that place a lot of responsibility on them.

Histological studies of early lesions demonstrate lymphocytes centered around a hair follicle, with keratinocytes within the external hair root sheath and surrounding epidermis showing extensive cell necrosis.

The etiology is unknown; however, an abnormal inflammatory reaction to components of the hair follicle has been postulated, particularly to commensal or pathogenic microorganisms, such

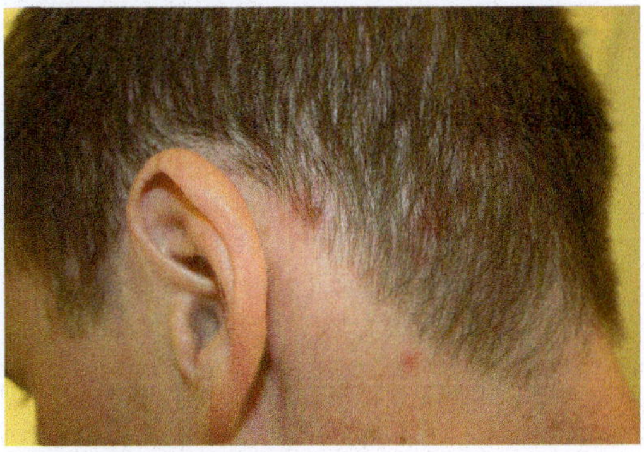

Fig. 5.1 Acne necrotica miliaris

as *Propionibacterium acnes*, *Malassezia* spp., *Demodex folliculorum*, and, in the more severe cases, *Staphylococcus aureus*.

Additionally extreme mechanical manipulation of the scalp due to scratching may be to blame.

The condition usually responds well to oral antibiotics, particularly long-term tetracyclines, in combination with a topical corticosteroid cream, and a shampoo treatment alternating an antiseptic shampoo containing povidone-iodine with an antidandruff shampoo containing ketoconazole. Mild cases may be treated with topical antibiotics such 0.5–1.0 g tetracycline in 70 % isopropyl alcohol (at 100.0 g), 1 % clindamycin solution, or 4 % erythromycin gel. Refractory cases usually can be managed with long-term low-dose oral isotretinoin (start with 20 mg daily and taper to the individually required minimal dosage). In particularly tense patients, the addition of oral doxepin hydrochloride 10–50 mg in the evening may be helpful in alleviating the itch–scratch cycle.

5.3 Primary Psychiatric Disorders

The term primary psychiatric disorders refers to cases in which there is no real skin condition. Everything that is seen on the scalp is self-induced, or there are no objective signs of complaints relating to the condition of the scalp and hair. This category includes conditions such as trichotillomania, neurotic excoriations, factitial dermatitis, delusions of parasitosis, and psychogenic pseudoeffluvium.

Since the dermatologic presentations are quite stereotypic, but the underlying psychopathology varies, a critical step in psychodermatology is to try to ascertain the nature of the underlying psychopathologic condition.

Any one of the numerous psychopathologies listed in the Diagnostic and Statistical Manual of Mental Disorders, 5th edition (DSM-V) and in the International Statistical Classification of Diseases and Related Health Problems, 10th edition (ICD-10) can be presented by these patients. In general, one of the following four types of underlying psychopathology is present:

1. Generalized anxiety disorder
2. Depressive disorder
3. Delusional disorder
4. Obsessive–compulsive disorder

Generalized Anxiety Disorder. Generalized anxiety disorder is characterized by a sustained, increased free floating anxiety, which is not orientated toward a certain object or situation. It expresses itself in the form of anxious expectations and enhanced alertness, combined with hypertension and, as a physiological correlate, vegetative hyperreactivity. Subjective symptoms include feelings of restlessness, irritability, feeling "on edge," tension, dizziness, agitation, and an inability to relax. These are frequently associated with physiological correlates such as muscle tension, sweating, shortness of breath, dry mouth, palpitations, abdominal complaints, and frequent urination. The uninhibited breakthroughs of tremendous anxiety show that the anxiety defense mechanisms have failed in the affected individuals. The causes of anxiety are repressed, but the ongoing arousal and fear are overwhelming. The patient's appearance is clinging and helpless. The patients signify a strong demand to be guided and assisted in their surroundings. The fixation toward fear of love deprivation may lead to attachments to strong "father figures," e.g., a physician, and strong emotional reactions on parting situations: a change of physician can cause severe separation anxiety and may therefore seem unbearable.

When patients with psychophysiological disorders complain that they are "stressed," they are usually referring to an underlying sense of anxiety. In the United States, anxiety disorder represents the most common mental health problem, especially in the over 55 years age group, where the prevalence is approximately one in ten.

Depressive Disorder. In a depressive disorder, the affected individual suffers from the symptoms of a depressive syndrome, which may be interspersed with shorter or longer periods of normal mood. Depression is characterized by subjective symptoms, such as depressed mood, crying spells, anhedonia (inability to experience pleasure), a sense of helplessness, hopelessness and worthlessness, excessive guilt, and suicidal ideation. Frequently associated physiological correlates are psychomotor retardation or agitation, insomnia or hypersomnia, loss of appetite or hyperphagia, and, especially in older patients, complaints of constipation. In a depressive character disorder, affected individuals appear humble, unambitious, and sacrificing. They have high self-expectations and avoid close approaches from others; they would rather give up their own intentions and become subordinate to others. Usually there are coexisting wishes of dependency that others shall acknowledge the sacrifice and turn their attention and love to them. In others this may provoke an aggressive defense mechanism, which may appear as a hostile dissociation. These mismatched expectations mainly affect the patient's partnerships, when self-sacrifice and the excessive demand of love become overbearing.

Depression is especially common among patients seen in a medical setting. In turn, it may affect patient motivation toward recovery and is associated with poorer medical outcomes.

Delusional Disorder. The presence of delusion defines psychosis. A delusion is a false idea on which the patient is absolutely fixed. A delusion is deemed to be a basic psychotic phenomenon, in which the objective falseness and impossibility of the delusional content are usually easy to realize. Delusional convictions are not simple misbeliefs; they are constitutions of an abnormal mind that refer to the individual's cognitive experiences of his or her environment – their ego–environment relationship. Delusions are not voluntarily invented by the patients: they are caused by psychotic experiences. From the psychodynamic point of view, a delusional disorder is a special consequence of abnormal self-development. The delusion derives from the patient's desire to be in a safe place, away from the tension caused by the brittleness and contradictoriness of the patient's ego–environment relationship. The subjective certainty of the delusion's content causes its incorrectability: patients consistently keep their convictions, without considering their incompatibility with reality. Neither contrary experiences nor logical arguing can influence them. By definition, delusional patients have no insight, and others cannot talk them out of their belief system.

The type of delusional patient most often seen by the dermatologist is not the schizophrenic, but the patient with monosymptomatic hypochondriacal psychosis. Monosymptomatic hypochondriacal psychosis is characterized by a delusional ideation held by a patient that revolves around one particular hypochrondriacal concern, while with schizophrenia, many other mental functions become compromised, besides the presence of delusional ideation.

Obsessive–Compulsive Disorder. Obsessive–compulsive symptoms may be seen across the whole spectrum of psychopathology. In early childhood, they may occur as a temporary phenomenon in response to stress or anxiety, e.g., trichotillomania; they may occur as a psychoneurotic symptom in a person with an obsessive–compulsive personality configuration, e.g., onychophagia or acne excoriée; they may occur as a feature of the obsessive–compulsive disorder; or they may also occur in patients with psychosis. Individuals with an obsessive–compulsive personality configuration are rigid, perfectionist, and indecisive for fear of making a mistake; they lack self-confidence, are sensitive to criticism, and are socially reserved. Perhaps most importantly, they have profound difficulty in handling anger and aggression, which sometimes is explosive and at other times is displaced into self-destructive picking of the skin rather than being expressed directly in a modulated fashion. The essential feature of obsessive–compulsive disorder required for diagnosis is recurrent obsessions or compulsions that are severe enough to be time-consuming or cause impairment in relationships, employment, school, or social activities. An obsession is a persistent idea, thought, impulse, or image that intrudes into a person's consciousness uncontrollably and causes distress, anxiety, and often feelings of shame. The individual with obsessive–compulsive disorder realizes that the obsession is inappropriate and irrational but cannot resist. The obsessional concerns often lead to compulsive acts. Compulsions are repetitive, stereotyped motor acts, often ritualized, and designed to reduce intolerable anxiety or distress. Obsessions may involve themes of aggression (harming self or others), contamination (dirt, germs, body secretions), sex (forbidden thoughts or impulses), religion (concern with blasphemy or sacrilege), or somatic concerns.

Patients suffering from obsessive–compulsive disorder have insight into their condition, whereas delusional patients do not.

The clinical manifestations on the hair and scalp of the respective psychopathologic conditions are listed in Table 5.1.

Table 5.1 Psychopathologic conditions and their clinical manifestations on the hair and scalp

Manifestations of generalized anxiety disorder:
Neurotic excoriations of the scalp
Scalp dysesthesia
Manifestations of depressive disorder:
Neurotic excoriations of the scalp
Scalp dysesthesia
Imaginary hair loss (psychogenic pseudoeffluvium)
Manifestations of delusional disorder:
Delusions of parasitosis
Imaginary hair loss (psychogenic pseudoeffluvium)
Manifestations of obsessive–compulsive disorder:
Trichotillomania
Neurotic excoriations of the scalp
Factitial dermatitis of the scalp

5.3.1 Neurotic Excoriations of the Scalp

The term neurotic excoriations refers to patients with self-inflicted excoriations of the scalp in the absence of an underlying specific dermatologic disease condition. The etiology is varied, and psychiatrically, patients with neurotic excoriations are not a homogenous group, each requiring an individual therapeutic approach.

The condition may occur at any time from childhood to old age, with the most severe and recalcitrant cases reportedly starting in the third to fifth decade.

Because the patients, by definition, can inflict lesions only on those areas of the body that can be reached, and because patients tend to excoriate areas that are easily accessible, the clinical distribution of lesions besides the scalp can give a clue to the diagnosis. The lesions may affect the scalp in an isolated manner or may be associated with excoriations of the face and/or of the upper trunk and extensor aspects of the arms. The excoriations may be initiated by minor irregularities of the skin surface, such as a keratin plug, insect bite, acne papule (acne excoriée), or irritated hair follicle, or may start de novo. There is a decreased threshold for itch with tendency to habitual or neurotic scratching. Picking activity may start inadvertently as the hand comes across on an irregularity of the skin, or it may occur in an organized and ritualistic manner, sometimes using an auxiliary instrument, such as the point of a knife, etc. Tissue damage itself may again trigger itching, and the itch–scratch cycle may take on a life of its own. This activity typically takes place when the patient is unoccupied, and precipitating psychosocial stressors are usually present.

Neurotic excoriations occur across the spectrum of psychopathology. In mild and transient cases, it may be a response to stress, particularly in the younger patient, such as examination stress (thinker's itch), mainly in someone with obsessive–compulsive personality traits. In the more severe and sustained cases, psychiatric evaluation may diagnose a generalized anxiety disorder, depression, or obsessive–compulsive disorder.

The inflicted lesions are rather nonspecific. Varying in size from a few millimeters to several centimeters in the well-developed case, lesions are seen in all stages of evolution, from small superficial saucerized excoriations, to deep scooped-out skin defects (Fig. 5.2), to thickened hyperpigmented nodules, and finally to hypopigmented atrophic scars. Secondary bacterial infection may lead to regional lymphadenopathy. The histology is that of an excoriation with nonspecific inflammatory changes. Microbiological studies may reveal secondary bacterial infection, usually with *S. aureus*.

Since other dermatologic conditions can lead to similar lesions as neurotic excoriations of the scalp, clinicians must be careful not to make this diagnosis on the basis of the morphology of lesions alone. Specifically, pruritic skin conditions of dermatologic or other origins need to be excluded.

Examples are atopic dermatitis, folliculitis necrotica, chronic cutaneous lupus erythematosus, pemphigus vulgaris, pemphigoid, parasitic infestation, neurologic disorders, and other psychiatric disorders, such as cocaine intoxication, delusions of parasitosis, and factitial dermatitis.

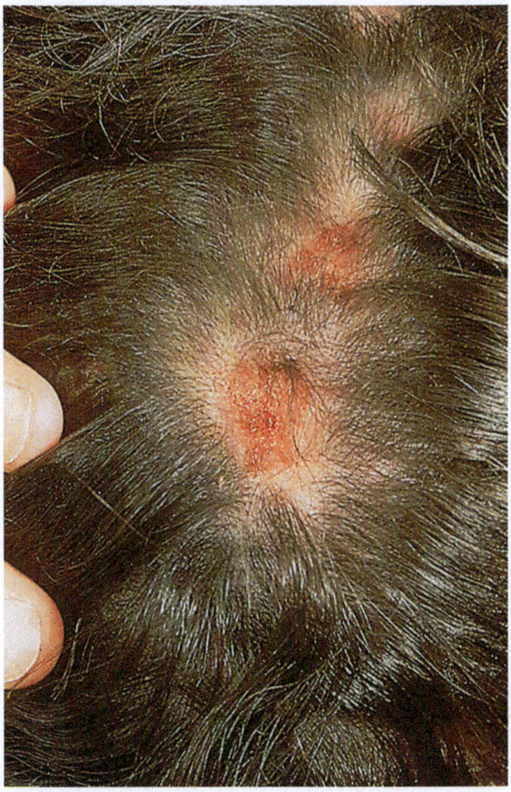

Fig. 5.2 Neurotic excoriations of the scalp

Most importantly, one needs to confirm the diagnosis by ascertaining the presence of psychopathology through both clinical observation and direct patient questioning.

Dermatologic treatment includes the prescription of non-irritating or "sensitive" shampoos, topical glucocorticoid–antibiotic cream preparations, and sedative antihistamines, such as hydroxyzine or doxepin, preferably given at nighttime. Cool compresses are soothing, provide hydration, and facilitate debridement of crusts. When followed by the application of an emollient, they reduce any contribution that xerosis makes to itching. When present, secondary bacterial infection must be treated appropriately, usually with a short course of oral antibiotics.

Psychiatric treatment includes nonpharmacologic and pharmacologic therapeutic options. In both, the choice of the appropriate technique or pharmacologic agent depends on the underlying mental disorder.

Although behavioral modification, cognitive psychotherapy, psychodynamic psychotherapy, and an eclectic approach have met variable success, many patients who present to the dermatologist are reluctant to agree to the psychiatric nature of their skin disorder and lack insight into the circumstances that trigger the drive to excoriate. Unless the patient is managed in a liaison clinic where dermatologists and psychiatrists can confer, it is the dermatologist who will take the responsibility for treatment.

If the patient is suffering from excessive stress, there are specific and nonspecific approaches. Those individuals who can find specific, real-life solutions to the difficulties they report are the more fortunate ones. Many patients experience stress from work or home relationships for which there is no easy way out. For these patients, a nonspecific solution to the stress can still be beneficial. Among the nonspecific solutions to stress, there are nonpharmacologic and pharmacologic means. The nonpharmacologic means include exercise, biofeedback, yoga, self-hypnosis, progressive relaxation, and other techniques learned in stress-management courses. Some patients do not have time to take stress-management courses, and others have special difficulty benefiting from this type of approach, for example, those who are not psychologically minded. For these patients, cautious use of antianxiety agents may be an alternative. In general, there are two types of anxiolytics: a quick-acting benzodiazepine type that can be sedating and produce dependency, such as alprazolam, and a slow-acting non-benzodiazepine type that is nonsedating and does not produce dependency, such as buspirone. Alprazolam differs from the older benzodiazepines such as diazepam and chlordiazepoxide because its half-life is short and predictable. Another advantage is that it has an antidepressant effect, whereas most other benzodiazepines generally have a depressant effect. Because of the possible risk of addiction with long-term use, the most prudent way of using alprazolam would be to restrict its use to 2–3 weeks. If the patient requires long-term therapy for anxiety, buspirone may be considered. However, it must be kept in mind that the effect of buspirone is usually not experienced by the patient for the first 2–4 weeks of treatment. Also, buspirone cannot be used on an "as-needed" basis. If buspirone does not work for a patient with chronic anxiety disorder, an alternative would be the use of low-dose doxepin. Even though doxepin is a tricyclic antidepressant, in low doses, it has been compared to benzodiazepines in terms of its anxiolytic effects. Sometimes, also a low dose of a low-potency antipsychotic agent such as thioridazine can be used.

Although there are a number of nonpharmacologic treatment options for depression, most dermatologists have neither the time nor the training to execute these treatment modalities. Nonetheless, it is advantageous to be conscious of these options, especially for those patients who agree to a referral to a mental health professional. Individual psychotherapy can be useful if there are definable psychological issues to be discussed, e.g., frustrations at work, a maladaptive style in interpersonal relationships, and the presence of maladaptive views of oneself, such as unrealistic expectations or fear of failure. Other patients have neurobiological predispositions to depression, and their depressive episodes may not be associated with any identifiable psychosocial difficulties. For these patients, the use of specific psychopharmacologic agents may in fact correct the primary cause of their depression. There are a number of antidepressants to choose from for the treatment of depression pharmacologically. Among the tricyclic antidepressants, again doxepin is probably the most suitable for the treatment of depressed patients with neurotic excoriations. If the patient cannot tolerate the sedative side effect of doxepin, desipramine or one of the newer, nontricyclic antidepressants such as fluoxetine, sertraline, and paroxetine are alternatives.

Finally, for the obsessive–compulsive patient with neurotic excoriations, there are, once again, nonpharmacologic and pharmacologic therapeutic options. However, if the dermatologist were to follow a nonpharmacologic approach for patients who reject referral to a mental health professional, it would have to be a technique that is simple enough to perform in a dermatologic setting. One such technique is the invocation of a "1- or 5-minute rule," a simple behavioral technique to try to interrupt the progression from obsessive thoughts to compulsive behavior. The patient is asked to try to put an interval of 1–5 min between the occurrence of the obsessive thought and the execution of the compulsive behavior. Once the patient is successful in refraining for 1 min, the time is gradually increased to 5, 10, or even 15 min, and, eventually, with such a long interruption between the obsessive thought and the compulsive behavior, one anticipates to break the natural progression from one to the other. In a dermatologic setting, the pharmacologic approach may be most feasible for patients who refuse to be referred elsewhere. Moreover, the recognition that serotonin pathways are involved and that the SSRI group of antidepressant agents reduces compulsive activity has made it more likely that the dermatologist will meet with success. Frequent short visits should be scheduled for supervision of the dermatologic regimen and for emotional support, and either clomipramine (an older antidepressant with extensive documentation about its anti-obsessive–compulsive efficacy in the medical literature) or one of the newer SSRIs (fluoxetine or fluvoxamine maleate) should be prescribed.

5.3.2 Imaginary Hair Loss (Psychogenic Pseudoeffluvium)

Patients with imaginary hair loss or psychogenic pseudoeffluvium are frightened of the possibility of going bald or are convinced they are going bald without any objective findings of hair loss. Basically they suffer from what Cotterill has termed "dermatologic nondisease." Although dermatologists are used to seeing patients with minor skin and hair problems in significant body areas that cause disproportionate anxiety and cosmetic distress, with dermatologic nondisease, there is no dermatologic pathology.

> It is important to realize that imaginary hair loss only makes up for a minority of patients complaining of hair loss and that patients with psychogenic pseudoeffluvium have varied underlying mental disorders.

The most common underlying psychiatric problems present are depressive disorder and body dysmorphic disorder. The clinical spectrum is wide, and the majority of patients are at the neurotic end of the spectrum and merely have overvalued ideas about their hair, whereas a minority of patients are truly deluded and suffer from delusional disorder. These patients lie at the psychotic end of the psychiatric spectrum. Those parts of the body that are important in body image are the focus of the preoccupation and concern.

True telogen effluvium resulting from androgenetic alopecia, telogen effluvium, or involutional alopecia must carefully be excluded.

> Differential diagnosis of psychogenic pseudoeffluvium is particularly challenging, since there is a considerable overlap between hair loss and psychological problems. Patients with hair loss have lower self-confidence, higher depression scores, greater introversion, and higher neuroticism and feelings of being unattractive.

A careful medical history, including medications, hormones, and crash diets, clinical examination of the hair and scalp (no alopecia, normal scalp), hair calendar (normal counts of hairs shed), trichogram (normal anagen and telogen rates), and laboratory work-up should be performed to exclude real effluvium and if necessary repeated.

In addition to the relentless complaint of hair loss, patients suffering from body dysmorphic disorder adopt obsessional, repetitive ritualistic behavior and may come to spend the majority of the day in front of a mirror, repeatedly checking their hair. Another aspect of this behavior is a constant need for reassurance about the hair, not only from the immediate family but also from the medical profession and from dermatologists in particular. These patients may become the most demanding types of patient to try to manage. The first step in the treatment is to establish a good rapport with the patient.

> It is important to recognize that patients with psychogenic pseudoeffluvium are expecting the clinician to treat them with respect as a trichologic patient and not as a psychiatric case. The most effective approach to psychogenic pseudoeffluvium is to take the chief complaint seriously and give the patient a complete trichologic examination.

Patients with overvalued ideas may respond to a sympathetic and unpatronizing dermatologist.

Psychotherapy is aimed at any associated symptomatology of depression, regardless of whether there is a causal relationship between the psychiatric findings and the imagined hair loss, because it is possible that patients who are depressed perceive even normal hair shedding in an exaggerated manner.

Patients with anxiety related to the fear of hair loss may also benefit from anxiolytic therapy with alprazolam or buspirone.

Many different treatments have been advocated to treat patients with body dysmorphic disorder: a wide variety of psychotropic agents (including tricyclic antidepressants and benzodiazepines) and antipsychotic drugs (including pimozide and thioridazine) have been tried in this condition, with poor results. Although there have been no controlled clinical trials of the treatment of patients with body dysmorphic disorder, preliminary data indicate that SSRIs, such as fluoxetine and fluvoxamine maleate, may be effective, though the effective dosage of the SSRI drugs needs to be higher than the dosage conventionally employed to treat depression, and the duration of treatment is long term. Response to this group of drugs takes up to 3 months, and not all patients with body dysmorphic disorder will respond to treatment with SSRIs. In patients who fail to respond to SSRIs given for 3 months, it has been suggested to add either buspirone to the SSRIs or, if the patient has delusional body dysmorphic disorder, to add an antipsychotic agent such as pimozide.

> Patients with body dysmorphic disorder expect the solutions to their problems in dermatologic (trichotropic agents) or surgical terms (hair transplantation).

Accordingly, following an initial consultation, it is common for a patient with body dysmorphic disorder to be given dermatologic treatment for alopecia. After repeated consultations with the patient, the dermatologist realizes that he or she is dealing with dermatologic nondisease. The result is often a frustrated dermatologist and a patient who eventually defaults from follow-up. The long and tough consultations, repeated telephone calls, and constant need for reassurance can put a significant strain on the dermatologist involved. Finally, a minority of patients with dysmorphic body disorder are angry, and these patients can direct this anger not only at themselves but also at the attending physician, with reproachful letters (Fig. 5.3), threats, and even physical violence. It is important not to reject these patients and treat them mechanistically, but to adopt an empathetic approach.

The prognosis depends on the underlying psychopathology, its appropriate treatment, and the attending physician's capability to reassure and guide the patient.

5.3.3 Dorian Gray Syndrome

The recently proposed *Dorian Gray syndrome* denotes a cultural and societal phenomenon characterized by extreme pride in one's own appearance accompanied by difficulties coping with the

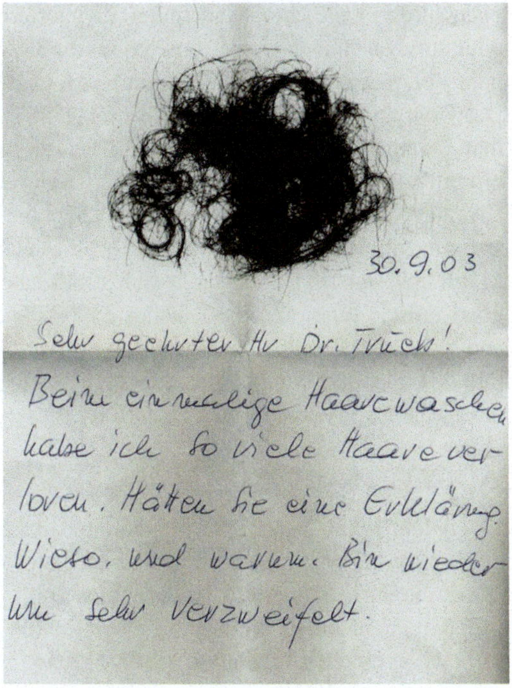
30.9.03

Sehr geehrter Hr. Dr. Trüeb!
Beim einmalige Haarwaschen habe ich so viele Haare verloren. Hätten Sie eine Erklärung Wieso, und warum. Bin wiederum sehr verzweifelt.

Fig. 5.3 Letter from a patient with overvalued ideas concerning hair shedding

aging process. Sufferers of Dorian Gray syndrome are by definition users of cosmetic medical procedures and products in an attempt to preserve their youth, including hair growth restorers.

The syndrome was first described on the occasion of a symposium on lifestyle drugs and aesthetic medicine and is named after Oscar Wilde's famous gothic horror novel "The Picture of Dorian Gray," in which the protagonist, a beautiful young aesthete, exclaims in front of his portrait:

> Why should it keep what I must lose? Every moment that passes takes something from me, and gives something to it. Oh, if it were only the other way! If the picture could change, and I could be always what I am now! For that - for that - I would give everything! Yes, there is nothing in the whole world I would not give! I would give my soul for that!

The syndrome probably represents a variant of body dysmorphic disorder. Body dysmorphic disorder represents a condition in which sufferers are intensely preoccupied with an imagined or grossly exaggerated defect in some aspect of their physical appearance. They are more likely to consult physicians for correction of the "defect" than to seek help from mental health professionals. The particularity of the Dorian Gray syndrome is that patients wish to remain forever young and seek lifestyle drugs and surgery to deter the natural aging process (Table 5.2).

Table 5.2 Criteria for the diagnosis of Dorian Gray syndrome

Signs of body dysmorphic disorder
Inability to mature and to progress in terms of psychological development
Use of at least two of the following medical/surgical lifestyle treatments (different groups required):
1. Hair growth-promoting agents
2. Weight-reducing agents
3. Agents to treat erectile dysfunction
4. Mood-modifying agents
5. Minimal invasive cosmetic dermatologic procedures
6. Cosmetic surgery

From Brosig et al (2001) The "Dorian Gray Syndrome": psychodynamic need for hair growth restorers and, other "fountains of youth." *Int J Clin Pharmacol Ther* 39: 279–283

An estimated 3 % of the total population in Western society displays features of the syndrome. Disastrous results of excessive plastic surgery and cosmetic dermatologic procedures are found under www.oddee.com/item_96587.aspx. Among the ten worst male celebrity examples are Michael Jackson (1958–2009) and Pete Burns (of "Dead or Alive"). If the defensive "acting out" character of the syndrome is not understood properly and the patient incessantly uses lifestyle products without understanding the underlying psychodynamics, a chronic state of narcissistic emptiness may develop. Depressive episodes and suicidal crisis are often observed if medical and surgical lifestyle treatments as means of defense are not sufficient to preserve the patient's idea of beauty.

Beauty is an abstract concept and has been an object of interest and discussion both of philosophers since Ancient Greece and of evolutionary scientists. The earliest Western theory on beauty can be found in the records of early

Greek philosophers from the pre-Socratic period, such as Pythagoras (570–495 BC). The Pythagorean school believed in a strong association between mathematics and beauty; in particular, they noted that objects proportioned according to the *golden ratio* seemed more attractive. Plato (428–348 BC) considered beauty to be the idea (form) above all other ideas. Aristotle (384–322 BC) saw a relationship between the beautiful and virtue, arguing that "virtue aims at the beautiful." The classical Greek noun for beauty was *kállos*, and the Koine Greek word for beautiful was *hōraios*, an adjective etymologically coming from the word *hōra*, meaning "hour." In Koine Greek, beauty was thus associated with "being of one's hour."

Therefore, a ripe fruit (of its time) was considered beautiful, whereas a young being trying to appear older or an older being trying to appear younger would not be considered beautiful.

Beauty has been understood as an individual's subjective appraisal of attractiveness that is influenced by cultural standards. Sociocultural images of beauty are best reflected in a variety of popular beauty icons. However, despite some unique cultural variabilities in aesthetic judgements, evidence has shown that similar patterns emerge across different cultures. Moreover, a set of convincing studies confirm that our perception of attractiveness predate cultural influences. Studies in infants have suggested that the ability to discriminate attractive from unattractive faces may be an innate abilities or at least one acquired at an earlier age than previously believed. For the International Mate Selection Project, 50 scientists studied 10,047 people in 37 cultures located on 6 continents and 5 islands and found that without exception, physical signs of youth and health were perceived as attractive. In his seminal "The Descent of Man and Selection in Relation to Sex," Charles Darwin (1809–1882) reflected on the physical characteristics that seemed to act as open lures to predators and therefore interfere with survival. For example, how could the brilliant plumage of peacocks have evolved? Darwin's answer was *sexual selection*, that is, that certain characteristic evolved because of reproductive advantage rather than survival advantage. The evolutionary argument hypothesizes that physical signs of youth and health, such as full lips, smooth skin, clear eyes, lustrous hair, good muscle tone, animated facials expression, and high energy level, are at the top of every culture's beauty list, simply because they are the most reliable physical signals for fertility.

Contemporary research has attempted to identify the physical features that account for the attractiveness of an individual and has recognized several factors: facial and body symmetry, averageness of appearance (koinophilia), body-size ratios, and youthfulness.

Youthfulness in particular marks an extended period of reproductive potential. Looking young may be more important than actually being young, and altering facial features in the direction of youth results in higher ratings of attractiveness.

In the 1990s, *body image* became one of the hottest topics covered by numerous professional textbooks and hundreds of journal articles. In a landmark publication, "Exacting Beauty," Thompson et al. pointed out that at least 14 terms are used with reference to body image and that body image is akin to *self-esteem*. Thompson et al. suggested that body image has come to be accepted as the internal representation of our own outer appearance and plays a significant role in how people feel about both their appearance and themselves. While there is little agreement to the exact definition of body image, there is a consensus that body image is a multidimensional construct: *perceptual influences* account for an individual's capacity to determine the physical features of a specific body part; *developmental influences* take the influence of childhood and adolescent experiences, such as appearance-related teasing, into consideration; and *sociocultural influences* relate to the interaction of the mass media and cultural ideas of appearance, which frequently portray unrealistic or exaggerated iconic images of beauty.

Finally, the issue of *body image dissatisfaction* determines behaviors to improve body image, from cosmetic to cosmetic surgical procedures.

> Body image dissatisfaction falls into a continuum from a dislike of a specific appearance feature to psychopathological dissatisfaction.

Sarwer et al. suggested that attitudes toward the body condition have two dimensions: The first consists of *valence*, defined as the degree of importance of body image to one's self-esteem, and the second consists of *value*, which is understood as the degree of satisfaction or dissatisfaction with the body image. The theory of body image can be used to understand physical appearance concerns and the relentless pursuit of an improved body image through respective behaviors.

In contrast to the substantial literature on the psychology of physical appearance and attractiveness, relatively little has been published on the impact of androgenetic alopecia. In the earliest study, published in 1971, sketches of balding men were rated as weak, inactive, and least potent; those of bald men were considered as most unkind, bad, ugly, and hard; while men with a full head of hair were seen as most handsome, virile, and active. Because of the limited validity of a study design with sketches of men, Cash subsequently conducted a controlled study on the first impressions brought forth by photographs of 18 men with visible androgenetic alopecia compared with 18 men with a full head of hair, who were matched on age, facial expression, attire, and other physical features. Adults of both sexes judged balding men as older and less physically and socially attractive that their non-balding peers. When the physical attractiveness differences between balding and non-balding men were statistically removed, all other perceived differences disappeared as well.

> Further research corroborated that baldness diminishes perceived attractiveness and youthfulness.

Although androgenetic alopecia may initially influence social perceptions, the more important issue is whether hair loss affects the individual's own psychological well-being and quality of life. Patients' reactions to their hair loss relate more to self-perceptions of their alopecia than to objective clinical ratings. Extreme distress in some patients may involve body dysmorphic disorder, a condition in which sufferers are intensely preoccupied with an imagined or grossly exaggerated defect in some aspects of their physical appearance.

> Hair thinning and the fear of baldness are a focal preoccupation in 50 % of body dysmorphic disorder cases, second only to the skin at 65 %.

5.3.4 Delusions of Parasitosis (Ekbom's Disease)

In delusions of parasitosis or Ekbom's disease, there is an unshakable conviction that the skin is infested by parasites. In the older literature, this condition is also described as "parasitophobia" or "acarophobia." However, the terms with "phobia" attached to them are misnomers and should be omitted, because in classic phobia, patients are aware of the fact that their fearful reactions are both excessive and irrational, while in the case of delusions of parasitosis, the patient is truly convinced of the validity of his or her perceptions.

In dermatologic practice, the type of delusional patient most frequently seen is the patient with a delusional ideation that revolves around only one particular hypochondriacal concern. These patients are said to suffer from monosymptomatic hypochondriacal psychosis. These patients are different from other psychotic patients, such as schizophrenics or patients with a major depression, since the latter have many deficits in mental functioning, which is not the case in patients with monosymptomatic hypochondriacal psychosis. Moreover, a delusional disorder appears to run distinct from schizophrenia and mood disorders and does not appear to be a prodrome to either of these conditions. From a nosological point of view, delusions of parasitosis are classified as a delusional disorder of the somatic type/with predominantly somatic delusions.

In the medical literature, the typical patient with delusions of parasitosis is reported to be a middle-aged woman, though there seems to be a bimodal distribution of age group.

Delusion of parasitosis is frequently encountered in patients in their 20s and 30s of either sex who are at a lower socioeconomic status and who have a marginal existence in society, in work, and in interpersonal relationships.

Patients report cutaneous sensations such as crawling, biting, and stinging, which they relate to their unshakable conviction that their skin is infested by parasites. They often bring in bits of dry skin, debris, and other specimens to try to prove the existence of these "parasites" (Fig. 5.4). Sometimes secondary injury to the skin or infection such as cellulitis may result from excessive scratching or the attempt to remove the "parasites" from the skin.

Though the patient with delusions of parasitosis presenting to the dermatologist more frequently suffers from monosymptomatic hypochondriacal psychosis, it must be remembered that the presence of a delusional ideation may be one particular manifestation of a more global psychiatric derangement, such as schizophrenia or major depression.

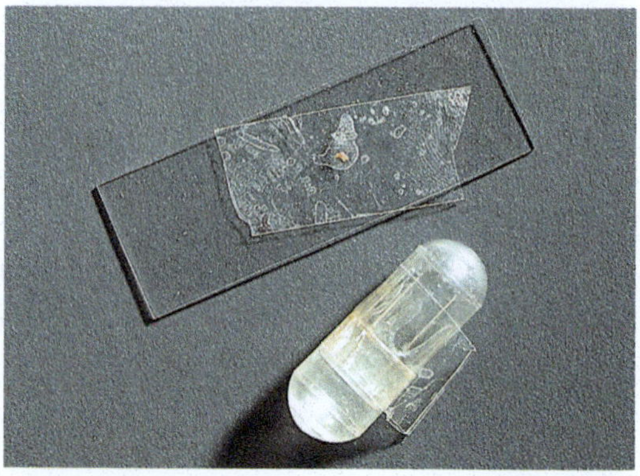

Fig. 5.4 Specimen brought in by a patient with delusion of parasitosis

Another subset of patients with delusions of parasitosis to consider are those who are substance abusers: drugs such as cocaine and amphetamine can induce formication and sometimes a delusional state that can be clinically identical to that of idiopathic delusions of parasitosis. Because the induction of formication is so well known among cocaine users, this phenomenon has been labeled cocaine bugs among substance abusers.

Also, neurologic disorders, such as multiple sclerosis, pernicious anemia, and especially in the elderly brain dysfunction with manifest encephalomalacia due to cerebral arteriosclerosis, should be considered in the differential diagnosis.

Chronic tactile hallucinosis describes those unusual cases in which patients develop chronic tactile sensations without delusions or other definable psychiatric disturbances and without associated medical or neurologic conditions.

Finally, the presence of inflammatory and pruritic skin disorders or real infestation, such as pediculosis capitis and furunculoid myiasis of the scalp, should not be overlooked.

Since trying to talk a patient out of a delusion is generally counterproductive, the most feasible way to have an impact on delusional ideation is to start the patient on an antipsychotic drug.

Traditionally, pimozide was prescribed. Newer agents include risperidone and olanzapine. The most challenging aspect of managing patients with delusions of parasitosis is to try to get their cooperation in taking one of these agents. This results from the discrepancy between the patient's belief system and the clinician's understanding of the situation. The first step is to establish a good rapport with the patient. In trying to do so, it is important to recognize that the patient with delusions of parasitosis is expecting the clinician to treat him with respect as a skin patient, not as a psychiatric case. Therefore, the most effective approach is to take the chief complaint seriously, give the patient a good skin examination, and pay attention to whatever "specimens" are brought in.

However, one should not make any comment that may reinforce the patient's delusional ideation.

Once the clinician senses that a reasonable working relationship is established with the patient, psychopharmacological treatment is offered as an "empirical therapeutic trial," purposely avoiding any argument about the pathogenesis of the condition or the mechanism of action of the medication. No matter how skillful the clinician is, some delusional patients remain beyond reach. In this situation, the best the physician can do for the patient is simply to take on a supportive role and watch out for any secondary complication such as cellulitis, which may result from skin injury.

If untreated, the condition runs a chronic course. Many patients respond to pimozide, with symptomatic improvement occurring as early as 2 weeks after starting treatment, although several months of treatment may be needed for complete control. Most patients require ongoing maintenance therapy; some achieve remission; in a few, cure does occur. Remission is seldom associated with insight.

5.3.5 Trichotillomania

Trichotillomania involves the repetitive, uncontrollable pulling of one's hair, resulting in noticeable hair loss. It represents a disorder of impulse control. The disorder usually begins between early childhood and adolescence. It occurs six to seven times more frequently in children than in adults; before the age of 6, males predominate, thereafter females.

In younger children, trichotillomania results from a mild form of frustration in a climate of psychosocial stress and soon becomes a habitual practice.

From puberty onward, trichotillomania is related to more severe pathologic psychodynamics, and prognosis is more guarded, particularly in female patients.

Most commonly, scalp hair is pulled, resulting in ill-defined areas of incomplete hair loss. In the affected areas, there are different lengths of hair, short, longer, and normal (Fig. 5.5).

Associated features of trichotillomania may include excoriations of the scalp, nail biting (onychophagia), and eating of hairs (trichophagia) with the risk of gastrointestinal obstruction by a mass of hair (trichobezoar), a complication that has been termed the *Rapunzel syndrome*.

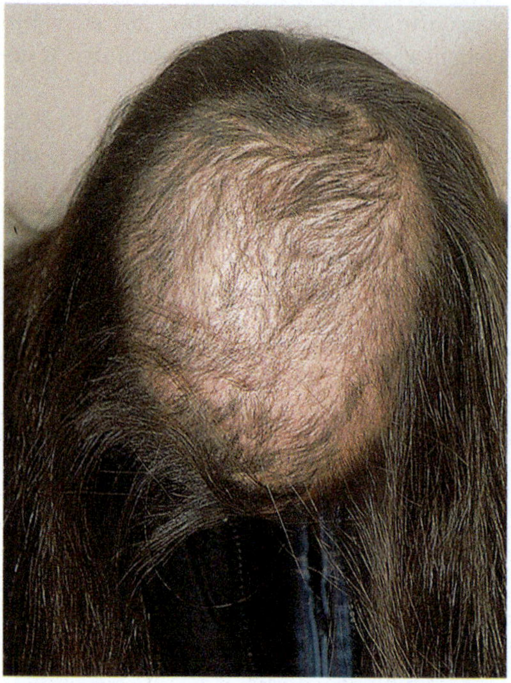

Fig. 5.5 Trichotillomania with tonsural pattern

Parents seldom notice their child's behavior, and most of them do not believe that their child would pull out his or her own hair. Once the diagnosis is suspected, it is confirmed in the following way:

1. With the parents out of the room, in a friendly way, ask the youngster to show you how this is done. This immediately tells the patient that you know what is going on and often initiates the disclosure or demonstration of how it is done.
2. If necessary, the next most simple way to prove the diagnosis is to perform a trichogram, which will typically show a significantly decreased telogen rate at the periphery of the area of hair loss (since the telogen hairs are more easily pulled out than the anagen hairs).
3. Finally, do a biopsy. This cannot rule out the diagnosis, but, if present, the following histopathologic findings will confirm it: wavy, wrinkled, corkscrew-shaped hair shaft (trichomalacia), the presence of many hairs in the catagen stage, and a lack of perifollicular inflammation (found in alopecia areata).

The most important differential diagnosis is alopecia areata. Moreover, trichotillomania may result from scratching at the site of alopecia areata that is symptomatic with pruritus, initiating a habit-forming behavior, and then poses a special diagnostic challenge. Alternatively, patients with a mental predisposition may artificially prolong the disfigurement as the hair on the bald patches of alopecia areata regrows, with the aim to maintain gratification of dependency needs, which were being met during alopecia areata.

Traumatic alopecia due to child abuse (battered child), though uncommon, is yet another differential diagnosis to take into consideration in a child with unexplained hair loss and other signs of physical trauma (Fig. 5.6).

Children with trichophagia should be screened for iron deficiency as part of their evaluation, since the association of *pica* – an unusual craving for nonfood items – and iron deficiency has been reported. The compulsive oral behavior characteristically resolved with the oral administration of therapeutic doses of iron. It must be kept in mind though that iron deficiency may either be a cause of trichophagia or result from gastrointestinal bleeding in the case of trichobezoar.

The primary treatment approach for trichotillomania is habit reversal combined with stress management and behavioral contracting. Parents can help by recognizing the problem in its early stages and getting involved in its treatment. Treatment may involve self-monitoring of hair-pulling episodes as well as the feelings and situations that are most likely to lead to hair pulling. Youngsters are then systematically introduced to new behaviors, for example, squeezing a ball or tightening their fist whenever they feel the urge to pull at their hair. Relaxation training and other stress-reduction techniques may also be used,

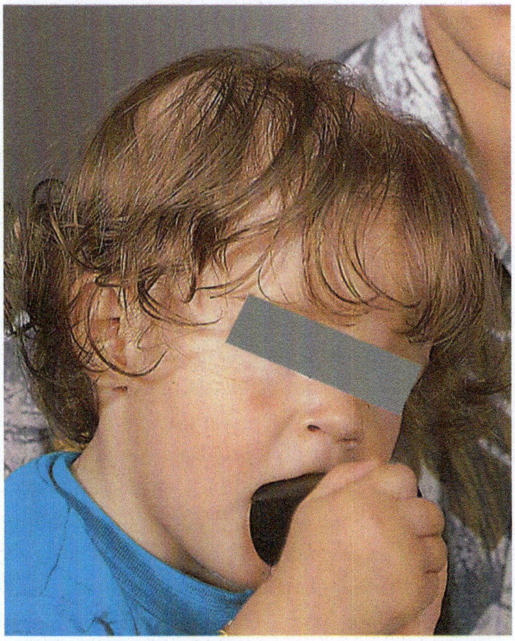

Fig. 5.6 Traumatic alopecia due to child abuse (battered child). Note hematoma in the face

including reward charts that help track and monitor a child's progress with the added incentive of earning small rewards for continued progress. In addition, cognitive therapy is found to be effective.

The younger the patient, the smaller the percentage of cases referred to a psychiatrist; the rest are treated by the dermatologist who applies his or her own psychiatric knowledge (liaison psychiatry). A proper follow-up is required to establish whether improvement has actually occurred. When the symptom is present in adolescents or adults, competent help from a psychiatrist should be sought.

In a dermatologic setting, a pharmacologic approach may be most feasible for patients who refuse to be referred elsewhere. Basically, the same pharmacologic agents are used for the treatment of trichotillomania as for obsessive–compulsive disorder: the older tricyclic antidepressants imipramine and clomipramine and the newer selective serotonin reuptake inhibitors (SSRIs) fluoxetine, fluvoxamine, sertraline, and paroxetine. Physicians using SSRIs for the treatment of patients with obsessive–compulsive disorders or trichotillomania are cautioned that the duration of treatment is critical in determining adequate treatment. Improvement continues to occur when the drugs are taken beyond 8- or 12-week trials. A patient showing a partial response after 4–6 weeks would be expected to continue to improve during the following weeks. Cessation of pharmacotherapy results in a relapse in the majority of patients. Despite success with SSRIs, patients with obsessive–compulsive disorders tend to respond to medication with only partial symptom reduction, suggesting that obsessive–compulsive disorders may be a neurobiological heterogeneous disorder that may require alternative treatment options in the individual patient. For example, successful treatment of five adult trichotillomania patients with a combination of the SSRI escitalopram with the anticonvulsant topiramate was originally reported. Subsequently, Lochner et al. performed an open-label pilot study to investigate the efficacy and safety of topiramate in 14 adults with trichotillomania. They found that topiramate may be useful in the treatment of trichotillomania and suggested that future studies should investigate the efficacy of topiramate in an appropriately powered randomized placebo-controlled trial.

An interesting new therapy is based on the glutamate modulator *N*-acetylcysteine. It is hypothesized that *N*-acetylcysteine, an amino acid, restores the extracellular glutamate concentration in the nucleus accumbens and, therefore, offers promise in the reduction of compulsive behavior. In a 12-week, double-blind, placebo-controlled study performed in 50 individuals with trichotillomania (45 women and 5 men with a mean age [SD] of 34.3 [12.1]), Grant et al. originally found that *N*-acetylcysteine (dosing range, 1,200–2,400 mg/day) demonstrated statistically significant reductions in trichotillomania symptoms. No adverse events occurred in the *N*-acetylcysteine group, and *N*-acetylcysteine was well tolerated.

To examine the efficacy of *N*-acetylcysteine for the treatment of trichotillomania in children, Bloch et al. again performed a double-blind, placebo-controlled (add-on) study with a total of 39 children and adolescents aged 8–17 years with trichotillomania randomly assigned to receive the active agent or matching placebo for 12 weeks. No significant difference between *N*-acetylcysteine and placebo was found on outcome measures. It is noteworthy that on several measures of hair pulling, subjects significantly improved with time regardless of treatment assignment: in the *N*-acetylcysteine group, 25 % of subjects were judged as treatment responders, compared with 21 % in the placebo group.

Dronabinol, a cannabinoid agonist, represents yet another novel pharmacologic approach, again studied by Grant et al. The authors hypothesized that dronabinol reduces the excitotoxic damage caused by glutamate release in the striatum, again offering promise in reducing compulsive behavior. Fourteen female subjects with a mean age of 33.3 ± 8,9 diagnosed with trichotillomania were enrolled in a 12-week open-label treatment study of dronabinol (dose ranging from 2.5 to 15 mg/day). The authors found that dronabinol demonstrated statistically significant reductions in trichotillomania symptoms, in the absence of negative cognitive effects.

5.3.6 Factitial Dermatitis of the Scalp

Factitial dermatitis or factitious disorder with physical symptoms is a condition in which the patient creates lesions on the skin to satisfy a psychological need of which he or she is not consciously aware, usually a need to be taken care of by assuming the sick role. Patients with factitious disorder or factitial dermatitis create the lesions for psychological reasons and not for monetary or other discrete objectives as in the case of malingering. Patients knowingly fake symptoms but will deny any part in the process. They desire the sick role and may move from physician to physician in order to receive care. They are usually loners with an early childhood background of trauma and deprivation. They are unable to establish close interpersonal relationships and generally have severe personality disorders. Unlike malingerers, they follow through with medical procedures and are at risk for drug addiction and for the complications of multiple operations. In the more severe form known as Munchhausen syndrome or *laparotomophilia migrans*, a series of successive hospitalizations becomes a lifelong pattern.

Little is known about the etiology of factitious disorder. Besides the difficulties involved in making the diagnosis, the reluctance of these patients to undergo psychological testing and the heterogeneity in the details of cases published in the literature lie at the origin of this situation. Some clinicians have remarked that patients with factitious disorder often present traumatic events, particularly abuse and deprivation, and numerous hospitalizations in childhood and as adults lack support from relatives and/or friends. The majority of patients suffer from borderline personality disorder. Because of emotional deficits in early life and a frequent history of physical or sexual abuse, patients have failed to develop a stable body image with clearly defined physical and emotional boundaries. For these patients, the factitial lesions serve many purposes: the excitement and stimulation ease the sense of emptiness and isolation, and skin sensation defines boundaries and helps establish personal and sexual identity, whereas the sick role gratifies dependency needs. In all reported series, females outnumber male patients from 3:1 to 20:1; onset is highest in adolescence and early adulthood, and a remarkably high number of patients work, or have a close family member working, in the health-care field.

Factitial dermatitis of the scalp is only one aspect of the whole picture of factitious disease. The condition for which dermatologists are consulted often has already occasioned many visits to other physicians. The patient typically presents a bundle of normal investigative findings and a shopping bag filled with oral and topical medications. The lesions themselves are as varied as the different methods employed to create them; on the scalp, there are usually ulcerations (Fig. 5.7) or areas of cutoff hair (trichotemnomania). They are bizarre in shape and distribution and usually appear on normal skin. Though the possibilities are limitless, consistent is a "hollow" history – a term that refers to the patient's vagueness and inability to give details of how the lesions evolved. Consistent also are the affects of both

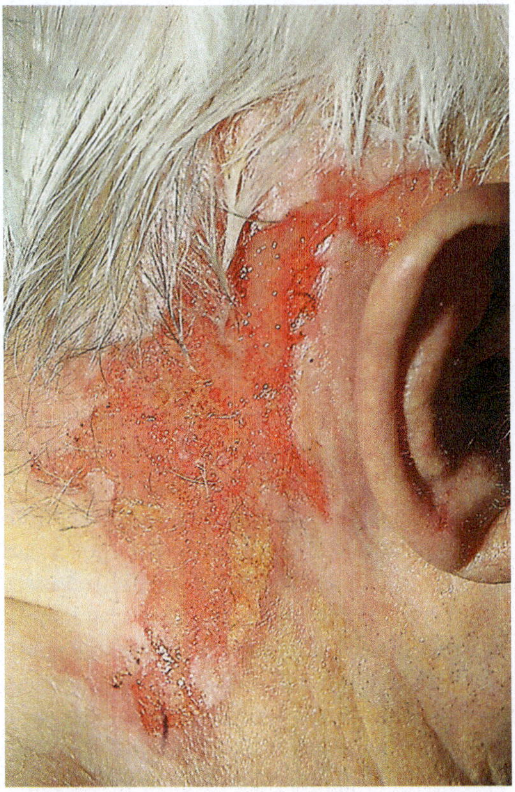

Fig. 5.7 Factitial dermatitis of the scalp

the patient and their family. Although the patient seems astonishingly unmoved by the lesions, the family is angry, accusatory, and critical of what they interpret as medical incompetence.

A number of dermatologic, neurologic, and mental disorders may share similar symptoms. Clinically the differential diagnostic considerations are determined by the morphology and cover the scope of clinical dermatology. Among the most important disorders affecting the scalp that have to be taken into consideration are necrotizing herpes zoster (shingles), temporal arteritis, angiosarcoma, neurotrophic ulcerations of the scalp, and neurotic excoriations of the scalp.

> With respect to the treatment of factitial dermatitis, the essential and probably most difficult step is to secure an enduring and stable patient–physician relationship.

For achieving this goal, most clinicians advocate a nonconfrontational strategy reframing the factitious manifestation as a "cry for help." An interesting approach is that of "contract conference." In this approach, the psychiatrist emphasizes the need for the patient to express himself/herself in the common language of difficult relationships, feelings, and problems in living instead of the (factitious) language of illness. After that, the patient and the clinician can focus their efforts on resolving those real problems. Once a stable relationship is installed, the management of the disorder must be oriented to avoid unnecessary hospitalizations and medical procedures.

Another important issue in the management of this condition is recognition and adequate treatment of frequently associated disorders, such as personality disorders, depression, drug and/or alcohol abuse and dependency, etc.

Dermatologic treatment is symptomatic and determined by the clinical presentation. The uses of occlusive dressings are a diagnostic tool rather than an effective therapeutic intervention, since success is only of a temporary nature. Because of the patient's intense emotional investment in their skin, it may be helpful to prescribe positive measures such as wet dressings, emollients, and other bland topicals to replace the prior destructive activity.

Some case reports focus on the use of pharmacological agents. A good response has been reported to the antipsychotic drug pimozide; other clinicians, because of the resemblance to the obsessive–compulsive disorder, advocate the use of clomipramine or the SSRIs fluoxetine and fluvoxamine maleate.

In the vast majority of patients, the condition remains chronic.

5.4 Chronic Cutaneous Sensory Disorders

Some patients only present with a cutaneous sensory complaint such as itching, burning, stinging, or other disagreeable sensations without any diagnosable dermatologic, neurologic, or medical diagnosis. Patients with chronic cutaneous sensory disturbance of unknown etiology can be divided into those with diagnosable psychiatric findings, such as a depression or anxiety, and those with no diagnosable psychiatric findings. The latter patients have been termed to be suffering from somatoform pain disorder.

In dermatology, the somatoform disorders consist of a heterogeneous pattern of differing clinical presentations based on a comparable emotional disorder, the characteristic of which is repeated presentation of physical symptoms in combination with a stubborn demand for medical examination, despite repeated negative results, and the physician's assurance that the symptoms have no physical basis. The term *dermatologic nondisease* has also been coined for this disorder.

The somatoform disorders have been further classified into:

1. Conversion disorder, also known as hysteria
2. Hypochondriacal and body dysmorphic disorder
3. Somatization disorder (Briquet's syndrome)
4. Somatoform pain disorder

Conversion Disorder. Conversion disorder is characterized by the loss of a bodily function. It is involuntary, and diagnostic testing does not show a somatic cause for the dysfunction. The patient with conversion disorder confronts an acute stressor, which creates a psychic conflict and the physical symptoms serve as the resolution of the conflict, while the patient may be unaware of the stressor. Conflicts or other stressors that precede the onset or worsening of the symptoms suggest that psychological factors are related to it. The disorder may be best thought of as disturbances of illness perception or need. They are paradigms of mind–body interactions and of the critical role that mental factors play in the production of illness. Again, the loss of function may symbolize the underlying conflict associated with it. Psychodynamic theory interprets the cause of the symptoms as a defense mechanism that absorbs and neutralizes the anxiety generated by an unacceptable impulse or wish. The patient doesn't consciously feign the symptoms for material gain or to occupy the sick role.

Hypochondriacal and Body Dysmorphic Disorder. Unlike conversion disorder, where the affected individual perceives a functional disorder and simply uses it to escape from uncomfortable situations, the patient with hypochondriacal disorder has no real illness but is overly obsessed over normal bodily functions. They read into the sensations of these normal bodily functions the presence of a feared illness. Because of misinterpreting bodily symptoms, they become preoccupied with ideas or fears of having a serious illness, while appropriate medical investigation and reassurance do not relieve these ideas. These ideas cause distress that is clinically important or impairs work, social, or personal functioning. They are not delusional (as in delusional disorder) and are not restricted to concern about appearance (as in body dysmorphic disorder). Hypochondriacal disorder usually develops in middle age or later and tends to run a chronic course. Patients typically seek many tests and much reassurance from their doctor.

Probably the more important group of problem patients for the dermatologist in practice is that with body dysmorphic disorder or "dysmorphophobia" (a term that is incorrect, since we are not dealing with a phobic disorder).

It is classified together with hypochondriacal disorder, though this classification will probably be abandoned in the future in favor of a new class of its own. This disorder tends to occur in younger adults. The patient becomes preoccupied with a nonexistent or minimal cosmetic defect and persistently seeks medical attention to correct it. Cases of body dysmorphic disorder can range from relatively mild to very severe. The patient is preoccupied with an imagined defect of appearance or is excessively concerned about a slight physical anomaly. This preoccupation causes clinically important distress or impairs work, social, or personal functioning. Another term used for body dysmorphic syndrome is *Thersites complex* (named after Thersites who was the ugliest soldier in Odysseus' army, according to Homer).

One of various theories attempting to make the onset of body dysmorphic disorder understandable is the "self-discrepancy theory," in which affected patients present conflicting self-beliefs with discrepancies between their actual and desired self. Patients have an unrealistic ideal as to how they should look. Media-induced factors are considered to predispose to body dysmorphic disorder by establishing role models for beauty and attractiveness.

Somatization Disorder. Somatization disorder presents with a pattern of recurrent, multiple somatic complaints that do not have an organic basis. Starting before the age of 30, the patient has usually had many physical complaints occurring over several years and sought treatment for them, or the complaints have materially impaired social, work, or personal functioning. Typically there is a combination of pain symptoms, related to different body sites or body functions, gastrointestinal symptoms, sexual dysfunction, and pseudoneurological symptoms. None of these are limited to pain (as in somatoform pain disorder). Physical or laboratory investigations determine that each of the symptoms cannot be fully explained by a general medical condition or by substance abuse, including medications and drugs of abuse, or if the patient does have a general medical condition, the impairment or complaint is greater than would be expected based on history and laboratory and physical examinations.

In dermatology, environment-related physical complaints, the so-called ecosyndromes, are noteworthy among the somatization disorders. The patients report multiple complaints in various organ systems, of which the purported cause is exposure to environmental toxins, without proof of any direct toxic causal relationship between exposure and symptomatology. Examples are the multiple chemical sensitivity syndrome and the amalgam-related complaint syndrome.

Occasionally, the complaint of hair loss is related to the amalgam in tooth fillings, and patients unnecessarily have all fillings removed and pay for expensive detoxification procedures.

Somatoform Pain Disorder. In somatoform pain disorder, by definition, pain is in the foreground. It is reported by the patient as clinically relevant, causes suffering and professional and/or social impairments, and cannot be adequately explained by either a somatic cause or another psychiatric disorder. In dermatology, mainly regional cutaneous or mucosal dysesthesias occur. Depending on their localization, specific names for the conditions are available, such as glossodynia (tongue), vulvodynia (vulva), and penodynia (penis).

5.4.1 Trichodynia

The term "trichodynia" was proposed for discomfort, pain, or paresthesia of the scalp related to the complaint of hair loss. Rebora found that 34.2 % of female patients, who had their hair consultation because of hair loss, complained of this phenomenon. In a subsequent survey, Grimalt et al. claimed that 22.1 % of their female patients reported trichodynia.

The cause of trichodynia is not understood, though it has been proposed that it is probably polyetiologic.

The most prevalent speculations with respect to the pathogenesis of trichodynia are perifollicular inflammation, increased expression of neuropeptide substance P localized in the vicinity of hair follicles, and underlying psychiatric disorders.

Originally, trichodynia was reported to be more prevalent in female patients with chronic telogen effluvium and to a lesser extent in patients with androgenetic alopecia. Rebora et al. proposed the symptom to be distinctive for chronic telogen effluvium.

Willimann and Trüeb's study on 403 patients (311 females, 92 males) whose main complaint was hair loss confirms the previously published findings in the literature that trichodynia affects a significant proportion of patients complaining of hair loss. The aim of the study was to assess the frequency of trichodynia in patients complaining of hair loss and its correlation with gender, age, cause, and activity of hair loss. It was found that 17 % of patients complaining of hair loss, i.e., 20 % of female patients and 9 % of male patients, reported "hair pain," pain or discomfort of the scalp, not otherwise explained by the presence of a specific dermatologic disease, such as psoriasis or eczema, or neurologic disorder, such as migraine equivalent.

Statistical analysis failed to demonstrate any significant correlation between trichodynia, the extent of hair thinning, and hair loss activity, quantified by the hair pull, daily hair count, wash test, and trichogram. It is noteworthy though that trichodynia typically increases the anxiety related to the patient's preoccupation with hair loss or fear of hair loss.

As opposed to the suggestion of Rebora et al. that trichodynia would be typical for chronic telogen effluvium, the symptom did not allow any discrimination with respect to the cause of hair loss, and was found with similar frequencies in association with androgenetic alopecia, chronic telogen effluvium, or a combination of both.

The cause of trichodynia remains obscure. Rebora et al. proposed a possible role of perifollicular microinflammation. Hoss and Segal interpreted scalp dysesthesia as a cutaneous dysesthesia syndrome related to underlying psychiatric disorders, with affected individuals either suffering from depressive, generalized anxiety, or somatoform disorder. Hordinsky and collaborators found localization of the neuropeptide substance P in the scalp of patients with painful scalp, suggesting a causal relationship between the presence of substance P and trichodynia. Substance P represents a neuropeptide involved in nociception and neurogenic inflammation.

Willimann and Trüeb proposed that trichodynia probably is polyetiologic. Though only a small number of patients with trichodynia in the studied patients showed telangiectasia of the scalp, this finding strongly correlated with the presence of trichodynia.

An interesting analogy is the observation of Lonne-Rahm et al. who found that patients with the telangiectatic variant of rosacea respond more frequently with stinging sensations to the topical application of 5 % lactic acid on the cheeks than patients with the papulopustular type of rosacea or normal controls. On the basis of these findings, they concluded that the blood vessels are of importance in stinging sensations and a connection exists between sensory or subjective irritation and cutaneous vascular reactivity. Also the observation of the development of cutaneous allodynia during a migraine attack provides clinical evidence for the relation of vascular changes and pain.

In this context, it is interesting to note that substance P not only represents an important mediator of nociception and neurogenic inflammation but also exerts a potent vasodilatory effect. The role of substance P and related substances (neuropeptides) in the pathogenesis of trichodynia and especially its relation to the nervous system and emotional stress need further elucidation.

> By the virtue of their bidirectional effects on the neuroendocrine and immune systems, substance P and other neuropeptides may well represent key players in the interaction between the central nervous system and the skin immune and microvascular system.

Such mechanisms would explain the noxious effects not only of external stimuli (mechanical, thermal, chemical) but also of emotional distress on cutaneous nociception through the release of neuropeptides, such as substance P. Interestingly, Paus and collaborators have recently demonstrated that stress-induced immune changes of the hair follicles in mice could be mimicked by injection of substance P in nonstressed animals and were abrogated by selective substance P receptor antagonism in stressed animals.

> A lower prevalence of male patients suffering from trichodynia might be connected to gender-related differences in pain perception, inasmuch as increase of pain perception in relation to anxiety scores has been found to be more pronounced in females.

Trichodynia tends to affect the centroparietal area of the scalp, seemingly surprising since the pain threshold of the centroparietal scalp is otherwise considered to be higher.

In the absence of any other specific morphologic changes of the scalp or correlation with quantitative parameters of hair loss, management of trichodynia remains empiric and empathetic, tailored to the individual patient's needs. The therapeutic choice includes non-irritating shampoos, topical antipruritic or anesthetic agents, topical capsaicin, corticosteroids, tricyclic antidepressants, gabapentin, and pregabalin. The efficacy of oral substance P (neurokinin 1 receptor) antagonists such as aprepitant in the treatment of pain and depression has so far not been convincing.

> As a general rule, topical overtreatment of the scalp is to be avoided. Most importantly, the patient needs to be reassured that trichodynia does not reflect hair loss activity, which may ease the patient's anxiety and in our experience also may beneficially influence cutaneous nociception.

Ultimately, the treatment of trichodynia with botulinum toxin (BTX) seems a rational approach, since there is increasing evidence that BTX decreases the mechanical sensitivity of nociceptors and inhibits neurogenic vasodilation through the inhibition of sensory neuropeptide release. BTX treatment can be done basically following the current migraine headache protocols.

5.4.2 Trichoteiromania

Trichoteiromania is the term originally coined by Freyschmidt-Paul et al. in 2001 for breakage of hair by forcefully rubbing an area of the scalp. The typical clinical presentation is that of a bald patch with broken hairs (Fig. 5.8). Subsequently, Reich and Trüeb reported four patients with trichoteiromania and further characterized them on the basis of clinical, morphological, and psychopathological criteria.

In contrast to trichotillomania, trichoteiromania has no diagnostic histopathological features and a normal trichogram. Traumatic changes to the hair shaft are more conspicuous, with splitting at the ends of the hairs, giving the impression of white tips.

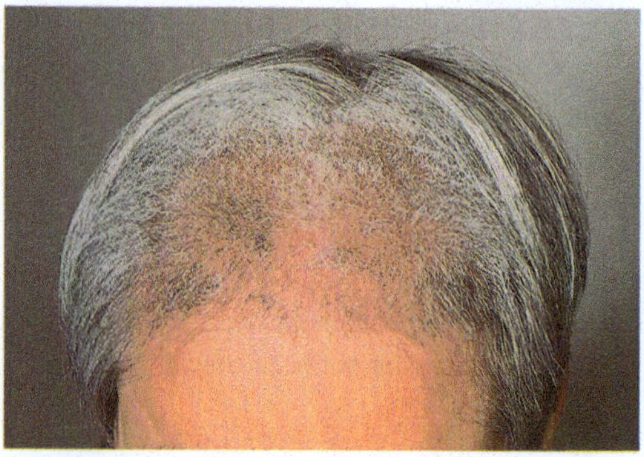

Fig. 5.8 Trichoteiromania

The underlying mental disorder in trichoteiromania varies among the patients, though an underlying cutaneous sensory disorder, not explained through any specific dermatologic disorder, is a common denominator in all cases.

While trichotillomania is considered to be an obsessive–compulsive disorder, the underlying mental disorder in trichoteiromania represents a more heterogeneous group, including anxiety, depression, or somatoform disorder.

Cooperation with the psychiatrist is indicated, in as much as the management and prognosis of trichoteiromania again will depend on the recognition of the underlying mental disorder and its specific psychotherapeutic and pharmacological treatment.

5.5 Adjustment Disorders

Even though most patients with hair disorders experience significant psychological impact, it is usually not of an intensity to qualify as a mental illness. Nevertheless, the impact that hair disorders have on body image significantly contributes to the overall impact on the patient's quality of life. If one appreciates the psychosocial impact of hair disease, there is no doubt that appropriate treatment frequently has a huge bearing on the patients' quality of life. The clinician should keep in mind that the distress the patient feels from having a hair disease can be handled both dermatologically and psychologically.

Some patients have difficulties adjusting to hair loss. As a result, the individual may have difficulty with his or her mood and behavior. From a psychopathological point of view, adjustment disorders may result from the stressful event of hair loss, depending on its acuity, extent, and prognosis. An adjustment disorder is a debilitating reaction to a stressful event or situation. These symptoms or behaviors are clinically significant as evidenced by either of the following: distress that is in excess of what would be expected or significant impairment in social, occupational, or educational functioning. Adjustment disorder subtypes include:

- Adjustment disorder with depressed mood
- Adjustment disorder with anxiety
- Adjustment disorder with mixed anxiety and depressed mood
- Adjustment disorder with disturbance of conduct
- Adjustment disorder with mixed disturbance of emotions and conduct

Associated features may be somatic and/or sexual dysfunction, feelings of guilt, and/or obsession.

The best way to alleviate the emotional distress caused by hair disease is to eliminate the hair disease that is causing the problem.

In other words, the intensity of the distress that the patient feels should be part of the clinician's formula in deciding how aggressively to treat the hair disease. For example, a decision to use or not to use topical minoxidil or oral finasteride in a patient with a borderline clinical state of androgenetic alopecia, or to recommend or not to recommend hair surgery to a patient with permanent alopecia, may hinge on the amount of distress the patient feels from the alopecia.

> Besides being a sympathetic and concerned professional, a dermatologist may give a referral to a support organization, such as the National Alopecia Areata Foundation.

First, many of these support organizations specialize in providing educational materials to patients and their relatives so they have an opportunity to inform themselves with respect to the nature and prognosis of their hair problem. Second, being part of such an organization breaks the sense of isolation patients often feel. Finally, by learning more about different treatment options, there is less risk that the patients will prematurely give up on treatment in despair and resign themselves to having uncontrolled alopecia. Keeping up hope is critical in not losing a positive outlook, in spite of having a chronic or recurrent condition.

5.6 Personality Disorders

In the Oxford Dictionary, *personality* is defined as the combination of characteristics or qualities that form an individual's distinctive character. From a psychological point of view, personality encompasses the organized pattern of behavioral characteristics of an individual.

The modern sense of individual personality is a result of the shifts in culture originating in the Renaissance. In contrast, Medieval Europe's sense of self was linked to a network of social roles that represented the building blocks of personhood: household, kinship network, or guild. There has been much debate over the subject of studying personality in a cross-cultural context, since some believe that personality comes entirely from culture, while others think that some elements are shared by all cultures and have made the effort to demonstrate the cross-cultural applicability of the *Big Five*, which are openness to experience, conscientiousness, extroversion, agreeableness, and neuroticism or emotionality.

Some ideas in the psychological and scientific study of personality include personality genetics, personality development (the concept that personality is affected by various sources), personality types (the patterns of relatively enduring characteristics of behavior that occur with sufficient frequency), personality traits (enduring personal characteristics that are revealed in a particular pattern of behavior in a variety of situations), personality psychology (the theory and study of individual differences, traits, and types), personality pathology (characterized by adaptive inflexibility, vicious cycles of maladaptive behavior, and emotional instability under stress), and the personality disorders.

Personality disorders (sometimes also called character disorders) refer to a group of mental disorders characterized by deeply ingrained maladaptive patterns of behavior and personality style, defined by the fourth edition, text revision (2000) of the Diagnostic and Statistical Manual of Mental Disorders (DSM) as sufficiently rigid and deep-seated to bring a person into repeated conflicts with his or her social and occupational environment. Personality disorders have their onset in adolescence or early adulthood, are stable over time, and cause significant emotional pain by the virtue of difficulties in relationships and occupational performance. In addition, the patient usually sees the disorder as being consistent with his or her self-image and may blame others for his or her social, educational, or work-related problems. In addition, DSM-IV specifies that these dysfunctional patterns must be regarded as nonconforming or deviant by the person's culture.

The study of human personality started in antiquity with Hippocrates' (460–370 BC) *four humors* and gave rise to *four temperaments*. The explanation was further refined by Galen (129–216 AD) during the second century AD. The four humors theory held that a person's personality was based on the balance of bodily humors: yellow bile, black bile, phlegm, and blood. Choleric people were characterized as having an excess of yellow bile, making them irascible. High levels of black bile were indicative of melancholy and pessimism. Phlegmatic people were thought to have an excess of phlegm, leading to their sluggish, calm temperament. Finally, people thought to have high levels of blood were said to be sanguine and were characterized by their cheerful, passionate dispositions. In his *Characters*, Theophrastus (371–287 BC) divided the people of the Athens of the fourth century BC into 30 different personality types. The *Characters* exerted a strong influence on subsequent studies of human personality such as those of Thomas Overbury (1581–1613) in England and Jean de la Bruyère (1645–1696) in France. The concept of personality disorder itself is much more recent and tentatively dates back to 1801 with French psychiatrist Philippe Pinel's (1745–1826) description of *manie sans délire*, a condition which he characterized as outbursts of rage and violence (*manie*) in the absence of any signs of psychotic illness such as delusions and hallucinations (*délires*). In 1896, German psychiatrist Emil Kraepelin (1856–1926) delineated seven forms of antisocial behavior under the umbrella of *psychopathic personality*. The term was later broadened by Kraepelin's younger colleague Kurt Schneider (1887–1967) to include those who suffer from their abnormality. Schneider's seminal volume, *Psychopathic Personalities* (1923), still forms the basis of current classifications of personality disorders such as that contained in DSM-IV.

Official criteria for diagnosing personality disorders are listed in the DSM, published by the American Psychiatric Association, and in the mental and behavioral disorders section of the International Statistical Classification of Diseases (ICD) and Related Health Problems, published by the World Health Organization (WHO). The DSM-V published in 2013 now lists personality disorders in exactly the same way as other mental disorders, rather than on a separate axis as previously.

DSM lists ten personality disorders classified into three clusters based on symptom similarities:

- *Cluster A* (paranoid PD, schizoid PD, schizotypal PD): patients appear odd or eccentric to others.
- *Cluster B* (antisocial PD, borderline PD, histrionic PD, narcissistic PD): patients appear overly emotional, unstable, or self-dramatizing to others.
- *Cluster C* (avoidant PD, dependent PD, obsessive–compulsive PD): patients appear tense and anxiety-ridden to others.

Some psychiatrists maintain that the classification is inadequate and should be expanded to include three additional categories:

- *Passive–aggressive PD*, characterized by a need to control or punish others through frustrating them or sabotaging plans
- *Cyclothymic PD*, characterized by intense mood swings alternating between high spirits and moroseness or gloom
- *Depressive PD*, characterized by a negative and a pessimistic approach to life

Finally, there is an '*Others*' *category* involving conditions characterized as:

Eccentric, haltlos (derived from German which means drifting, aimless, and irresponsible), immature, and psychoneurotic

An additional category is for *unspecified PD*, including:

Character neurosis and pathological personality

PD = personality disorder

The DSM clustering system does not mean that all patients can be fitted neatly into one of the three clusters. It is possible for patients to have symptoms of more than one personality disorder or to have symptoms from different clusters. Since the criteria for personality disorders include friction or conflict between the patient and his or her social environment, these syndromes are open to redefinition as societies change. Successive editions of DSM have tried to be sensitive to cultural differences, including changes over time, when defining personality disorders. One criticism that has been made of the general category of personality disorder is that it is based on Western notions of individual uniqueness. Its applicability to people from cultures with different definitions of human personhood is thus open to question.

Therefore, DSM recommends taking a patient's background, especially recent immigration, into account before deciding that he or she has a personality disorder.

To meet the diagnosis of personality disorder, the individual's problematic behaviors must appear in two or more of the following areas:

- Perception and interpretation of the self and other people
- Intensity and duration of feelings and their appropriateness to situations
- Relationships with others
- Ability to control impulses

These behavioral patterns are typically associated with significant disturbances in some behavioral tendencies of an individual, usually involving several areas of the personality, and are nearly always associated with considerable personal and social disruption. Personality disorders are inflexible and pervasive across many situations, due in large part to the fact that such behaviors are perceived to be appropriate by that individual. This behavior can result in maladaptive coping skills, which may lead to personal problems that induce extreme anxiety, distress, or depression.

Psychologist Theodore Millon (1928–2014), who has written numerous popular works on personality, proposed the following description of personality disorders:

Paranoid
Guarded, defensive, distrustful and suspiciousness. Hypervigilant to the motives of others to undermine or do harm. Always seeking confirmatory evidence of hidden schemes. Feels righteous, but persecuted.

Schizoid
Apathetic, indifferent, remote, solitary, distant, humorless. Neither desires nor needs human attachments. Withdrawal from relationships and prefer to be alone. Little interest in others, often seen as a loner. Minimal awareness of feelings of self or others. Few drives or ambitions, if any.

Schizotypal
Eccentric, self-estranged, bizarre, absent. Exhibits peculiar mannerisms and behaviours. Thinks can read thoughts of others. Preoccupied with odd daydreams and beliefs. Blurs line between reality and fantasy. Magical thinking and strange beliefs.

Antisocial
Impulsive, irresponsible, deviant, unruly. Acts without due consideration. Meets social obligations only when self-serving. Disrespects societal customs, rules, and standards. Sees self as free and independent.

Borderline
Unpredictable, manipulative, unstable. Frantically fears abandonment and isolation. Experiences rapidly fluctuating moods. Shifts rapidly between loving and

hating. Sees self and others alternatively as all-good and all-bad. Unstable and frequently changing moods.

Histrionic
Dramatic, seductive, shallow, stimulus-seeking, vain. Overreacts to minor events. Exhibitionistic as a means of securing attention and favors. Sees self as attractive and charming. Constant seeking for others' attention.

Narcissistic
Egotistical, arrogant, grandiose, insouciant. Preoccupied with fantasies of success, beauty, or achievement. Sees self as admirable and superior, and therefore entitled to special treatment.

Avoidant
Hesitant, self-conscious, embarrassed, anxious. Tense in social situations due to fear of rejection. Plagued by constant performance anxiety. Sees self as inept, inferior, or unappealing. Feels alone and empty.

Dependent
Helpless, incompetent, submissive, immature. Withdraws from adult responsibilities. Sees self as weak or fragile. Seeks constant reassurance from stronger figures.

Obsessive–compulsive
Restrained, conscientious, respectful, rigid. Maintains a rule-bound lifestyle. Adheres closely to social conventions. Sees the world in terms of regulations and hierarchies. Sees self as devoted, reliable, efficient, and productive.

Depressive
Somber, discouraged, pessimistic, brooding, fatalistic. Presents self as vulnerable and abandoned. Feels valueless, guilty, and impotent. Judges self as worthy only of criticism and contempt.

Passive–aggressive (*negativistic*)
Resentful, contrary, skeptical, discontented. Resists fulfilling others' expectations. Deliberately inefficient. Vents anger indirectly by undermining others' goals. Alternately moody and irritable, then sullen and withdrawn.

Sadistic
Explosively hostile, abrasive, cruel, dogmatic. Liable to sudden outbursts of rage. Feels selfsatisfied through dominating, intimidating and humiliating others. Is opinionated and close-minded

Self-defeating (*masochistic*)
Deferential, pleasure-phobic, servile, blameful, self-effacing. Encourages others to take advantage. Deliberately defeats own achievements. Seeks condemning or mistreatful partners.

Diagnosis of personality disorders is complicated by the fact that affected persons rarely seek help until they are in serious trouble or until their families and the law pressure them to get treatment. The reason for this slowness is that the problematic traits are so deeply entrenched that they seem normal to the affected individual. Doctors rarely give a diagnosis of personality disorder to children on the grounds that children's personalities are still in the process of formation and may change considerably by the time they are in their late teens. In retrospect, however, many individuals with personality disorders could be judged to have shown evidence of the problems in childhood. Some patients are not diagnosed until later in life because their symptoms had been modified by the demands of their job or by marriage. After retirement or the spouse's death, however, these patients' personality disorders become fully apparent. In general, however, it is unusual for people to develop personality disorders out of the blue in midlife or late life. If so, substance abuse or personality change caused by medical or neurological problems must be ruled out before considering the diagnosis of a personality disorder.

It is difficult to give close estimates on the prevalence of personality disorders in the general community. The majority of people with a personality disorder never come into contact with mental health services. While patients with antisocial and borderline disorders are more likely to get into trouble with the law or otherwise attract attention, individuals with narcissistic or obsessive–compulsive personality disorders may be outwardly successful because their symptoms are useful within their particular occupations.

> It has, however, been estimated that about 15 % of the general population of the United States has a personality disorder.

The causes of personality disorders are the subject of considerable debate and controversy. Some experts believe that personality disorders are caused by early experiences that prevented the development of normal thought and behavior patterns. Other researchers believe that biological or genetic influences are the root cause of personality disorders. A study of almost 600 male college students, averaging almost 30 years of age and who were not drawn from a clinical sample, examined the relationship between childhood experiences of sexual and physical abuse and currently reported personality disorder symptoms. Childhood abuse histories were found to be definitively associated with greater levels of symptomatology. Child abuse and neglect consistently evidence themselves as antecedent risks to the development of personality disorders in adulthood. In a following study, efforts were taken to match retrospective reports of abuse with a clinical population that had demonstrated psychopathology from childhood to adulthood who were later found to have experienced abuse and neglect. In a study of 793 mothers and children, researchers asked mothers if they had screamed at their children and told them that they did not love them or threatened to send them away. Children who had experienced such verbal abuse were three times as likely as children who did not experience such verbal abuse to have borderline, narcissistic, obsessive–compulsive, or paranoid personality disorders in adulthood. The sexually abused group demonstrated the most consistently elevated patterns of psychopathology. Officially verified physical abuse showed an extremely strong correlation with the development of antisocial and impulsive behavior.

Treatment. At one time, psychiatrists thought that personality disorders did not respond well to treatment. This opinion was derived from the notion that human personality is fixed for life once it has been molded in childhood and from the belief among people with personality disorders that their own views and behaviors are correct and that others are the ones at fault.

> More recently, however, it has been recognized that humans can continue to grow and change throughout life.

Most patients with personality disorders are now considered to be treatable, although the degree of improvement may vary. The type of treatment recommended depends on the personality characteristics associated with the specific disorder. There are many different modalities of treatment used for personality disorders: Individual psychotherapy has been a mainstay of treatment. Group therapy is probably the second most used. Psychological education may be used as an addition. Self-help groups may provide resources for personality disorders. Milieu therapy is a kind of group-based residential approach. Finally, psychiatric medications are used for treating symptoms of personality dysfunction.

Maffei et al. found the prevalence of personality disorders in subjects with androgenetic alopecia to be significantly higher than in the general population and found the existence of three distinct personality profiles:

- Suspicious, with grandiose sense of self-importance, obsessive, and socially withdrawn
- Impulsive, identity disordered, and socially maladjusted
- Dramatic, emotional, and dependent

The psychological effects of hair loss may be hard to differentiate clinically from preexisting psychopathology. Nevertheless, patients with personality disorders tend to experience more distress from hair loss than nondisordered patients, since these individuals lack a secure sense of self and effective coping skills and therefore may be especially vulnerable to the adverse effects of androgenetic alopecia.

Ultimately, patients with personality disorders tend to be more difficult to handle with respect to the treatment of hair loss.

Patient compliance issues are a problem in patients with paranoid, avoidant, or passive–aggressive (negativistic) personality disorders; nocebo reactions are more frequent in patients with paranoid, passive–aggressive (negativistic), or histrionic personality disorders; and overvalued ideas are typical for patients with histrionic or narcissistic personality disorders.

The physician should be careful not to be judgmental or to scold because this may rapidly close down communication. Sometimes the difficult patient gains therapeutic benefit just from venting concerns in a safe environment with a caring physician.

Further Reading

Psychopathological Disorders: Classification

Koblenzer CS (1993a) Psychiatric syndromes of interest to dermatologists. Int J Dermatol 32:82–88

Koblenzer CS (1993b) Pharmacology of psychotropic drugs useful in dermatologic practice. Int J Dermatol 32:162–168

Koo J (1995) Psychodermatology: a practical manual for clinicians. Curr Prob Dermatol VII:199–234

Psychophysiological Disorders

Griesemer RD (1978) Emotionally triggered disease in a dermatology practice. Psychiat Ann 8:49–56

Folliculitis Necrotica

Frank SB, Minkin W (1969) Folliculitis with scarring simulating acne varioliformis. Arch Dermatol 100(4):51

Hersle K, Mobacken H, Möller A (1979) Chronic nonscarring folliculitis of the scalp. Acta Derm Venereol 59(3):249–253

Kossard S, Collins A, McCrossin I (1987) Necrotizing lymphocytic folliculitis: the early lesion of acne necrotica (varioliformis). J Am Acad Dermatol 16:1007–1014

Maibach H (1989) Acne necroticans (varioliformis) versus Propionibacterium acnes folliculitis. J Am Acad Dermatol 21:323

Milde P, Goerz G, Plewig G (1993) Acne necrotica (varioliformis). Necrotizing lymphocytic folliculitis. Hautarzt 44(1):34–36

Zirn JR, Scott RA, Hambrick GW (1996) Chronic acneiform eruption with crateriform scars. Acne necrotica (varioliformis) (necrotizing lymphocytic folliculitis). Arch Dermatol 132(11):1367, 1370

Primary Psychiatric Disorders: Neurotic Excoriations of the Scalp

Fruensgaaard K (1986) Neurotic excoriations: a controlled psychiatric examination. Act Psychiatr Scand Suppl 69:1–52

Fruensgaaard K (1991a) Psychotherapeutic strategy and neurotic excoriations. Int J Dermatol 30:198–203

Fruensgaaard K (1991b) Psychotherapy and neurotic excoriations. Int J Dermatol 30:262–265

Harris BA, Sherertz EF, Flowers FP (1987) Improvement of chronic neurotic excoriations with oral doxepin therapy. Int J Dermatol 26:541–543

Primary Psychiatric Disorders: Imaginary Hair Loss (Psychogenic Pseudoeffluvium)

Cotterill JA (1996a) Dermatologic nondisease. Dermatol Clin 14:439–445

Cotterill JA (1996b) Body dysmorphic disorder. Dermatol Clin 14:457–463

Harth W, Hermes B, Seikowski K, Gieler U (2007) Nihilodermia in psychodermatology. Hautarzt 58(5): 427–434

Primary Psychiatric Disorders: Dorian Gray Syndrome

Brosig B, Kupfer J, Niemeier V et al (2001) The "Dorian Gray Syndrome": psychodynamic need for hair growth restorers, and other "fountains of youth". Int J Clin Pharmacol Ther 39:279–283

Cash TF (1990) Losing hair, losing points? The effects of male pattern baldness on social impression formation. J Appl Soc Psychol 20:154–167

Muscarella F, Cunningham MR (1996) The evolutionary significance and social perception of male pattern baldness and facial hair. Ethol Sociobiol 17:99–117

Phillips KA (1996) The broken mirror: understanding and treating body dysmorphic disorder. New York, Oxford

Roll S, Verinis JS (1971) Stereotypes of scalp and facial hair as measured by the semantic differential. Psychol Rep 28:975–980

Sarwer DB, Wadden TA, Pertschuk MJ et al (1998) The psychology of cosmetic surgery: a review and reconceptualization. Clin Psychol Rev 18:1–22

Sarwer DB, Grossbart TA, Didie ER (2003) Beauty and society. Semin Cutan Med Surg 22:79–92

Thompson JK, Heinberg LJ, Altabe M et al (1990) Exacting beauty: theory, assessment and treatment of body image disturbance. American Psychological Association, Washington DC, pp 19–47

Primary Psychiatric Disorders: Delusions of Parasitosis (Ekbom's Disease)

Damiani JT, Flowers FP, Pierce DK (1990) Pimozide in delusions of parasitosis. J Am Acad Dermatol 22:312–313

Gould WM, Gragg TM (1976) Delusions of parasitosis. An approach to the problem. Arch Dermatol 112:1745–1748

Lyell A (1983) Delusions of parasitosis. Br J Dermatol 108:485–499

Marneros A, Rohde A, Deister A (1987) Most delusional parasitosis are organic mental disease. Clin Psych News 15:23

Pope FM (1970) Parasitophobia as the presenting symptom of vitamin B12 deficiency. Practitioner 204:421–422

Reilly TM, Batchelor DH (1986) The presentation and treatment of delusional parasitosis. Int Clin Psychopharmacol 1:340–353

Van Moffaert M (1991a) Localization of self-inflicted dermatological lesions: what do they tell the dermatologist. Acta Derm Venereol Suppl (Stockh) 156:23–27

Wykoff RF (1987) Delusions of parasitosis: a review. Rev Infect Dis 9:433–437

Primary Psychiatric Disorders: Trichotillomania

Bloch MH, Panza KE, Grant JE, Pittenger C, Leckman JF (2013) N-acetylcysteine in the treatment of pediatric trichotillomania: a randomized, double-blind, placebo-controlled add-on trial. J Am Acad Child Adolesc Psychiatry 52:231–240

Blum NJ, Barone VJ, Friman PC (1993) A simplified behavioral treatment of trichotillomania: report of two cases. Pediatrics 91:993–995

Delsmann BM, Nikolaidis N, Schomacher PH (1993) Trichobezoar als seltene Ursache eines Dünndarmileus. Dtsch Med Wochenschr 118:1361–1364

Grant JE, Odlaug BL, Kim SW (2009) N-acetylcysteine, a glutamate modulator, in the treatment of trichotillomania: a double-blind, placebo-controlled study. Arch Gen Psychiatry 66(7):756–763

Grant JE, Odlaug BL, Chamberlain SR, Kim SW (2011) Dronabinol, a cannabinoid agonist, reduces hair pulling in trichotillomania: a pilot study. Psychopharmacology (Berlin) 218:493–502

Lochner C, Seedat S, Niehaus DJ, Stein DJ (2006) Topiramate in the treatment of trichotillomania: an open-label pilot study. Int Clin Psychopharmacol 21:255–259

McGehee FT, Buchanan GR (1980) Trichophagia and trichobezoar: etiologic role of iron deficiency. J Pediatr 97:946–948

Meiers HG, Rechenberger HG, Rechenberger I (1973) Trichotillomanie. Untersuchungen zur Ätiologie, Diagnostik und Therapie. Hautarzt 24:248–252

Muller SA (1990) Trichotillomania: a histopathologic study in sixty-six patients. J Am Acad Dermatol 23:56–62

Oranje AP, Peereboom-Wynia JDR, de Raeymaecker DMJ (1986) Trichotillomania in childhood. J Am Acad Dermatol 15:614–619

Pericin M, Kündig TM, Trüeb RM (1996) Trichotillomanie in Verbindung mit Alopecia areata. Z Hautkrankh 12:921–924

Reinhardt V, Reinhardt A, Houser D (1986) Hair pulling and eating in captive rhesus monkey troops. Folia Primatol (Basel) 47:158–164

Sheikha SH, Wagner KD, Wagner RF (1993) Fluoxetine treatment of trichotillomania and depression in a prepubertal child. Cutis 51:50–52

Shome S, Bhatia MS, Gautam RK (1993) Culture-bound trichotillomania. Am J Psychiatr 150:674

Swed SE, Lenane MC, Leonard HL (1993) Long-term treatment of trichotillomania (hair pulling). N Engl J Med 329:141–142

Tribó MJ, Ros S, Toll A et al (2005) Trichotillomania: about five cases. 11th international congress dermatology and psychiatry abstract book. 84 p

Trüeb RM (1993) Differential diagnosis in pediatric dermatology: trichotillomania/battered child syndrome. Eur J Pediatr Dermatol 3:134–139

Trüeb RM, Cavegn B (1996) Trichotillomania in connection with alopecia areata. Cutis 58:67–70

Weller EB, Weller RA, Carr S (1989) Imipramine treatment of trichotillomania and co-existing depression in a seven-year-old. J Am Acad Child Adolesc Psychiatry 28:952–953

Primary Psychiatric Disorders: Factitial Dermatitis of the Scalp

Braun-Falco O, Vogel PG (1968) Trichotemnomanie. Eine besondere Manifestation eines hirnorganischen Psychosyndroms. Hautarzt 119:551–553

Fabisch W (1980) Psychiatric aspects of dermatitis artefacta. Br J Dermatol 102:29–34

Gandy DT (1953) The concept and clinical aspects of factitious dermatitis. South Med J 46:551–555

Hollender MH, Abram HS (1973) Dermatitis factitia. South Med J 66:1279–1285

Lyell A (1979) Cutaneous artifactual disease. A review amplified by personal experience. J Am Acad Dermatol 1:391–407

Sneddon I, Sneddon J (1975) Self-inflicted injury: a follow-up study of 43 patients. Br Med J 2:527–530

Taylor S, Hyler SE (1993) Update on factitious disorders. Int J Psychiatry Med 23:81–94

Van Moffaert M (1991b) Localization of self-inflicted dermatological lesions: what do they tell the dermatologist. Acta Derm Venereol Suppl (Stockh) 156:23–27

Chronic Cutaneous Sensory Disorders: Trichodynia

Arck PC, Handjiski B, Hagen E et al (2001) Indications for a 'brain-hair follicle axis (BHA)': inhibition of keratinocyte proliferation and up-regulation of keratinocyte apoptosis in telogen hair follicles by stress and substance P. FASEB J 15:2536–2538

Burstein R, Cutrer MF, Yarnitsky D (2000) The developmental of cutaneous allodynia during a migraine attack clinical evidence for the sequential recruitment of spinal and supraspinal nociceptive neurons in migraine. Brain 123:1703–1709

Chizh BA, Göhring M, Tröster A, Quartey GK, Schmelz M, Koppert W (2007) Effects of oral pregabalin and aprepitant on pain and central sensitization in the electrical hyperalgesia model in human volunteers. Br J Anaesth 98:246–254

Ericson M, Gabrielson A, Worel S et al (1999) Substance P (SP) in innervated and non-innervated blood vessels in the skin of patients with symptomatic scalp. Exp Dermatol 8:344–345

Gazerani P, Au S, Dong X, Kumar U, Arendt-Nielsen L, Cairns BE (2010) Botulinum neurotoxin type A (BoNTA) decreases the mechanical sensitivity of nociceptors and inhibits neurogenic vasodilation in a craniofacial muscle targeted for migraine prophylaxis. Pain 151:606–616

Grimalt R, Ferrando J, Grimalt F (1998) Trichodynia (letter). Dermatology 196:374

Hafizi S, Chandra P, Cowen J (2007) Neurokinin-1 receptor antagonists as novel antidepressants: trials and tribulations. Br J Psychiatry 191:282–284

Hoss D, Segal S (1998) Scalp dysesthesia. Arch Dermatol 134:327–330

Kramer MS, Cuttler N, Feighner J et al (1998) Distinct mechanism for antidepressant activity by blockade of central substance P receptors. Science 281: 1640–1645

Lonne-Rahm SB, Fischer T, Berg M (1999) Stinging rosacea. Acta Derm Venereol 79:460–461

Lucioni A, Bales GT, Lotan TL, McGehee DS, Cook SP, Rapp DE (2008) Botulinum toxin type A inhibits sensory neuropeptide release in rat bladder models of acute injury and chronic inflammation. BJU Int 101: 366–370

Mustafa G, Anderson EM, Bokrand-Donatelli Y, Neubert JK, Caudle RM (2013) Anti-nociceptive effect of a conjugate of substance P and light chain of botulinum neurotoxin type A. Pain 154(11):2547–2553, pii: S0304-3959(13)00409-0

Panconesi E, Hartmann G (1996) Psychophysiology of stress in dermatology. The psychologic pattern of psychosomatics. Dermatol Clin 14:399–421

Rebora A (1997) Telogen effluvium. Dermatology 195:209–212

Rebora A, Semino MT, Guarrera M (1996) Trichodynia (letter). Dermatology 192:292–293

Rebora A, Semino MT, Guarrera M (1998) Reply to Trüeb RM. Telogen effluvium and trichodynia (letter). Dermatology 196:374–375

Rollman GB, Lautenbacher S, Jones KS (2000) Sex and gender differences in responses to experimentally induced pain in humans. Sex, gender, and pain. In: Fillingim RB (ed) Progress in pain research and management, vol 17. IASP Press, Seattle

Trüeb RM (1997) Trichodynie. Hautarzt 48:877–880

Trüeb RM (1998) Telogen effluvium and trichodynia (letter). Dermatology 196:374–375

Willimann B, Trüeb RM (2002) Hair pain (trichodynia): frequency and relationship to hair loss and patient gender. Dermatology 205:374–377

Chronic Cutaneous Sensory Disorders: Trichoteiromania

Freyschmidt-Paul P, Hoffmann R, Happle R (2001) Trichoteiromanie. Eur J Dermatol 11:369–371

Reich S, Trüeb RM (2003) Trichoteiromanie. J Dtsch Dermatol Ges 1:22–28

Adjustment Disorders

Cash TF (1992) The psychological effects of androgenetic alopecia in men. J Am Acad Dermatol 26:926–931

Cash TF (1999) The psychosocial consequences of androgenetic alopecia: a review of the research literature. Br J Dermatol 141:398–405

Cash TF, Price VH, Savin RC (1993) Psychological effects of androgenetic alopecia on women: comparisons with balding men and with female control subjects. J Am Acad Dermatol 29:568–575

Personality Disorders

American Psychiatric Association (2013) Diagnostic and statistical manual of mental disorders, 5th edn. American Psychiatric Publishing, Arlington, pp 646–649. ISBN 978-0-89042-555-8

http://en.wikipedia.org/wiki/Personality_disorder

Maffei C, Fossati A, Rinaldi F, Riva E (1994) Personality disorders and psychopathologic symptoms in patients with androgenetic alopecia. Arch Dermatol 130(7): 868–872

Millon T, Davis RD (1996) Disorders of personality: DSM-IV and beyond. Wiley, New York, p 226. ISBN 0-471-01186-X

6 Tackling Adverse Effects

I think of my body as side effect of my mind.
Carrie Fisher (1956–)

A side effect is an effect that is secondary to the one intended. The term is primarily used to describe unwanted or adverse effects. In the broader sense, the term can also apply to unintended, but beneficial effects from the use of the drug. An example is the hair growth-promoting effect of minoxidil that was originally a drug intended to lower the blood pressure but proved to be a powerful trichotrophic agent.

> Occurrence or fear of adverse effects is a major barrier to patient compliance. Therefore, it is of upmost importance to inform patients on potential adverse effects, their frequencies, and appropriate management.

Some adverse effects are directly related to the pharmacological effect of the drug and others to a patient's individual allergic or idiosyncratic disposition, to drug–drug interactions, or to simply not following instructions for proper use of the medication. Patients should be aware of possible allergies to active ingredients or additives, and report other medical conditions and medications. Therefore, it is highly recommended, even when treatment can be purchased without a doctor's prescription, that the patient visits a physician for proper indication, exclusion of contraindications, instructions for proper use, and follow-up.

Topical minoxidil and oral finasteride are the most frequently used drugs for treatment of alopecia. For a comprehensive list of reported adverse reactions to other drugs used for treatment of hair loss and related disorders, the readers are encouraged to refer to the respective information for consumers and healthcare professionals accompanying the drug.

6.1 Adverse Reactions to Topical Minoxidil

Topical minoxidil solution and foam are used to promote hair growth in the treatment of androgenetic alopecia. Minoxidil is not indicated for treatment of telogen effluvium or alopecia areata, lest androgenetic alopecia represents a comorbidity. Efficacy and safety data are not available before the age of 18 years and after the age of 65 years. Nevertheless, minoxidil can be safely used before 18 or after

R.M. Trüeb, *The Difficult Hair Loss Patient: Guide to Successful Management of Alopecia and Related Conditions*, DOI 10.1007/978-3-319-19701-2_6

65 years at the discretion of the prescriber (off-label use).

Children are at higher risk of adverse cardiovascular effects of topical minoxidil solution.

Therefore, before the age of 12 years, the dosage should be halved. Any of the following health problems should caution to the use of topical minoxidil: active diseases of the scalp, e.g., eczema, infection, and cuts, as well as heart problems, e.g., chest pain, heart attack, and heart failure.

Before applying minoxidil to the scalp, the area should be clean and dry. The product may be applied to damp hair. To use the solution, the applicator is filled with 1 ml of medication. The hair in the area of thinning is parted, and the solution is applied evenly to the affected area of the scalp and gently rubbed in. The solution or foam is applied twice a day. The solution is allowed to dry completely before using other styling products, e.g., gels or mousse, or before going to bed. If a dose is missed, the missed dose is to be skipped and the usual dosing schedule resumed. The dose should not be doubled to catch up.

Upon initiation of treatment with topical minoxidil, patients may experience temporary increased shedding of hair (shedding phase). Patients should be prepared and informed that this represents a physiological response to treatment, since minoxidil not only increases the duration of anagen in the hair cycle but also triggers an immediate telogen release.

The best thing to do is to continue treatment until the shedding stops (usually within 6 weeks) and new hair growth is seen (usually at 3 months). Patients should also be aware that it takes time for hair to regrow. Most people need to use this medication regularly for at least 8 weeks to see a benefit. If the condition does not improve or worsens after using this medication for 3–6 months, the condition and treatment need to be reevaluated by the physician. The effect of minoxidil builds up until 12 months of treatment. Once it is established that minoxidil is effective, treatment should thereafter continue indefinitely since positive results will be reversed within 6 weeks to 3 months once treatment is stopped.

Another common adverse effect of minoxidil is elongation, thickening, and enhanced pigmentation of fine facial hair and rarely of body hair (hypertrichosis). This develops relatively early in the course of treatment (usually within 6 weeks after starting therapy). It is usually first noticed on the temples (Fig. 6.1a.), between the hairline and the eyebrows, or in the sideburn area of the upper lateral cheek (Fig. 6.1b). Upon discontinuation of minoxidil, new hair growth stops, but up to 12 months may be required for restoration to pretreatment appearance.

Minoxidil-induced hair growth may be especially disturbing to women. Patients should therefore be carefully informed about this possible effect before treatment is started.

The risk is significantly higher with 5 % topical minoxidil, in women with preexistent hypertrichosis, especially those of Mediterranean or Indian origin. Disturbing hairs may be bleached, clipped, or waxed.

Itching, redness, or irritation at the treated area are far more frequently due to an irritant dermatitis to propylene glycol or the alcohol-based solution of minoxidil.

If irritant scalp dermatitis is a problem, either minoxidil foam or a minoxidil compound should be used that are free of propylene glycol.

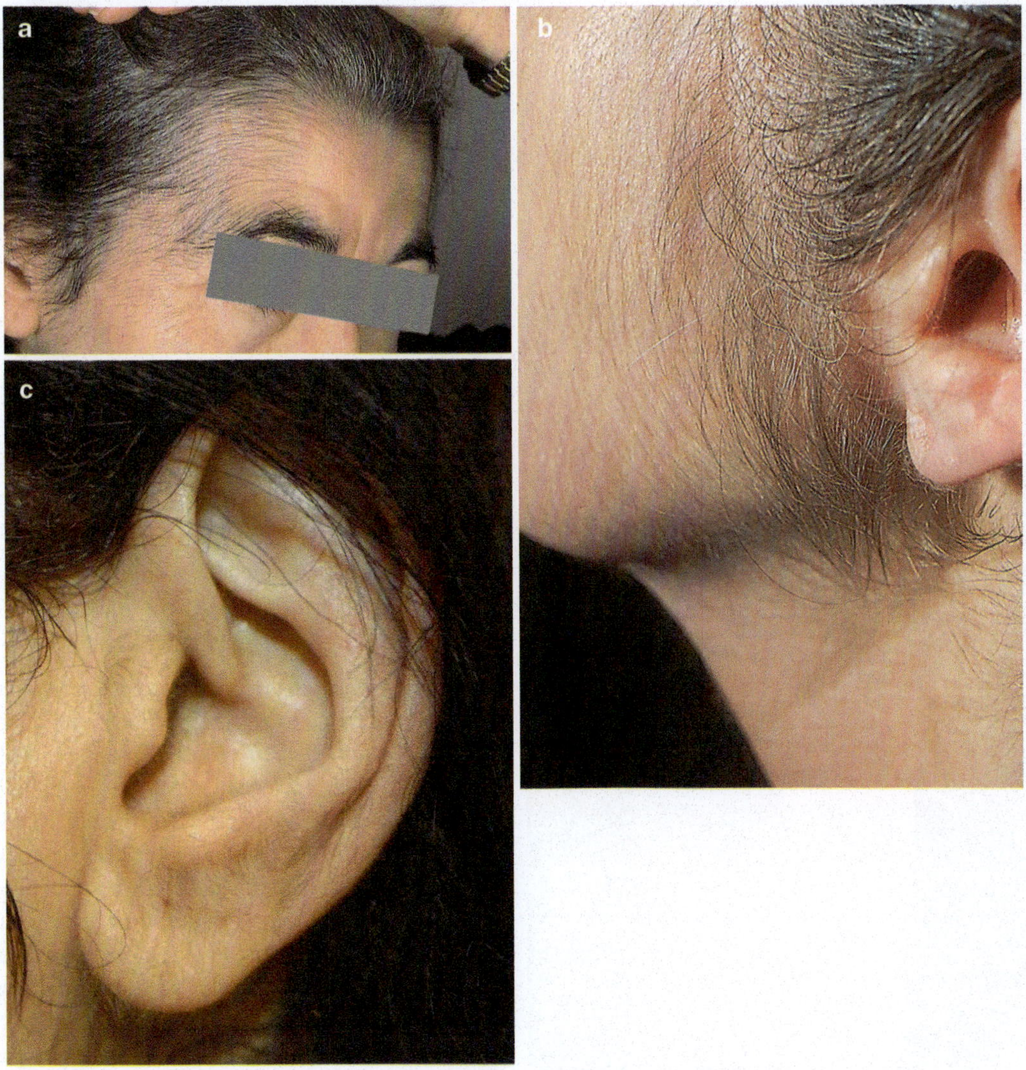

Fig. 6.1 (**a–c**) Minoxidil-induced hypertrichosis. (**a**) On the temple. (**b**) Of the sideburn area and lateral cheek. (**c**) Of the ear

Rp.	
Minoxidil	2.0, 3.0, or 5.0 g
Glycerin	10.0 g
Water	20.0 g
Ethanol 96 %	ad 100.0 g
M(isce).D(a).S(igna). Apply twice daily 1 ml to the affected area	

After applying minoxidil onto the scalp, exposure to the sun should be avoided, since it may cause sunburns. Minoxidil should not be used on skin that is red, painful, irritated, scraped, cut, or infected, since doing so may cause the drug to be absorbed into the body and result in systemic side effects. Hands should be thoroughly washed after application. Caution is to be given to avoid getting the medication in eyes. If this occurs, eyes should be rinsed with large amounts of cool water.

Very few minoxidil users are truly allergic to the active ingredient. While irritant dermatitis usually develops early in the course of treatment, allergic reactions are usually acquired later.

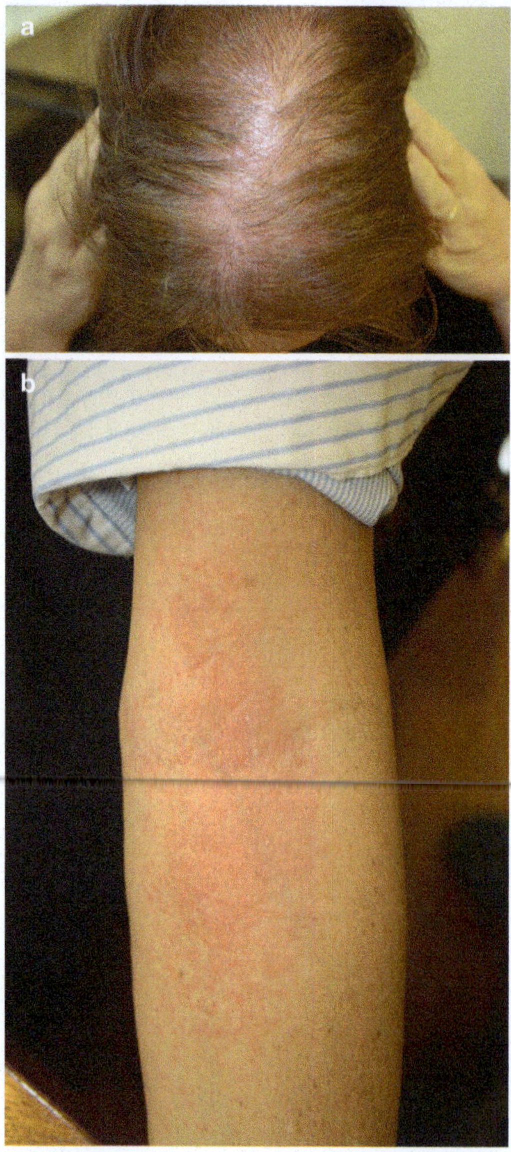

Fig. 6.2 (**a**, **b**) Allergic contact dermatitis to minoxidil. (**a**) Of the application area and (**b**) positive ROAT

If an allergic reaction to minoxidil is suspected (Fig. 6.2a), this can be clarified by performing a repeated open application test (ROAT) to the forearm: minoxidil is applied twice daily to an area of 5 × 5 cm on the inner aspect of the forearm for a duration of 7 days. In the event of a contact allergic reaction, an erythematous rash with papules will become apparent usually within 48–72 h (Fig. 6.2b).

While most of patients with allergic contact dermatitis described in the literature showed a positive sensitization to the vehicle substance propylene glycol evaluated by patch testing, reactions to the active ingredient minoxidil are rare. Hagemann et al. reported a case of allergic sensitization to minoxidil, which they evaluated and differentiated from an irritative reaction by a combination of patch testing and lymphocyte transformation test (LTT).

> The differentiation of allergic and irritative adverse effects of topical minoxidil solutions and the identification of the causative agent are of major relevance for the proceeding and adjustment of therapy.

Patients with sensitizations against propylene glycol are candidates for preparations with alternative solvents but can proceed treatment with minoxidil. In contrast, patients with allergies to the active ingredient itself are no longer candidates for treatment with minoxidil and should undergo alternative therapeutic options.

Other reported adverse reactions to topical minoxidil solution include migraine headache, erosive pustular dermatosis of the scalp, pustular allergic contact dermatitis, pigmented contact dermatitis, leukoderma, central chorioretinopathy, severe hypertrichosis of the external ear canal, and trichostasis spinulosa of the forehead (Fig. 6.3). Adverse reactions to topical minoxidil are summarized in Table. 6.1.

Cases of fetal malformation (brain, heart, and vascular), of caudal regression syndrome, and of hypertrichosis of the infant were reported from the use of topical minoxidil during pregnancy.

Eight deaths occurred during the original Upjohn-sponsored clinical trials with topical minoxidil and 2 deaths in subjects who used extemporaneous formulations of the drug. Of the 8 patients, 5 had cardiovascular abnormalities, 2 had acquired immunodeficiency

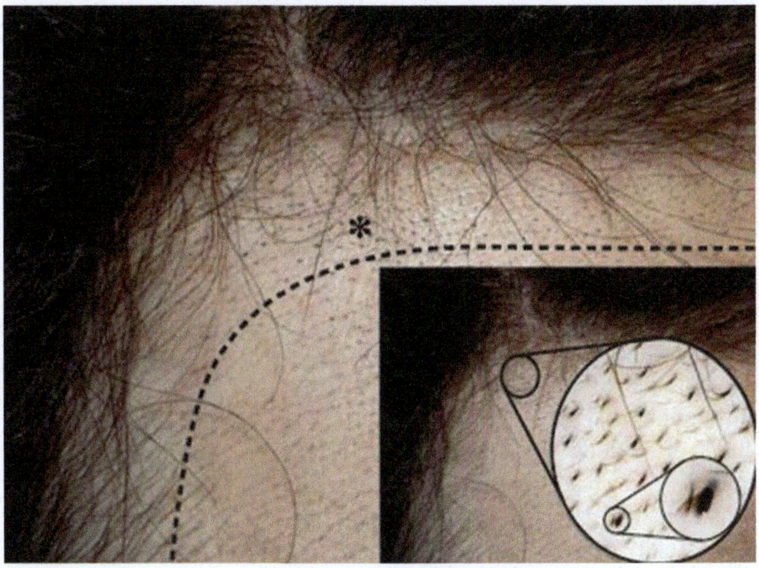

Fig. 6.3 Minoxidil-induced trichostasis spinulosa. The temporal region shows multiple small blackish spines extruding from hair follicle openings. The *dotted line* indicates the approximate area of minoxidil application. The *asterisk* indicates the region evaluated by dermoscopy shown in the inset at original magnification × 10 (From Navarin A, Ziegler M, Kolm I et al (2010) *Arch Dermatol* 146:1434–1435)

Table 6.1 Adverse reactions to 2 or 5 % topical minoxidil solution

Common:
Hair shedding (during initial 4–6 weeks of treatment)
Unwanted hair growth elsewhere on the body (usually facial in women, within 3–6 weeks of treatment: Fig. 6.2)
Itching, redness, or irritation at the treated area (usually due to propylene glycol)
Changes in hair color or texture
Burning or irritation of the eye
Rare (treatment should be withheld immediately):
Severe allergic reactions: rash, hives, itching, difficulty breathing, tightness in the chest, swelling of the mouth, face, lips, or tongue
Cardiovascular effects: chest pain; dizziness; fainting; increased heart rate; pounding heartbeat; sudden, unexplained weight gain; swollen hands or feet
Unexplained: breast tenderness, changes in vision or hearing
Thrombocytopenia and leukopenia (WBC < 3,000/mm^3) and toxic epidermal necrolysis (TEN) have very rarely been reported with oral minoxidil

syndrome-related pneumonia, and one patient died of a self-inflicted gunshot wound. Of the subjects who were using extemporaneous topical minoxidil, one had hypertension and arteriosclerotic disease, and the other died of myocardial infarction.

There is a little likelihood of serious adverse effects from the proper use of topical minoxidil in otherwise healthy, adult patients, and the evidence suggests that reported deaths were the result of causes other than the use of minoxidil because of its low systemic absorption.

The percutaneous absorption and excretion of 5 % solution of minoxidil labeled with carbon 14 were measured in adult male subjects, who received nine topical applications to a bald area on the scalp, with the radioactive solutions applied on days 1 and 9. Urinary excretion of radioactivity was low, with mean values ranging from 1.6 to 3.9 % of applied dose. No radioactivity was detected in fecal samples. Recovery of radioactivity from the skin surface and from scalp and pillowcase washes was in the range of 41–45 % of applied dose.

Although minoxidil is poorly absorbed through the skin, systemic doses in the range of 2.4–5.4 mg/day can be anticipated if application is made to the entire scalp. Therefore, it is recommended to refrain from the use of topical minoxidil in patients with significant and arrhythmogenic cardiovascular disease.

Healthy male volunteers completed a four-way, multiple-dose, randomized crossover study to determine the relationship between contact time of applied drug on the scalp and minoxidil absorption from a 2 % topical solution. One milliliter of solution was applied twice daily over 150 cm^2 of bald scalp to each subject for 6 days. Unabsorbed drug was washed off the scalp after 1, 2, 4, and 11.5 h of contact time in each of four treatments. Cumulative urinary excretion profiles within steady-state, 12-h dosing intervals were well described by straight lines for all treatments, indicating that systemic minoxidil elimination was rate controlled by constant, zero-order percutaneous drug absorption. The extent of minoxidil absorption, expressed as steady-state urinary excretion of unchanged minoxidil, minoxidil glucuronide, or the sum of these, increased in a disproportionate manner with increase in contact time of drug on the scalp.

Relative to the amount of topical minoxidil absorbed after a contact time of 11.5 h, absorption was approximately 50 % complete by 1 h and greater than 75 % complete by 4 h.

This suggests that minoxidil absorption from the vehicle into skin occurs rapidly relative to diffusion through skin. The rate of minoxidil absorption from vehicle into skin was characterized as nonlinear, whereas minoxidil excretion into urine was rate controlled by diffusion from one or more components of the skin which apparently serve as a reservoir, or depot, for minoxidil.

The effect of application frequency on the systemic absorption of topical minoxidil was studied in 52 normal men. Subjects received 1 ml 3 % minoxidil solution applied four, six, or eight times daily to the scalp. Serum and urine were collected and analyzed for minoxidil. No systemic minoxidil accumulation occurred from increasing application frequency to the scalp.

Systemic minoxidil accumulation resulting from frequent application is unlikely. The initial dose probably saturates the skin for a period of time longer than the dosing intervals examined.

Since the efficacy of combining topical 5 % minoxidil with 0.01 % tretinoin once daily was demonstrated to be equivalent to that of conventional 5 % topical minoxidil solution twice daily, a combination of topical minoxidil with tretinoin in a compound has been suggested for treatment of androgenetic alopecia.

However, healthy male volunteers completed a three-way, randomized, crossover study to determine the effect of tretinoin on percutaneous absorption of minoxidil. Subjects received, for 20 days, twice-daily administrations of 1 ml aqueous 2 % topical minoxidil solution either alone, with once-daily applications of a 0.05 % tretinoin cream, or with once-daily applications of a vehicle control cream.

When minoxidil was co-administered with tretinoin, minoxidil absorption was increased nearly threefold, increasing the risk of systemic adverse effects.

Transepidermal water loss measurements, which are sensitive to changes in stratum corneum function, were also significantly increased with tretinoin. No treatment-related changes in stratum corneum thickness were observed on the basis of skin biopsy analysis. The findings indicate that percutaneous minoxidil absorption is enhanced by tretinoin as a result of increased stratum corneum permeability.

> Moreover, the combination of topical minoxidil with tretinoin enhances the risk of irritant contact dermatitis of the scalp.

6.2 Adverse Reactions to Oral Finasteride

One milligram oral finasteride received FDA approval for treatment of male pattern baldness in 1997. In several clinical studies, oral finasteride, like topical minoxidil solution, was shown to work on both the crown area and the hairline, but is most successful in the crown area. Again, finasteride is effective only for as long as it is taken. The hair gained or maintained is lost within 6–12 months of stopping treatment.

In a more recent 10-year study of 118 men between 20 and 61 years of age treated with 1 mg oral finasteride daily for androgenic alopecia, Rossi et al. found that 86 % of men continued to benefit from treatment over the entire course of 10 years. In the opinion of the authors, the result after the first year could help in predicting the effectiveness of the treatment; however, many of those unchanged after 1 year of treatment were found to improve later on. Interestingly, better improvements were observed in patients older than 30 years with Hamilton–Norwood grades IV and V. Treatment efficacy was not reduced over time (including those over 40 years of age). Adverse effects were reported in 5.9 % of patients; however, some of them went on with treatment because of the good results.

In the most recent study published in 2012, Sato and Takeda reported on efficacy and safety of 1 mg oral finasteride for treatment of male androgenetic alopecia in the so far largest population study. The study enrolled 3,177 Japanese men treated with oral finasteride from January 2006 to June 2009 at the Tokyo Memorial Clinic Hirayama Department of Plastic and Aesthetic Surgery, School of Medicine, Kitasato University, Tokyo, Japan. Efficacy was evaluated by global photographic assessment, and safety data were assessed by interviews and laboratory tests. The overall effect on hair growth was seen in 87.1 %, in whom hair increased greatly in 11.1 %, moderately in 36.5 %, and slightly in 39.5 %. The response rate improved with increasing duration of treatment. Adverse reactions occurred in 0.7 % of men. Seven men discontinued treatment based on risk–benefit considerations. No specific safety problems associated with long-term use were observed. The authors concluded that in Japanese men with androgenetic alopecia, 1 mg oral finasteride used for long-term treatment maintains progressive hair regrowth without recognized side effect.

Nevertheless, since the original report of persistent diminished libido, erectile dysfunction, and depression among former users of oral finasteride by Traish et al. in 2011, there have been several reports on sexual side effects that may persist despite discontinuation of finasteride medication. These subjects also reported a wide range of symptoms including changes in cognition, ejaculate quality, and genital sensations. Ultimately, Irwig reported depressive symptoms and suicidal thoughts among former users of finasteride with persistent sexual side effects. The author concluded that prescribers of finasteride and men contemplating its use should be made aware of these potential adverse medication effects.

With respect to finasteride and male fertility, early studies did not show any significant influence of finasteride on parameters of semen quality, whereas some later case reports suggested that in subfertile patients, the effects of the drug might be amplified. Therefore, respective counseling may be particularly challenging for male partners of couples who are attempting to become pregnant.

Some users, in an effort to save money, buy 5 mg finasteride tablets instead of the original 1 mg pill and split them into several parts to approximate the 1 mg dosage. Also, finasteride 1 mg capsules formulated with an active ingredient of unknown origin are marketed unofficially to treat androgenetic alopecia in men.

Navarro Guerrero et al. performed a galenic-pharmaceutical study of pieces of Proscar® (5 mg finasteride) tablets and finasteride 1 mg capsules *versus* Propecia® in the treatment of androgenetic alopecia, with the effort to ascertain the pharmaceutical quality of these alternative preparations. The results obtained demonstrated a high variability in the dosage of pieces of tablets ranging from 0.49 mg to 1.81 mg of finasteride, only 10 % being within the dosage range, which is ±5 %, as compared with the authorized 1 mg dose. Applying the criteria of the mass uniformity test, set down in the European Pharmacopoeia, to the set of Proscar® pieces and to the value of the standard deviation percentage (18 %) obtained, the batch would have to be rejected. The finasteride 1 mg capsules showed variable in vitro availability values between 51 and 86 % as compared to Propecia®, which has 92 % availability. Some of these formulations again do not meet the availability specifications established by standard pharmacopeias. Furthermore, the dissolution efficiency of the capsules (from 27 to 76 %) was significantly lower than that of the reference proprietary drug with 82 % (unpublished data).

Finally, the 1 mg finasteride pills are coated to prevent contact with the active ingredient during handling, and the dust or crumbs from broken 5 mg finasteride tablets should be kept away from pregnant women or women who may become pregnant due to teratogenicity.

> Splitting 5 mg finasteride tablets to treat androgenetic alopecia is an inappropriate practice from the point of view of safety and dosage variability. With regard to the finasteride 1 mg capsules marketed unofficially, any finasteride formulation purportedly similar to the reference proprietary drug must prove its bioequivalence or interchangeability with respect to the availability of the active ingredient.

Due to interference with doping assays, many sports organizations had banned oral finasteride because it could be misused to mask steroid abuse. Not until 2009, finasteride was removed from the World Anti-Doping Agency's list of banned substances.

The Prostate Cancer Prevention Trial (PCPT) was a landmark study that sought to reduce the morbidity and mortality of prostate cancer with the use of oral finasteride to prevent disease. The investigators randomly assigned 18,882 men 55 years of age or older with a normal digital rectal examination and a prostate-specific antigen (PSA) level of 3.0 ng per milliliter or lower to treatment with finasteride (5 mg per day) or placebo for 7 years. Prostate biopsy was performed if the annual PSA level, adjusted for the effect of finasteride, exceeded 4.0 ng per milliliter or if the digital rectal examination was abnormal. Prostate cancer was detected in 803 of the 4,368 men in the finasteride group who had data for the final analysis (18.4 %) and 1,147 of the 4,692 men in the placebo group who had such data (24.4 %), for a 24.8 % reduction in prevalence over the 7-year period (95 % confidence interval, 18.6–30.6 %; $p<0.001$). Tumors of Gleason grade 7 or more were more common in the finasteride group (280 of 757 tumors [37.0 %] or 6.4 % of the 4,368 men included in the final analysis) than in the placebo group (237 of 1,068 tumors [22.2 %], $p<0.001$ for the comparison between groups, or 5.1 % of the 4,692 men included in the final analysis, $p=0.005$ for the comparison between groups). Sexual side effects were more common in finasteride-treated men, whereas urinary symptoms were more common in men receiving placebo.

To seek to alleviate the concern of the increase of number of high-grade cancers detected in the original PCPT, Thompson et al. examined long-term all-cause mortality among PCPT participants. The results were reassuring with an overall 15-year rate of death of 22 % in both the finasteride group and the control group. The investigators were unable to report prostate-cancer-specific mortality.

Adverse effects to oral finasteride are listed in Table 6.2.

In men 55 years or older, 5 mg oral finasteride prevents or delays the appearance of prostate cancer, but this possible benefit and a reduced risk of urinary problems must be weighed against sexual side effects. The increased risk of high-grade prostate cancer detected with finasteride in the original Prostate Cancer Prevention Trial did not prove to affect the overall 15-year rate of death in both the finasteride and the control group in a subsequent study, and the investigators were unable to report prostate-cancer-specific mortality.

Table 6.2 Adverse reactions to 1 mg oral finasteride

Common (frequency between ≥1/100 and 1/10):
Sexual dysfunction (finasteride 3.8 % vs. 2.1 % within first 12 months of treatment; 1 % of men withdrew finasteride because of sexual dysfunction within first 12 months of treatment; thereafter, frequency decreased to 0.6 % during following 4 years of treatment)
Diminished libido (finasteride 1.8 % vs. placebo 1.3 %)
Erectile dysfunction (finasteride 1.3% vs. placebo 0.7%)
Occasional (frequency between (≥1/1,000 and <1/100):
Abnormal ejaculation
Decreased ejaculatory volume
Rare (frequency between ≥1/10,000 and <1/1,000):
Testicular pain
Breast tenderness
Gynecomastia (may persist for months to years after cessation of finasteride treatment)
Allergic reactions: rash, itching, hives, swelling of the mouth, face, lips, or tongue (angioedema)
Very rare (frequency <1/10,000):
Depression
Male breast cancer
Unknown (frequency cannot be estimated from existing data):
Persistent diminished libido or erectile dysfunction (after cessation of finasteride treatment)
Male infertility (usually in association with preexistent subfertility)
Decrease in quality of semen (there are reports on normalization or improvement of semen quality following withdrawal of drug)
Post-finasteride syndrome
Cause-relationship unresolved:
High Gleason grade tumor (7–10) in the event of prostate carcinoma in men >55 years treated with 5 mg oral finasteride daily for benign prostatic hyperplasia (finasteride 6.4 % vs. placebo 5.1 %)

6.3 Post-Finasteride Syndrome

The post-finasteride syndrome has been claimed to occur in men who have taken oral finasteride to treat either hair loss or benign prostatic hyperplasia. Reported symptoms include loss of libido, erectile dysfunction, reduction in penis size, penile curvature or reduced sensation, gynecomastia, muscle atrophy, cognitive impairment, severely dry skin, and depression. The condition allegedly may have a life-altering impact on sufferers and their families, such as job loss and the breakup of romantic relationships or marriages while also being linked to suicides.

As yet, the condition is not recognized by the scientific community, although individuals who suffer from the syndrome do present with very distinctive and relatively homogenous symptoms.

While the incidence of persistent sexual, mental, and physical side effects which continue despite quitting finasteride is unknown, it is likely that over 1,000 men worldwide are experiencing the effects. This estimate is based on the number of registered users on the Internet forum (www.propeciahelp.com).

Persistent neurological effects from other drugs are well recognized, such as the tardive dyskinesias related to the use of phenothiazines for treatment of chronic schizophrenia. There is a growing body of scientific evidence from studies in rodents that finasteride may reduce the concentration of several neuroactive steroids important for neurogenesis and neuronal survival. An important neurosteroid is allopregnanolone (ALLO), a metabolite of dihydroprogesterone. ALLO is a potent ligand of the inhibitory GABA–barbiturate receptor. $GABA_A$ receptors have variable sensitivities to ALLO in the settings of neurosteroid withdrawal, stress, social isolation, and aging. Less ALLO, as a consequence of finasteride treatment, could alter GABAergic transmission with implications for neuronal progenitors and young neurons. Interestingly, the mechanisms of irreversible tardive dyskinesias from phenothiazines may be similar to the mechanisms underlying the persistent side effects of finasteride: in rats treated with haloperidol to induce orofacial dyskinesias, co-administration of progesterone prevented this side effect, while pretreatment of the rats with finasteride reversed this protective effect, demonstrating an important role of the progesterone pathway and its metabolites.

The Post-Finasteride Syndrome Foundation (www.pfsfoundation.org) is a nonprofit organization dedicated to helping fund research on the characterization, underlying biologic mechanisms, and treatments of the post-finasteride syndrome while improving public awareness of the condition.

Up to date there are no predictive factors for the risk of development of post-finasteride syndrome and no known treatment for the disorder. For the time being, as a general rule:

- Refrain from prescribing oral finasteride to a patient with a personal history of depression, sexual dysfunction, or fertility problems.
- When fertility is an issue, one may consider performing a sperm count before and during treatment with oral finasteride.
- In any case of adverse effects, stop oral finasteride treatment.
- In all men 45 and over, perform PSA before and after starting therapy with oral finasteride and thereafter on twice-yearly basis. The level should drop by ca. 50 % upon initiation of therapy. In case of increase >0.4 ng/ml per year, refer to urologist to check prostate condition.
- For men who choose regular prostate-cancer screening, the use of oral finasteride meaningfully reduces the risk of prostate cancer.

6.4 Adverse Reactions from Hair Transplantation Surgery

Autologous hair transplantation remains the only treatment option for advanced patterned baldness both in males and in females and may be performed in selected cases of cicatricial alopecia. With the advent of total micrografting and a sharp decline in scalp reduction procedures, hair restoration surgery has become more satisfying than in the recent past. Modern techniques use the visual qualities of hair and varying design patterns to create the optical illusion of more hair than is actually present. The main advances in hair restoration surgery have been the use of one to four hair grafts, which allows a natural, undetectable hairline, and the transplantation of large numbers of these small grafts during a single session.

Careful patient selection and newer techniques are geared toward naturalness and undetectability for the lifetime of the patient.

In the majority of patients, hair transplantation is performed under local anesthesia. Lidocaine is the most commonly used anesthetic. The key to success is superficial infiltration of the dermis, which allows both better pain control and hemostasis for the patient. The patient is placed in either a prone position or a seated position for donor site removal. The amount of hair in the donor area is the only limiting factor in hair transplant surgery. Therefore, efficiency in harvesting follicular groupings is critical. There are two types of methods for harvesting donor hair: strip harvesting and follicular unit extraction.

Strip harvesting has been standard methods for ages. On the posterior scalp, a donor ellipse contains hundreds to thousands of follicular groupings that can be utilized for hair transplantation. Once the donor ellipse is removed, the wound is closed with either staples or sutures. The size of the donor ellipse depends on the amount of grafts that are needed for the particular patient. As with any cutaneous excision, strip harvesting will create a scar on the scalp.

Follicular unit extraction (FUE) utilizes the steel punch technique that was used to extract donor hairs. Recently, 0.75–1.25 mm steel punches are used to harvest individual follicular units. These punches are so small that they usually do not leave visible scars. More recently, robotic follicular unit extraction has been introduced into the field. The robot is able to skillfully remove large numbers of follicular units with minimal transection. This technology is a major advance in the harvesting of individual follicular units with minimizing visible scars.

After either method of harvesting, the follicular units obtained must be trimmed under microscopic visualization using a razor blade. Under microscopic visualization, follicles are dissected out in order to produce intact follicular units.

Various techniques are utilized to create and prepare recipient sites for subsequent transplantation of follicular units. Although various types of graft implanter may be conveniently used for the insertion of the grafts, creating slits has been widely used for ages. In creating slits over the recipient area, important considerations include slit size, depth of incision and angle, and direction. Blades may be cut to match the size of the follicular units to be inserted. Hypodermic needles may be used to make incisions for subsequent graft placement. For the frontal hairline, to frame the face well and to create a natural-looking hairline, the slits are made in an irregular pattern to try to mimic natural hairlines, which are mostly very irregular and slightly asymmetric. Twenty-five to forty follicular unit grafts per square centimeter are the transplanted densities made by most hair restoration surgeons. This density goal shows a cosmetically acceptable outcome over the recipient area with most patients being satisfied by the results.

Jeweler forceps or similar non-toothed forceps are generally used to gently place the grafts into recipient sites. Transplanted hair follicle viability is maximized by minimizing mechanical trauma to the follicle. This is accomplished by handling the subcutaneous tissue along the base of the graft rather than the graft itself.

> Hair transplantation surgery can be performed in any person with androgenetic alopecia with a good donor area, good general health status, and reasonable expectations.

Caution should be exercised in very young patients whose early alopecia is still evolving, patients with Norwood grade VI or VII with poor density, patients with unrealistic expectations, and patients with significant systemic health problems. Unrealistic expectations or body dysmorphic disorder represents contraindications for hair transplantation surgery.

> In women, hair transplantation is most appropriate in patients with pronounced hair loss of limited extent, e.g., the frontal Olsen or Christmas tree pattern, and who retain good hair density in the donor site. Hair transplantation is ideally combined with medical treatment to prevent further hair loss and to improve hair growth, density, and texture.

Complications of hair transplantation may occur both in the donor site and in the recipient area and may be due to surgical or other causes.

In a retrospective analysis of male patients who underwent hair transplantation surgery for androgenetic alopecia, Loganathan et al. collected data from registers, telephonic inquiry, and electronic mails and recorded complications during and after surgery and the subjective feeling of patients about hair growth. Seventy-three patients were included in the analysis. The majority of patients had undergone follicular unit transplantation. Postoperative edema was found in 42.47 % of patients, followed by sterile folliculitis in 23.29 %, wide donor scar in 15.07 %, bacterial folliculitis and numbness/paresthesia in 10.96 %.

In another study, Salanitri et al. analyzed complications in 425 consecutive patients undergoing 533 hair transplantations. Patients with androgenetic alopecia (407 men and 17 women), cicatricial alopecia (9 men and 8 women), and malformations (1 man and 3 women) with a mean age of 36.9 years (standard deviation, 10.4 years) underwent hair transplantation between 1995 and 2006 and were followed up postoperatively for at least 1 year. Data on surgical complications were retrospectively analyzed. The overall complication rate was 4.7 %, including enlarged scar (1.2 %), folliculitis (1.0 %), necrosis in the donor area (0.8 %), keloids (0.4 %), bleeding (0.2 %), infection (0.2 %), and pyogenic granuloma (0.2 %). The frequency of enlarged scar increased proportionally according to the number of surgical procedures.

> As a result of impaired circulation and wound healing, smoking status has been implicated to represent a risk factor for a higher complication rate of hair restoration surgery.

Following a review of the operative technique for a single-stage vertical flap for reconstruction of the frontal hairline, Dardour et al. originally presented a series of 156 such flaps with a minimum follow-up of 6 months. Risk factors for necrosis or alopecia of the distal end of the flap included retroauricular design and cigarette smoking. There was not a single case of necrosis in nonsmokers with flaps shorter than 16 cm.

A peculiar adverse effect following hair transplantation surgery is *recipient-area folliculitis* (Fig. 6.4a): postoperative recipient-area folliculitis may be a cause of less or delayed growth of transplanted hair and an obvious cause of distress to the patient. Bunagan et al. performed a study of the clinical features and possible factors that may be associated with the development of recipient-area folliculitis after follicular unit transplantation (FUT) in a retrospective analysis of 27 patients who developed folliculitis after FUT and 28 patients without such complication. They found that lesion onset ranged from 2 days to 6 months after FUT (mean 1.44 months).

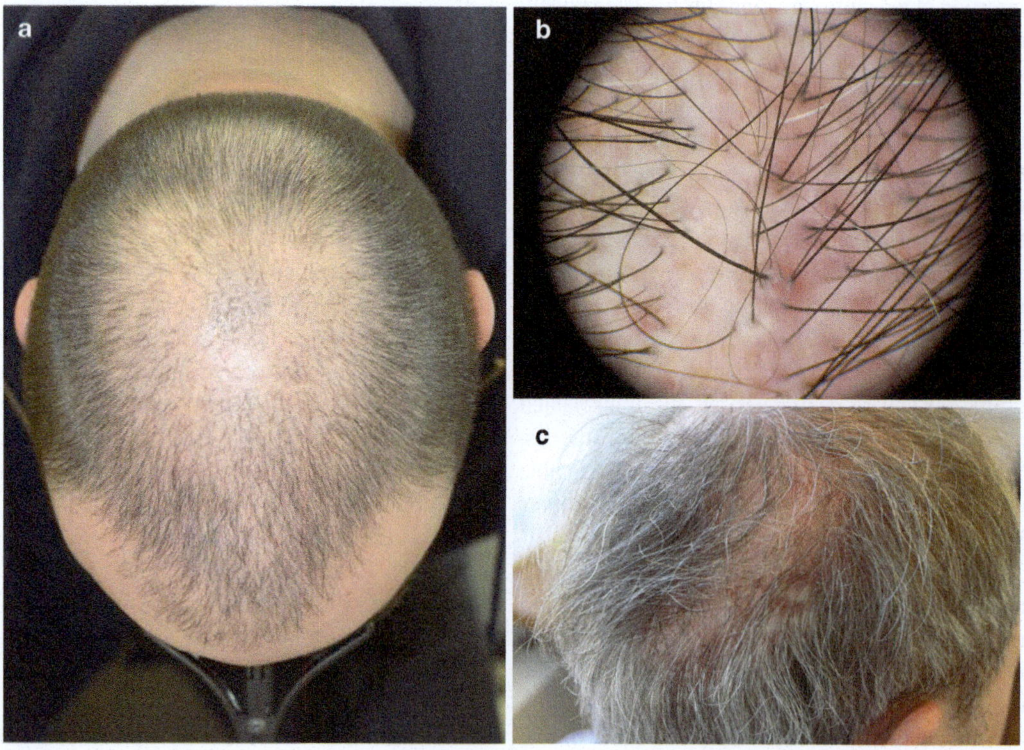

Fig. 6.4 (**a–c**) Adverse reactions from hair transplantation surgery. (**a, b**) Recipient-area folliculitis. (**b**) Dermoscopic finding. (**c**) Folliculitis decalvans

Lesions were mostly pustules that resolved without sequelae. Statistical analysis showed that, in terms of patient characteristics (e.g., hair features, scalp condition) and the number of grafts transplanted, there was no statistically significant difference in assessed parameters between those with and without folliculitis ($p < 0.05$). Ultimately, regardless of management, lesions healed without scarring and without affecting graft growth. Important differential diagnoses include folliculitis decalvans and lichen planopilaris developing after hair transplantation.

Otberg et al. reported *folliculitis decalvans developing after hair restoration surgery in punch grafts* (Fig. 6.4b) after 20 years. The relationship may be either causal or fortuitous. Nevertheless, the presence of bacterial biofilms in the infrainfundibular part of hair follicles has been identified and proposed to be pathogenic in folliculitis decalvans. A biofilm represents any group of microorganisms in which cells stick to each other within a self-produced matrix of extracellular polymeric substance on living or nonliving surfaces. Bacteria living in a biofilm have different properties from free-floating bacteria of the same species, as the dense and protected environment of the film allows them to cooperate and interact in various ways. One benefit of this environment is increased resistance to antibiotics. Biofilms have been found to be involved in a wide variety of microbial infections in the body. Typical examples are catheter infections; formation of dental plaque with gingivitis; coating contact lenses; infections of permanent indwelling devices, such as joint prostheses and heart valves; and more recently complications from dermal fillers.

> No matter the sophistication, biofilms are known to develop on all medical devices and tissue engineering constructs.

In the case of folliculitis decalvans, bacterial biofilms form at the interface of the hair shaft. Biofilms are usually found on solid substrates submerged in or exposed to an aqueous solution. Biofilms can contain many different types of microorganism; however, some organisms will form single-species films under certain conditions. In folliculitis decalvans following hair transplantation, it is conceivable that bacteria, usually *S. aureus*, are introduced in the course of the procedure.

Crisóstomo et al. originally reported two cases of *posttransplantation lesions compatible with lichen planopilaris* of both recipient and donor areas. The quality of the hair follicles in the donor area was apparently compromised by lichen planopilaris, the probable cause of hair loss in their cases. Chiang et al. subsequently reported a case series of lichen planopilaris following cosmetic scalp surgery: seven patients developed lichen planopilaris following hair transplantation, and three patients developed frontal fibrosing alopecia following face-lift surgery. In all cases there was no previous history of lichen planopilaris or frontal fibrosing alopecia. Therefore, there lacks the evidence to link the respective surgical procedures to the development of lichen planopilaris or frontal fibrosing alopecia. Nevertheless, the clinical observations suggest a possible common underlying pathogenic process. Explanations include the Koebner phenomenon induced by surgical trauma or an autoimmune process targeting an as yet unidentified hair follicle antigen liberated during surgery or perhaps a postsurgery proinflammatory milieu inducing hair follicle immune privilege collapse and follicular damage in susceptible individuals. Finally, Donovan provided further support for an association between hair transplant surgery and the development of lichen planopilaris: in a retrospective review of the records of patients referred for evaluation of suboptimal growth after hair transplantation, 17 patients (15 male, 2 female) were diagnosed with LPP after hair transplant surgery. The most common symptom was itching. Patients' scalps were evaluated using dermoscopy, and scalp biopsies were performed in all patients to confirm the diagnosis. Perifollicular erythema or perifollicular scale was present in 12 patients (70 %). The timing of disease occurrence was variable (4–36 months after hair transplantation). The author concluded that traumatic skin injury from recipient site creation may be relevant to the pathogenesis.

The incidence of lichen planopilaris following hair transplantation surgery and risk factors remain to be clarified. When lichen planopilaris is suspected, a biopsy of the scalp must be performed to avoid transplantation during disease activity.

Nirmal et al. evaluated evidence of perifollicular inflammation of donor area during hair transplantation in androgenetic alopecia in comparison with normal controls. A total of 21 male patients with androgenetic alopecia and 7 matched controls participated in the study. Histopathological analysis of biopsy specimens from donor strip of patients during hair transplantation and of two 4 mm punch biopsies from controls was performed. Nearly 76 % of androgenetic alopecia patients had evidence of significant perifollicular fibrosis, and 33.33 % of androgenetic alopecia patients showed moderate to dense perifollicular lymphocytic infiltrates, whereas none of the controls did. The authors propose histopathological evaluation of donor area during hair transplantation to evaluate the extent of perifollicular inflammation and achieve better results by following it up with treatment directed to decrease the inflammation.

6.5 Adverse Effects from Cosmetic Hair Treatments

Besides hair weathering, there exist a number of peculiar adverse effects resulting from inappropriate cosmetic hair treatments. These are:

- Hair matting (from inappropriate hair washing)
- Bubble hair (from inappropriate hair drying)
- Cosmetic hair beads (from inappropriate hairstyling)
- Allergic contact dermatitis (from contact sensitivity)

Patients sometimes blame shampoos for their hair loss. Diffuse hair loss due to an inhibition of mitosis associated with long-term use of shampoos containing keratostatic anti-dandruff agents, such as selenium sulfide, has been discussed in the older literature and remains controversial. More frequently, the impression of increased hair shedding is created through the detachment of scales containing groups of trapped telogen hairs.

The absence of effects of dimethicone- and non-dimethicone-containing shampoos on hair loss rates has systematically been demonstrated.

6.5.1 From Inappropriate Washing: Hair Matting

Hair matting or acute felting of the hair represents a rare condition of irreversible tangling of scalp hair with dramatic onset. It is not a primary hair disorder: physical conditions, chemical agents, and behavioral factors play the main roles. There is invariably a history of previous chemical hair treatment.

Damaged hair, e.g., permanently waved hair, is particularly prone to sudden entanglement, which can occur with the use of viscous fluids such as undiluted shampoo. The piling of long hair on the top of the head while shampooing and the repeated friction of wet hair facilitate the process of matting. The raised cuticle cells of the damaged hair interlock as a result of excessive friction and static electricity, and the hair becomes tangled. Accordingly, microscopy reveals twisting and bending of the hairs through 180°. An irreversible knot, sometimes referred to as a "bird's nest," forms over a limited area (Fig. 6.5).

Since the structure of the hair is significantly damaged, the only alternative is to cut off the tangled portion.

The best means of preventing hair matting in damaged hair is to follow the instructions for using shampoo products and to regularly use a conditioner, especially for permed hair.

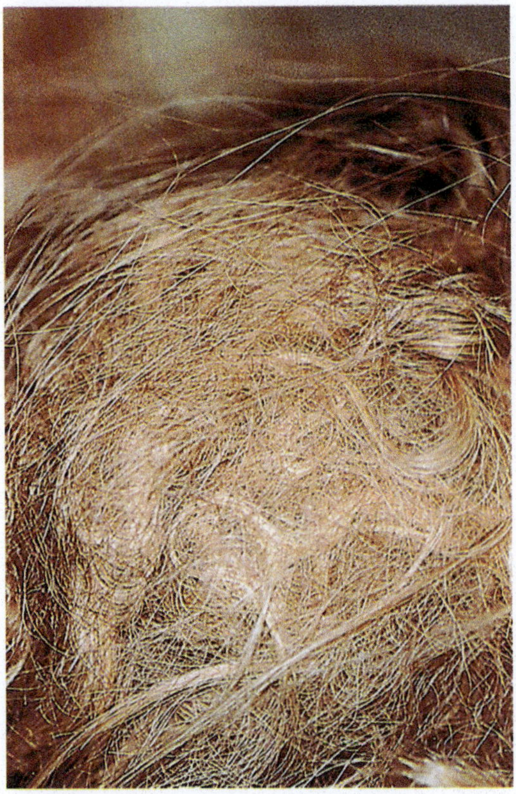

Fig. 6.5 Bird's nest hair

6.5.2 From Inappropriate Drying: Bubble Hair

Bubble hair is an acquired hair shaft abnormality characterized by a localized area of weak, dry, and brittle hair which breaks easily and bubble-like areas in the hair shaft seen with light microscopy. The overall texture of the hair may change from soft and naturally curly to straight and stiff. Bubble hair is a reproducible hair shaft defect caused by heat. Brief, focal heating of damp hair is sufficient to cause bubbles to form inside the hair fibers (Fig. 6.6a, b).

> The use of overheating hair dryers, or any other hair care equipment that overheats, should be avoided.

6.5.3 From Inappropriate Styling: Cosmetically Induced Hair Beads

Cosmetically induced hair beads present as monilethrix-like appearance of hair shafts through buildup of polymers (PVP, vinyl acetate, methacrylates) on hair as a result of excessive use of hair lacquer and hairstyling gel. Light microscopy reveals that the hair is encircled by a material with a glassy appearance (Fig. 6.7a, b).

6.5.4 From Contact Sensitivity: Allergic Contact Dermatitis

Allergic contact dermatitis represents the manifestation of an allergic response of the skin

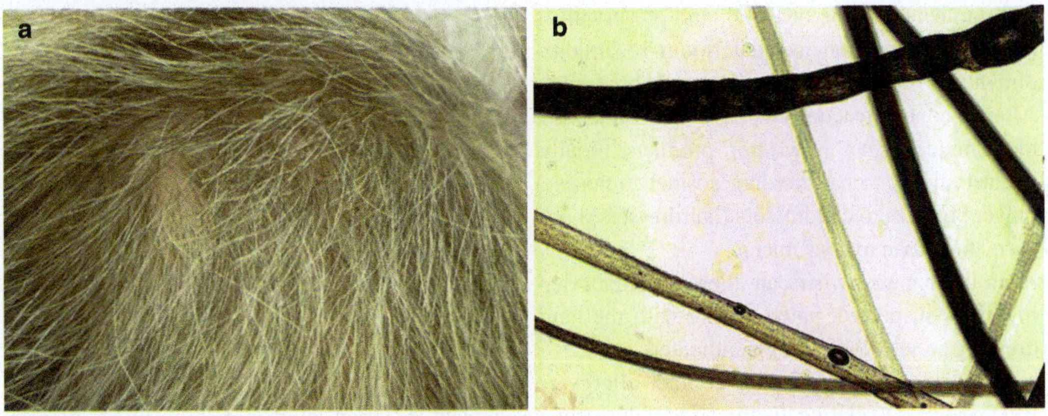

Fig. 6.6 (**a**, **b**) Bubble hair. (**a**) Localized area of brittle hair. (**b**) Bubbles inside hair fibers (light microscopy)

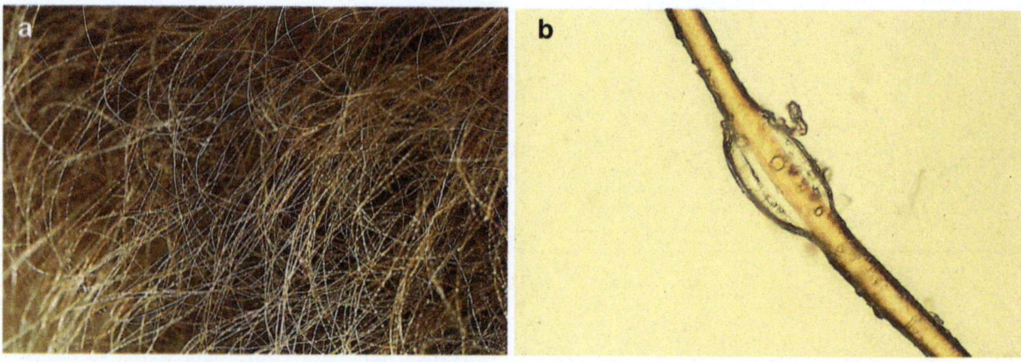

Fig. 6.7 (**a**, **b**) Cosmetic hair beads. (**a**) Monilethrix-like appearance of hair. (**b**) Buildup of polymers with glassy appearance on hair shaft (light microscopy)

caused by contact with a substance the individual is sensitized to.

> Allergic reactions to cosmetics are usually overestimated by consumers. Less than 10 % of the population report an intolerance reaction to a cosmetic product, and of those 1 % is caused by a contact allergen that is identified with patch testing.

In contrast to irritant contact dermatitis, allergic contact dermatitis represents a hypersensitivity reaction that is atypical within the general population. Common allergens in cosmetics implicated include the following (in order of frequency): fragrances, hair dyes (*p*-phenylenediamine or PPD and *p*-toluenediamine or PTD), and preservatives (formaldehyde, parabens, quaternium-15, imidazolinylurea, DMDM hydantoin, and bronopol). Allergic contact reactions to *leave-on* products are more frequent than to *wash-off* products. Finally, contact allergy to hairdressing cosmetics poses a bigger problem to hairdressers (hairdressers' hand dermatitis) than to consumers.

In those cases, where an allergic contact dermatitis is suspected, patch testing with the hairdressing series (Table 6.3) is indicated.

Most prevalent is allergic contact allergy to PPD and PTD relating to the use of hair dyes (Fig. 6.8a–c) that may result both in allergic contact dermatitis and an acute and diffuse (inflammatory) telogen effluvium following the allergic contact reaction approximately by 3 months. Contact allergy to ammonium thioglycolate relates to relaxers and contact allergy to ammonium persulfate to bleaching agents.

Table 6.3 Hairdressing series

1. *p*-Phenylenediamine (PPD)
2. Toluene-2,5-diamine sulfate
3. 2-Nitro-*p*-phenylendiamine
4. Ammonium thioglycolate
5. Ammonium persulfate
6. Formaldehyde
7. Nickel sulfate hexahydrate
8. Cobalt(II) chloride hexahydrate
9. Resorcinol
10. *m*-Aminophenol
11. *p*-Aminophenol
12. Hydrogen peroxide
13. Hydroquinone
14. Myroxylon pereirae resin
15. Chloroacetamide
16. Glyceryl monothioglycolate (glyceryl thioglycolate)
17. Cocamidopropyl betaine
18. Methylisothiazolinone + methylchloroisothiazolinone
19. 2-Bromp-2-nitropropane-1,3-diol (bronopol)
20. Captan
21. *p*-Chloro-*m*-cresol (PCMC)
22. Chloroxylenol (PCMX)
23. Imidazolidinyl urea
24. Quaternium-15 (Dowicil 200)
25. Zinc pyrithione (Zinc Omadine)
26. Diazolidinyl urea
27. Lauryl glucoside
28. Oleamidopropyl dimethylamine

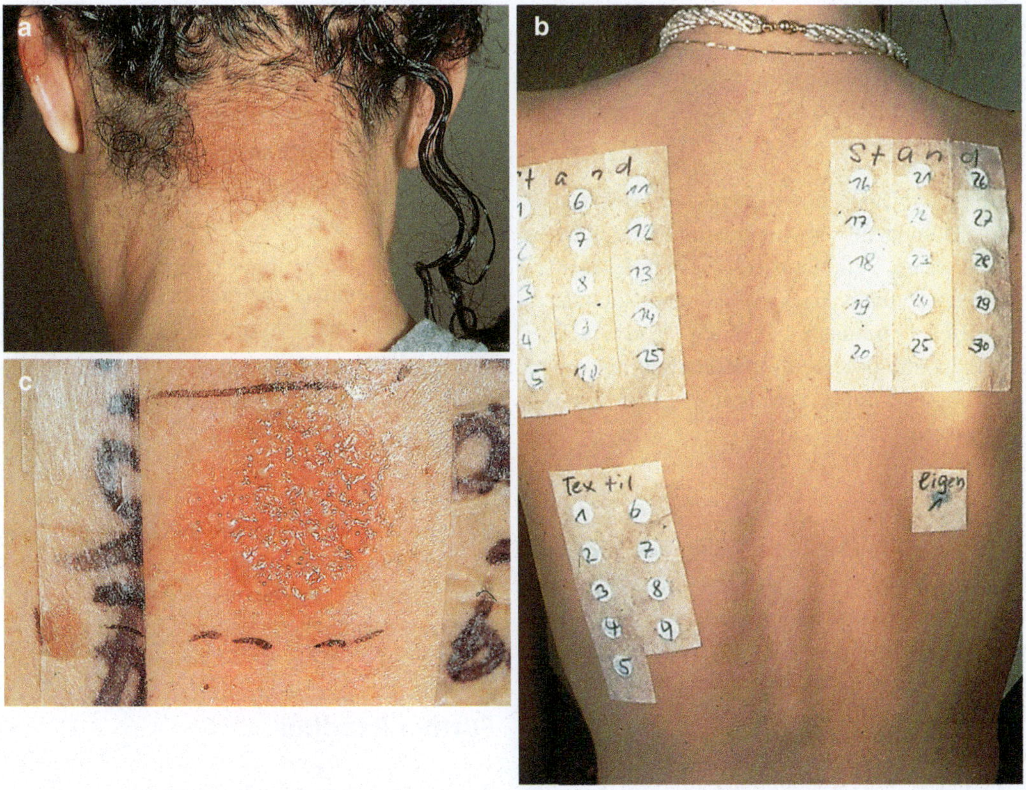

Fig. 6.8 (**a–c**) Allergic contact dermatitis. (**a**) Contact dermatitis to hair-coloring agent. (**b**) Patch testing. (**c**) Positive patch test

Severe cases of allergic contact dermatitis are best treated with oral corticosteroids which are tapered gradually, with various dosing schedules ranging from a total of 10–14 days to prevent recurrence of the rash. Sedating antihistamines such as oral hydroxyzine may be added to relieve the intense itching. Persons who develop contact sensitivity to a certain allergen are most likely to have it for the rest of their lives, and detecting the allergen by means of patch testing and avoiding it is mandatory in treating the condition and resolving its symptoms.

6.6 Nocebo Reaction

In a strict sense, a nocebo reaction refers to undesirable effects a subject experiences after receiving an inert dummy drug or placebo. Nocebo reactions are not chemically generated and are due only to the subject's pessimistic belief and expectation that treatment will produce negative consequences. In a wider sense, the term is being increasingly used for unexpected negative reactions to an active drug.

The term nocebo (from Latin for "I will harm") was originally coined in 1961 by W. Kennedy for the counterpart of placebo (from Latin for "I will please"), which refers to desirable effects a subject experiences after receiving an inert dummy drug. In both cases, there is no real pharmacologically active substance involved, but the actual negative or positive consequences, respectively, of the administration of the drug, which may be physiological, behavioral, emotional, or cognitive, are nonetheless real. Kennedy emphasized that his specific usage of the term nocebo does not refer to the iatrogenic action of the drug but insisted that a nocebo reaction is subject centered and that the term nocebo reaction specifically refers to a quality inherent in the patient rather than in the drug. Kennedy was precisely speaking of an outcome that is totally generated by a subject's negative expectation of a drug administration and is the exact counterpart of a placebo response that would be generated by a subject's positive expectation.

> In general, nocebo reactions are observed more frequently in women and in the older age group. Symptoms have a high level of psychosomatic background and include nausea, headaches, and drowsiness. Frequently observed objective findings are increased pulse frequency and blood pressure.

In 2007, Mondaini et al. addressed the question how many of sexual side effects associated with oral finasteride treatment are related to a nocebo phenomenon: 120 sexually active male patients with an International Index of Erectile Function-erectile function (IIEF-EF) domain ≥25 and a clinical diagnosis of benign prostatic hyperplasia were randomized to receive 5 mg oral finasteride concealed as an "X compound of proven efficacy for the treatment of benign prostatic hyperplasia" for 1 year with (group 2) or without (group 1) counseling on the drug sexual side effects. The phrase used to inform group 2 patients was "may cause erectile dysfunction, decreased libido, problems of ejaculation but these are uncommon." The estimation of side effects was conducted at 6 and 12 months using the male sexual function-4 (MSF-4 item) questionnaire and a self-administered questionnaire. 107 patients completed the study. Group 2 patients ($n=55$) reported a significant higher proportion of one or more sexual side effects as compared to group 1 ($n=52$) (43.6 % *vs.* 15.3 %, $p=0.03$). The incidence of erectile dysfunction, decreased libido, and ejaculation disorders were 9.6, 7.7, and 5.7 %, respectively, for group 1 and 30.9, 23.6, and 16.3 %, respectively, for group 2 ($p=0.02$, $p=0.04$, and $p=0.06$). The authors concluded that blinded administration of finasteride was associated with a significantly higher proportion of sexual dysfunction in patients informed on sexual side effects as compared to those in which the same information was omitted. A scenario is likely to occur in clinical practice, where the patient is counseled by the physician and has access to the drug information sheet. The burden of this nocebo effect has to be taken into account when managing finasteride sexual side effects.

> The influence of the prescribing physician should be kept in mind, since inspiring confidence *versus* skepticism and fear clearly impacts the outcome of treatment.

Ultimately, some patients with somatoform disorder and specific personality disorders, e.g., anxious, negativistic, histrionic, or paranoid, are more prone to nocebo reactions and should be recognized as such.

Further Reading

Adverse Reactions to Topical Minoxidil

Alomar A, Smandia JA (1988) Allergic contact dermatitis from minoxidil. Contact Dermatitis 18(1):51–52

Bamford JT (1987) A falling out following minoxidil: telogen effluvium. J Am Acad Dermatol 16(1 Pt 1):144–146

Baral J (1985) Scalp comedones after topical minoxidil. J Am Acad Dermatol 13(6):1051–1052

Baral J (1987) Deaths associated with topical minoxidil therapy. J Am Acad Dermatol 17(3):515–516

Cobos Toro LA, Ayani Almagia I (1994) Topical minoxidil and accompanying migraines. Aten Primaria 14(7):912

Corazza M, Borghi A, Ricci M, Sarno O, Virgili A (2010) Patch testing in allergic contact dermatitis from minoxidil. Dermatitis 21(4):217–218

Dawber RP, Rundegren J (2003) Hypertrichosis in females applying minoxidil topical solution and in normal controls. J Eur Acad Dermatol Venereol 17(3):271–275

Degreef H, Hendrickx I, Dooms-Goossens A (1985) Allergic contact dermatitis to minoxidil. Contact Dermatitis 13(3):194–195

Ebner H, Müller E (1995) Allergic contact dermatitis from minoxidil. Contact Dermatitis 32(5):316–317

Eller MG, Szpunar GJ, Della-Coletta AA (1989) Absorption of minoxidil after topical application: effect of frequency and site of application. Clin Pharmacol Ther 45(4):396–402

Ferry JJ, Forbes KK, VanderLugt JT, Szpunar G (1990a) Influence of tretinoin on the percutaneous absorption of minoxidil from an aqueous topical solution. Clin Pharmacol Ther 47(4):439–446

Ferry JJ, Shepard JH, Szpunar GJ (1990b) Relationship between contact time of applied dose and percutaneous absorption of minoxidil from a topical solution. J Pharm Sci 79(6):483–486

Fisher AA (1990) Use of glycerin in topical minoxidil solutions for patients allergic to propylene glycol. Cutis 45(2):81–82

Fisher AA (1993) Unusual acute, nonallergic eruptions of the scalp from combined use of minoxidil and retinoic acid. Cutis 51(1):17–18

Franz TJ (1985) Percutaneous absorption of minoxidil in man. Arch Dermatol 121(2):203–206

Friedman ES, Friedman PM, Cohen DE, Washenik K (2002) Allergic contact dermatitis to topical minoxidil solution: etiology and treatment. J Am Acad Dermatol 46(2):309–312

Georgala S, Befon A, Maniatopoulou E, Georgala C (2007) Topical use of minoxidil in children and systemic side effects. Dermatology 214:101–102

González M, Landa N, Gardeazabal J, Calderón MJ, Bilbao I, Díaz Pérez JL (1994) Generalized hypertrichosis after treatment with topical minoxidil. Clin Exp Dermatol 19(2):157–158

Guarneri C, Cannavò SP (2013) Erosive pustular dermatosis of the scalp from topical minoxidil 5% solution. Int J Dermatol 52(4):507–509

Hagemann T, Schlütter-Böhmer B, Allam JP, Bieber T, Novak N (2005) Positive lymphocyte transformation test in a patient with allergic contact dermatitis of the scalp after short-term use of topical minoxidil solution. Contact Dermatitis 53(1):53–55

Ingles RM, Kahn T (1983) Unusual hair changes with minoxidil therapy. Int J Dermatol 22(2):120–122

Kaler SG, Patrinos ME, Lambert GH, Myers TF, Karlman R, Anderson CL (1987) Hypertrichosis and congenital anomalies associated with maternal use of minoxidil. Pediatrics 79(3):434–436

Katz HI (1989) Topical minoxidil: review of efficacy and safety. Cutis 43(1):94–98

Kidwai BJ, George M (1992) Hair loss with minoxidil withdrawal. Lancet 340(8819):609–610

Leenen FH, Smith DL, Unger WP (1988) Topical minoxidil: cardiac effects in bald man. Br J Clin Pharmacol 26(4):481–485

Lorette G, Nivet H (1985) Diffuse hypertrichosis caused by minoxidil in a 2-and-a-half-year-old child. Ann Dermatol Venereol 112(6-7):527–528

Malakar S, Dhar S (2000) Leucoderma associated with the use of topical minoxidil: a report of two cases. Dermatology 201(2):183–184

McCormick MA, Forman MH, Manoguerra AS (1989) Severe toxicity from ingestion of a topical minoxidil preparation. Am J Emerg Med 7(4):419–2

Navarini AA, Ziegler M, Kolm I, Weibel L, Huber C, Trüeb RM (2010) Minoxidil-induced trichostasis spinulosa of terminal hair. Arch Dermatol 146(12):1434–1435

Peluso AM, Misciali C, Vincenzi C, Tosti A (1997) Diffuse hypertrichosis during treatment with 5% topical minoxidil. Br J Dermatol 136(1):118–120

Rebora A, Guarrera M (1989) Hair discoloration caused by minoxidil lotion. J Am Acad Dermatol 21(6):1314

Rodríguez-Martín M, Sáez-Rodríguez M, Carnerero-Rodríguez A et al (2007) Pustular allergic contact dermatitis from topical minoxidil 5%. J Eur Acad Dermatol Venereol 21(5):701–702

Rojansky N, Fasouliotis SJ, Ariel I, Nadjari M (2002) Extreme caudal agenesis. Possible drug-related etiology? J Reprod Med 47(3):241–245

Rossi A, Cantisani C, Melis L, Iorio A, Scali E, Calvieri S (2012) Minoxidil use in dermatology, side effects and recent patents. Recent Pat Inflamm Allergy Drug Discov 6(2):130–136

Ruas E, Gonçalo M, Figueiredo A, Gonçalo S (1992) Allergic contact dermatitis from minoxidil. Contact Dermatitis 26(1):57–58

Sánchez-Motilla JM, Pont V, Nagore E, Rodríguez-Serna M, Sánchez JL, Aliaga A (1998) Pustular allergic contact dermatitis from minoxidil. Contact Dermatitis 38(5):283–284

Satoh H, Morikaw S, Fujiwara C, Terada H, Uehara A, Ohno R (2000) A case of acute myocardial infarction associated with topical use of minoxidil (RiUP) for treatment of baldness. Jpn Heart J 41(4): 519–523

Scarinci F, Mezzana P, Pasquini P, Colletti M, Cacciamani A (2012) Central chorioretinopathy associated with topical use of minoxidil 2% for treatment of baldness. Cutan Ocul Toxicol 31(2):157–159

Scheman AJ, West DP, Hordinksy MK, Osburn AH, West LE (2000) Alternative formulation for patients with contact reactions to topical 2% and 5% minoxidil vehicle ingredients. Contact Dermatitis 42(4):241

Schmutz JL, Barbaud A, Tréchot P (2008) Systemic effects of topical minoxidil 2% in children. Ann Dermatol Venereol 135(8-9):62

Shapiro J (2003) Safety of topical minoxidil solution: a one-year, prospective, observational study. J Cutan Med Surg 7(4):322–329

Shin HS, Won CH, Lee SH, Kwon OS, Kim KH, Eun H (2007) Efficacy of 5% minoxidil versus combined 5% minoxidil and 0.01% tretinoin for male pattern hair loss: a randomized, double-blind, comparative clinical trial. Am J Clin Dermatol 8(5):285–290

Smorlesi C, Caldarella A, Caramelli L, Di Lollo S, Moroni F (2003) Topically applied minoxidil may cause fetal malformation: a case report. Birth Defects Res A Clin Mol Teratol 67(12):997–1001

Spindler JR (1987) Deaths occurring during clinical studies of topical minoxidil. J Am Acad Dermatol 16(3 Pt 2):725–729

Stern RS (1987) Topical minoxidil. A survey of use and complications. Arch Dermatol 123(1):62–65

Suzuki K, Suzuki M, Akamatsu H, Matsungaga K (2002) Allergic contact dermatitis from minoxidil: study of the cross-reaction to minoxidil. Am J Contact Dermat 13(1):45–46

Toriumi DM, Konior RJ, Berktold RE (1988) Severe hypertrichosis of the external ear canal during minoxidil therapy. Arch Otolaryngol Head Neck Surg 114(8):918–919

Tosti A, Bardazzi F, De Padova MP, Caponeri GM, Melino M, Veronesi S (1985) Contact dermatitis to minoxidil. Contact Dermatitis 13(4):275–276

Trattner A, David M (2002) Pigmented contact dermatitis from topical minoxidil 5%. Contact Dermatitis 46(4):246

Valsecchi R, Cainelli T (1987) Allergic contact dermatitis from minoxidil. Contact Dermatitis 17(1):58–59

van der Willigen AH, Dutrée-Meulenberg RO, Stolz E, Geursen-Reitsma AM, van Joost T (1987) Topical minoxidil sensitization in androgenic alopecia. Contact Dermatitis 17(1):44–45

Veyrac G, Chiffoleau A, Bailly C, Baudot S, Beaudouin S, Larousse C (1995) Cutaneous application of monoxidil during pregnancy: hairy infant. Therapie 50:474–476

Whitmore SE (1992) The importance of proper vehicle selection in the detection of minoxidil sensitivity. Arch Dermatol 128(5):653–656

Wilson C, Walkden V, Powell S, Shaw S, Wilkinson J, Dawber R (1991) Contact dermatitis in reaction to 2% topical minoxidil solution. J Am Acad Dermatol 24(4):661–662

Adverse Reactions to Oral Finasteride

Altomare G, Capella GL (2002) Depression circumstantially related to the administration of finasteride for androgenetic alopecia. J Dermatol 29:665–669

Canguven O, Burnett AL (2008) The effect of 5 alpha-reductase inhibitors on erectile function. J Androl 29:514–523

Finn DA, Long SL, Tanchuck MA, Crabbe J (2004) Interaction of chronic ethanol exposure and finasteride: Sex and strain differences. Pharmacol Biochem Behav 78:435–443

Glina S, Neves PA, Saade R, Netto NR Jr, Soares JB, Galuppo AG (2004) Finasteride-associated male infertility. Rev Hosp Clin Fac Med Sao Paulo 59:203–205

Gorin RE, Crabbe JC, Tanchuck MA, Long SL, Finn DA (2005) Effects of finasteride on chronic and acute ethanol withdrawal severity in the WSP and WSR selected lines. Alcohol Clin Exp Res 29:939–948

Irwig MS, Kolukula S (2011) Persistent sexual side effects of finasteride for male pattern hair loss. J Sex Med 8:1747–1753

Irwig MS (2012a) Depressive symptoms and suicidal thoughts among former users of finasteride with persistent sexual side effects. J Clin Psychiatry 73:1220–1223

Irwig MS (2013) Decreased alcohol consumption among former male users of finasteride with persistent sexual side effects: a preliminary report. Alcohol Clin Exp 37:1823–1826

Overstreet JW, Fuh VL, Gould J, Howards SS, Lieber MM, Hellstrom W, Shapiro S, Carroll P, Corfman RS, Petrou S, Lewis R, Toth P, Shown T, Roy J, Jarow JP, Bonilla J, Jacobsen CA, Wang DZ, Kaufman KD (1999) Chronic treatment with finasteride daily does not affect spermatogenesis or semen production in young men. J Urol 162:1295–1300

Ramot Y, Czarnowicki T, Zlotogorski A (2009) Finasteride induced gynecomastia: case report and review of the Literature. Int J Trichol 1:27–29

Ricci G, Martinelli M, Luppi S, Lo Bello L, De Santis M, Skerk K, Zito G (2012) Finasteride and fertility: case report and review of the literature. J Drugs Dermatol 11:1511–1513

Rossi A, Cantisani C, Scarnò M, Trucchia A, Fortuna MC, Calvieri S (2011) Finasteride, 1 mg daily administration on male androgenetic alopecia in different age groups: 10-year follow-up. Dermatol Ther 24:455–461

Sato A, Takeda A (2012) Evaluation of efficacy and safety of finasteride 1 mg in 3177 Japanese men with androgenetic alopecia. J Dermatol 39:27–32

Thompson IM, Goodman PJ, Tangen CM, Lucia MS, Miller GJ, Ford LG, Lieber MM, Cespedes RD, Atkins JN, Lippman SM, Carlin SM, Ryan A, Szczepanek CM, Crowley JJ, Coltman CA Jr (2003) The influence of finasteride on the development of prostate cancer. N Engl J Med 349:215–224

Thompson IM Jr, Goodman PJ, Tangen CM, Parnes HL, Minasian LM, Godley PA, Lucia MS, Ford LG (2013) Long-term survival of participants in the prostate cancer prevention trial. N Engl J Med 369:603–610

Traish AM, Hassani J, Guay AT, Zitzmann M, Hansen ML (2011) Adverse side effects of 5α-reductase inhibitors therapy: persistent diminished libido and erectile dysfunction and depression in a subset of patients. J Sex Med 8:872–884

Post-Finasteride Syndrome

Cecchin E, De Mattia E, Mazzon G, Cauci S, Trombetta C, Toffoli G (2014) A pharmacogenetic survey of androgen receptor (CAG)n and (GGN)n polymorphisms in patients experiencing long term side effects after finasteride discontinuation. Int J Biol Markers 29(4):e310–e316

Ganzer CA, Jacobs AR, Iqbal F (2014) Persistent sexual, emotional, and cognitive impairment post-finasteride: a survey of men reporting symptoms. Am J Mens Health 9:22–28

Irwig MS (2012b) Persistent sexual side effects of finasteride: could they be permanent? J Sex Med 9:2927–2932

LeFevre M (2013) A role for finasteride in the prevention of prostate cancer? N Engl J Med 369:670–671

www.pfsfoundation.org

www.propeciahelp.com

Singh MK, Avram M (2014) Persistent sexual dysfunction and depression in finasteride users for male pattern hair loss: a serious concern or red herring? J Clin Aesthet Dermatol 7(12):51–55

Adverse Reactions from Hair Transplantation Surgery

Bunagan MJ, Pathomvanich D, Laorwong K (2010) Recipient area folliculitis after follicular-unit transplantation: characterization of clinical features and analysis of associated factors. Dermatol Surg 36(7):1161–1165
Chiang YZ, Tosti A, Chaudhry IH et al (2012) Lichen planopilaris following hair transplantation and face-lift surgery. Br J Dermatol 166(3):666–370
Crisóstomo MR, Crisóstomo MC, Crisóstomo MG et al (2011) Hair loss due to lichen planopilaris after hair transplantation: a report of two cases and a literature review. An Bras Dermatol 86(2):359–362
Donovan J (2012) Lichen planopilaris after hair transplantation: report of 17 cases. Dermatol Surg 38(12): 1998–2004
Konior RJ (2013) Complications in hair-restoration surgery. Facial Plast Surg Clin North Am 21(3):505–520
Lam SM (2013) Complications in hair restoration. Facial Plast Surg Clin North Am 21(4):675–680
Loganathan E, Sarvajnamurthy S, Gorur D et al (2014) Complications of hair restoration surgery: a retrospective analysis. Int J Trichol 6(4):168–172
Matard B, Meylheuc T, Briandet R et al (2012) First evidence of bacterial biofilms in the anaerobe part of scalp hair follicles: a pilot comparative study in folliculitis decalvans. J Eur Acad Dermatol Venereol 27:853–860
Nirmal B, Somiah S, Sacchidanand SA, Biligi DS, Palo S (2013) Evaluation of perifollicular inflammation of donor area during hair transplantation in androgenetic alopecia and its comparison with controls. Int J Trichol 5(2):73–76
Otberg N, Wu WY, Kang H et al (2009) Folliculitis decalvans developing 20 years after hair restoration surgery in punch grafts: case report. Dermatol Surg 35(11): 1852–1856
Salanitri S, Gonçalves AJ, Helene A Jr, Lopes FH (2009) Surgical complications in hair transplantation: a series of 533 procedures. Aesthet Surg J 29(1):72–76

Adverse Effects from Cosmetic Hair Treatments

Adams RM, Maibach HI (1985) A five-year study of cosmetic reactions. J Am Acad Dermatol 13:1062–1069
Al-Ghani MA, Geilen CC, Blume-Peytavi U, Orfanos CE (2000) Matting of hair: a multifactorial enigma. Dermatology 20:101–104
Bolt HM, Golka K (2007) The debate on carcinogenicity of permanent hair dyes: new insights. Crit Rev Toxicol 37:521–536
Dawber R (1996) Hair: Its structure and response to cosmetic preparations. Clin Dermatol 14:105–112
Gathers RC, Jankowski M, Eide M, Lim HW (2009) Hair grooming practices and central centrifugal cicatricial alopecia. J Am Acad Dermatol 60:574–578
Gummer CL (1994) Bubble hair: a cosmetic abnormality caused by brief, focal heating of damp hair fibers. Br J Dermatol 131:9801–9903
Itin P, Schiller P, Mathys D, Guggenheim R (1997) Cosmetically induced hair beads. J Am Acad Dermatol 36:260–261
Kelsh MA, Alexander DD, Kalmes RM, Buffler PA (2008) Personal use of hair dyes and risk of bladder cancer: a meta-analysis of epidemiologic data. Cancer Causes Control 19:549–558
Khumalo NP, Gumedze F (2012) Traction: risk factor or co-incidence in central centrifugal cicatricial alopecia? Br J Dermatol 167(5):1191–1193
Kyei A, Bergfeld WF, Piliang M, Summers P (2011) Medical and environmental risk factors for the development of central centrifugal cicatricial alopecia: a population study. Arch Dermatol 147: 909–914
LoPresti P, Papa CM, Kligman AM (1968) Hot comb alopecia. Arch Dermatol 98:234–238
Rollison DE, Helzlsouer KJ, Pinney SM (2006) Personal hair dye use and cancer: a systematic literature review and evaluation of exposure assessment in studies published since 1992. J Toxicol Environ Health B Crit Rev 9:413–439
Swee W, Klontz KC, Lambert LA (2000) A nationwide outbreak of alopecia associated with the use of a hair-relaxing formulation. Arch Dermatol 136: 1104–1108
Tosti A, Piraccini BM, van Neste DJ (2001) Telogen effluvium after allergic contact dermatitis of the scalp. Arch Dermatol 137:187–190
Trüeb RM (2007) Shampoos: ingredients, efficacy and adverse effects. J Dtsch Dermatol Ges 5:356–365

Nocebo Reaction

Kennedy WP (1961) The Nocebo Reaction. Med World 95:203–205
Mondaini N, Gontero P, Giubilei G, Lombardi G, Cai T, Gavazzi A, Bartoletti R (2007) Finasteride 5 mg and sexual side effects: how many of these are related to a nocebo phenomenon? J Sex Med 4:1708–1712

7 Patient Noncompliance

We strive for error-free medicine in a world that is sometimes all too human.

Michael Burgess (1950–)

Even with a correct diagnosis of a hair condition and appropriate treatment for that specific condition, a proportion of patients do not get better. Urquhart proposed three categories of nonresponse to treatment: (1) pharmacodynamic (nonresponse), (2) pharmacokinetic (nonabsorption), and (3) pharmionic (noncompliance).

Pharmacodynamics involves problems due to deficient receptors or when the condition is too severe for the agent to work. Examples are the use of oral finasteride in some women or in men with advanced androgenetic alopecia.

Pharmacokinetic reasons include problems with drug absorption or with rates of drug metabolism, resulting in insufficient concentrations of the active drug. Examples are the use of oral methotrexate where bioavailability is unreliable or of topical minoxidil in patients with low sulfotransferase activity.

Finally, *pharmionic* refers to poor adherence to treatment. When it comes to topical treatments, poor adherence is the most likely reason for nonresponse. Quantitative studies of topical treatment have begun to reveal patients' less than ideal adherence behavior.

> Therefore, when we see nonresponse, we should consider the possibility of an adherence problem. Managing patient compliance may be just as important as making the correct diagnosis and prescribing the appropriate treatment.

Treatment success relies on patient compliance that, on its part, relies on confidence and motivation. Noncompliance is a major obstacle to the delivery of effective hair loss treatment. More often than being a failure of the patient, patient noncompliance results from failure of the physician to ensure that essential confidence and motivation for successful treatment.

Patient compliance describes the degree to which a patient correctly follows medical advice and instruction. It most commonly refers to drug prescriptions, but it can also apply to the use of medical devices, self-care, or therapeutic sessions. Patient perception of the balance between the necessity for treatment and concerns over its use is a powerful predictor of adherence with treatment.

R.M. Trüeb, *The Difficult Hair Loss Patient: Guide to Successful Management of Alopecia and Related Conditions*, DOI 10.1007/978-3-319-19701-2_7

This perception of the risk–benefit ratio of treatment explains why compliance with therapy for long-term conditions can be particularly poor. Since both the patient and the healthcare provider affect compliance, a positive physician–patient relationship and regular follow-up visits are the most important factor in determining the degree of patient compliance. The major barriers to compliance are listed in Table 7.1.

In general, efforts to improve compliance have been aimed at simplifying medication packaging, providing effective medication reminders, improving patient education including handouts, and limiting the number of medications prescribed simultaneously. Major recommendations for improvement of patient compliance are listed in Table 7.2.

Table 7.1 Major barriers to patient compliance

Denial of the problem
Lack of comprehension of treatment benefits
Occurrence or fear of side effects
Cost of the treatment
Complexity of treatment regimen
Poor previous experience
Poor communication and lack of trust
Neglect and forgetfulness

Table 7.2 Recommendations for improvement of patient compliance

Only recommending treatments that are effective in circumstances when they are required
Prescribing the minimum number of different medications, e.g., combining active ingredients into a single compound
Simplifying dosage regimen by selecting different treatment or using a preparation that needs fewer doses during the day
Selecting treatments with lower levels of side effects or fewer concerns for long-term risks
Discussing possible side effects and whether it is important to continue medication regardless of those effects
Advice on minimizing or coping with side effects
Regular follow-up for reassurance on drug safety and treatment benefits
Developing trust so patients don’t fear embarrassment or anger if unable to take a particular drug, allowing the doctor to propose a more acceptable alternative

In the treatment of alopecia, there are short-term compliance issues and long-term compliance issues to be taken into account. Accordingly, regular follow-up visits at 3, 6, and 12 months are recommended and later twice a year, typically in February and August, when due to seasonal variations of hair growth and shedding, telogen rates are the lowest and highest, respectively.

An additional visit at 1 month is optional in regard to drug tolerance issues, especially in the elderly put on topical minoxidil.

Short-term compliance issues that are addressed by the physician within the first 3 months of therapy are winning the patient’s confidence in the diagnosis and treatment plan and detecting problems relating to the prescribed treatment regimen or drug tolerance.

The overall goal is to gain short-term compliance as a prerequisite to long-term adherence to treatment.

Long-term compliance issues that are addressed at 6 and 12 months of follow-up and thereafter are treatment efficacy and sustainability, long-term toxicities, and treatment costs.

Ultimately, in the long-term treatment of an oligosymptomatic condition, neglect may become a problem, since the patient may take the pharmacologically induced condition for granted. On the other hand, forgetfulness is a frequent cause of noncompliance in the elderly.

Further Reading

Feldman SR (2007) Why don’t patients get better? The three ‘nons’. J Dermatol Treat 18:136–137

Keller V, White MK, Carroll JG, Segal E (1995) Difficult. In: Physician-patient relationships workbook. Bayer Institute for Health Care Communication, West Haven

Marinker M, Shaw J (2003) Not to be taken as directed. BMJ 326:348–349

Ngoh LN (2003) Health literacy: a barrier to pharmacist-patient communication and medication adherence. J Am Pharm Assoc 49:e132–e146

Stone MS, Bronkesh SJ, Gerbarg ZB, Wood SD (1998) Improving patient compliance. Strategic Medicine, www.patientcompliancemedia.com/Improving_Patient_Compliance_article.pdf

Urquhart J (2002) The odds of the three nons when an aptly prescribed medicine isn't working: non-compliance, non-absorption, non-response. Br J Clin Pharmacol 54(2):212–220

White MK, Keller V, Carroll JG (1995) Physician-patient communication workbook. Bayer Institute for Health Care Communication, West Haven

World Health Organization (2003) Adherence to long-term therapies: evidence for action. Geneva: WHO: http://www.who.int/chp/knowledge/publications/adherence_full_report.pdf.

8 Optimizing Therapy Beyond Evidence-Based Medicine

The human body experiences a powerful gravitational pull in the direction of hope. That is why the patient's hopes are the physician's secret weapon. They are the hidden ingredients in any prescription.

Norman Cousins (1915–1990)

Few dermatologic problems carry as much emotional overtones as the complaint of hair loss. The best way to alleviate the emotional distress related to hair loss is to effectively treat it. As with any medical problem, the patient complaining of hair loss requires a comprehensive medical and drug history, physical examination of the hair and scalp, and appropriate laboratory evaluation to identify the cause.

> Prerequisite for delivering appropriate therapy is an understanding of the underlying pathologic dynamics. Once the diagnosis is certain, therapy appropriate for that diagnosis is likely to control the problem.

Although testing medical interventions for efficacy had existed since the time of Avicenna's *The Canon of Medicine* in the eleventh century, it was only in the twentieth century that this effort evolved to impact almost all fields of health care and policy. In 1967, American physician and mathematician Alvan R. Feinstein published his seminal work *Clinical Judgment*, which together with Archie Cochrane's celebrated book *Effectiveness and Efficiency* (1972) led to an increasing acceptance of clinical epidemiology and controlled studies during the 1970s and 1980s and prepared the way for the institutional development of EBM in the 1990s. EBM seeks to assess the strength of the evidence of risks and benefits of diagnostic tests and treatments, using techniques from science, engineering, and statistics, such as the systematic review of medical literature, meta-analysis, risk–benefit analysis, and randomized controlled trials.

> EBM aims for the ideal that healthcare professionals should make conscientious, explicit, and judicious use of the best available evidence gained from the scientific method to clinical decision-making.

As EBM guidelines on hair loss are rare, a European consensus group was recently constituted to develop guidelines for treatment of androgenetic alopecia. The European consensus group conducted a systematic literature review in Medline, Embase, and Cochrane databases until August 2008. 1,370 publications were found and 51 added by hand search. 85 publications fulfilled the following inclusion criteria for the guideline: prospective study with a number of patients ≥20 (no minimal patient number required in twin studies), age ≥12 years, and with confirmed diagnosis of androgenetic alopecia (diagnosis either clinically or by further diagnostic evaluations, e.g., trichogram, TrichoScan, biopsy). Objective outcome measure of efficacy described for

R.M. Trüeb, *The Difficult Hair Loss Patient: Guide to Successful Management of Alopecia and Related Conditions*, DOI 10.1007/978-3-319-19701-2_8

Table 8.1 Overview of miscellaneous treatments with insufficient or lacking evidence for efficacy and proposed mechanisms of action in treatment of hair loss

Promotion of hair regrowth	Amino acids Iron supplements in the absence of deficiency Vitamins (biotin, niacin derivates) Proanthocyanidins Millet seed (silicic acid, amino acids, vitamins, minerals) Marine extract and silicea component Chinese herbals *Ginkgo biloba* *Aloe vera* Ginseng Bergamot Hibiscus Sorphora Caffeine Melatonin Retinoids Cyclosporine Electromagnetic/electrostatic field Low-level laser
Improved perifollicular vascularization	Prostaglandins (viprostol, latanoprost) Aminexil Glyceroloxyesters and silicium Minerals Niacin derivatives Mesotherapy
DHT inhibitory activity	Saw palmetto ß-sitosterol Polysorbate 60 Green tea *Cimicifuga racemosa*
Anti-inflammatory activity	Ketoconazole Zinc pyrithione Corticosteroids
Improved hair nutrition	Vitamins (biotin, niacin derivates) Trace elements (zinc, copper)
Others	Botulinum toxin

From: Blumeyer A et al. Evidence-based (S3) guideline for the treatment of androgenetic alopecia in women and in men. *J Dtsch Dermatol Ges*. 2011;9 Suppl 6:S1–S57

drug therapy was mean change from baseline hair count in target area or measurement of hair growth/loss in target area by global photography.

The guideline revealed excellent evidence levels for the therapeutic use of topical minoxidil and of oral finasteride, low evidence levels for hormonal treatments (in women), and insufficient, or lacking, evidence for a broad panel of miscellaneous treatments available claiming effectiveness for treatment of male or female androgenetic alopecia (Table 8.1).

Although EBM is becoming regarded as the gold standard for clinical practice, there are a number of limitations of its use.

> The limited success of evidence-based therapies points to a more important complexity of hair loss.

EBM guidelines do not remove the problem of extrapolation to different patient populations or longer time frames, and certain groups have been under-researched, such as people with comorbid diseases. Finally, EBM applies to groups of people, but this does not preclude clinicians from using their personal experience in deciding what is best for the individual at hand.

Therefore, good medical practice means integrating personal clinical expertise with the best available external clinical evidence from EBM.

By approaching the hair loss patient in a methodical way, commencing with objects the simplest and easiest to recognize, and ascending step by step to the knowledge of the more complex, an individualized treatment plan can be designed.

One must remain open-minded (1) for the possibility of a multitude of cause-relationships underlying hair loss and (2) to consider combination regimens for therapy that may act synergistic to enhance hair growth and quality. Both are too complex to be adequately included by the EBM method.

8.1 Impact of Seasonality of Hair Growth and Shedding

In 823 otherwise healthy women with telogen effluvium during an observational period of 6 years, Kunz et al. demonstrated the existence of an overall annual periodicity in the growth and shedding of hair, manifested by a maximal proportion of telogen hairs in July. Taking a scalp hair telogen phase duration of approximately 100 days into account, one would expect shedding of these hairs by autumn.

The authors pointed out that existence of seasonal fluctuations in hair growth and shedding complicates the assessment of pharmacological effects. Awareness of these fluctuations is prerequisite to providing the correct cause and prognosis to the patient and ensuring patient compliance with therapy and has potentially serious implications for investigations with new hair growth-promoting agents.

Depending on the stage of periodicity in growth and shedding of hair for a particular subject, the heterogeneity of included subjects relating to the season may be enough to distort clinical efficacy results of an investigational agent. In the active stage of seasonal telogen effluvium, the involved hair follicles would probably fail to respond to the therapeutic agent, which may cause a false-negative result. In the recovery stage, the increased amounts of spontaneous hair regrowth might be interpreted falsely as a positive result.

In her inaugural dissertation (University of Zurich, 2015), Hotzenköcherle Trüeb demonstrated the impact of seasonality of hair growth and shedding on study results through inhomogeneous inclusion of study patients in relation to the season. In a preceding double-blind placebo-controlled study using combining epiluminescence microscopy and digital imaging, efficacy of a specific oral hair growth-promoting agent for treating telogen effluvium in otherwise healthy women was demonstrated, and this is independent of patient age. Therefore, an open-label pilot study with the same agent was performed in 5 women aged between 64 and 84 years, which confirmed the former results with increase and normalization of anagen rates within 3 months of treatment (unpublished data). To further verify efficacy of the agent in women aged 60 years and more, Hotzenköcherle Trüeb performed a double-blind placebo-controlled study in 36 patients for a duration of 6 months. Unexpectedly, placebo showed similar improvement of hair growth as compared to active compound. A further subanalysis

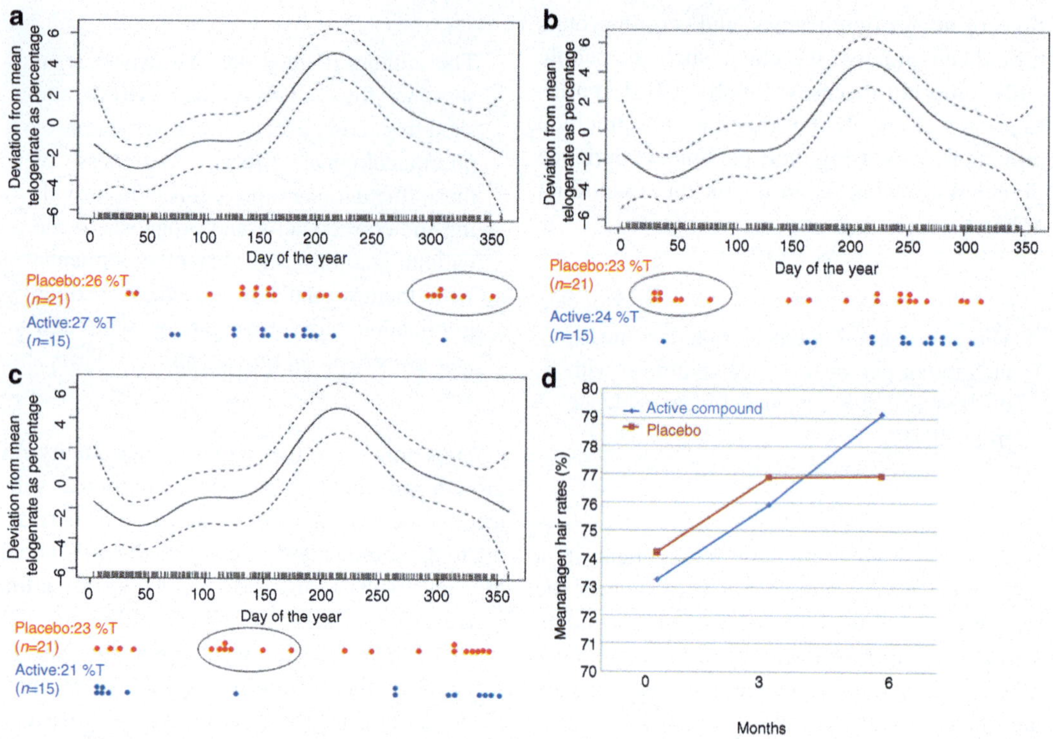

Fig. 8.1 (**a–d**) Inhomogeneous inclusion of study patients in relation to periodicity of hair growth and shedding: (**a**) at inclusion, (**b**) at 3 months, (**c**) at 6 months. Ellipse highlights cluster of patients in the placebo group that profited from seasonal hair growth within the first 3 months of treatment. (**d**) Improvement of anagen rates after 3 and 6 months of treatment (From Hotzenköcherle Trüeb. Inaugural Dissertation, University of Zurich 2015)

of patient data demonstrated that the result was falsified through inhomogeneous inclusion of study patients in relation to the season, with a cluster of patients on placebo profiting from the spontaneous recovery phase of seasonal hair growth and shedding (Fig. 8.1a–d).

> The impact of seasonality of hair growth and shedding on clinical trials with hair growth-promoting agents should always be taken into consideration, especially in studies with small numbers of patients and study durations <12 months, since heterogeneity of patient inclusion may be enough to distort clinical efficacy results.

Moreover, seasonal fluctuations in hair growth and shedding may be significant enough to be clinically apparent, specifically in women with patterned hair loss (Fig. 8.2a–c).

8.2 Concept of Multitargeted Treatment

Besides an understanding of the pathologic dynamics of hair loss as they relate to the hair growth cycle and integrity of the hair follicle, insight into the multitude of cause-relationships is prerequisite for delivering appropriate patient care. It must be borne in mind that hair loss often does not result from a single cause effect, but from a combination of internal and external factors that all need to be addressed simultaneously in an individualized manner for success, such as smoking and UV radiation, nutritional factors, medications, inflammatory phenomena and scarring, age-related phenomena, and ultimately the

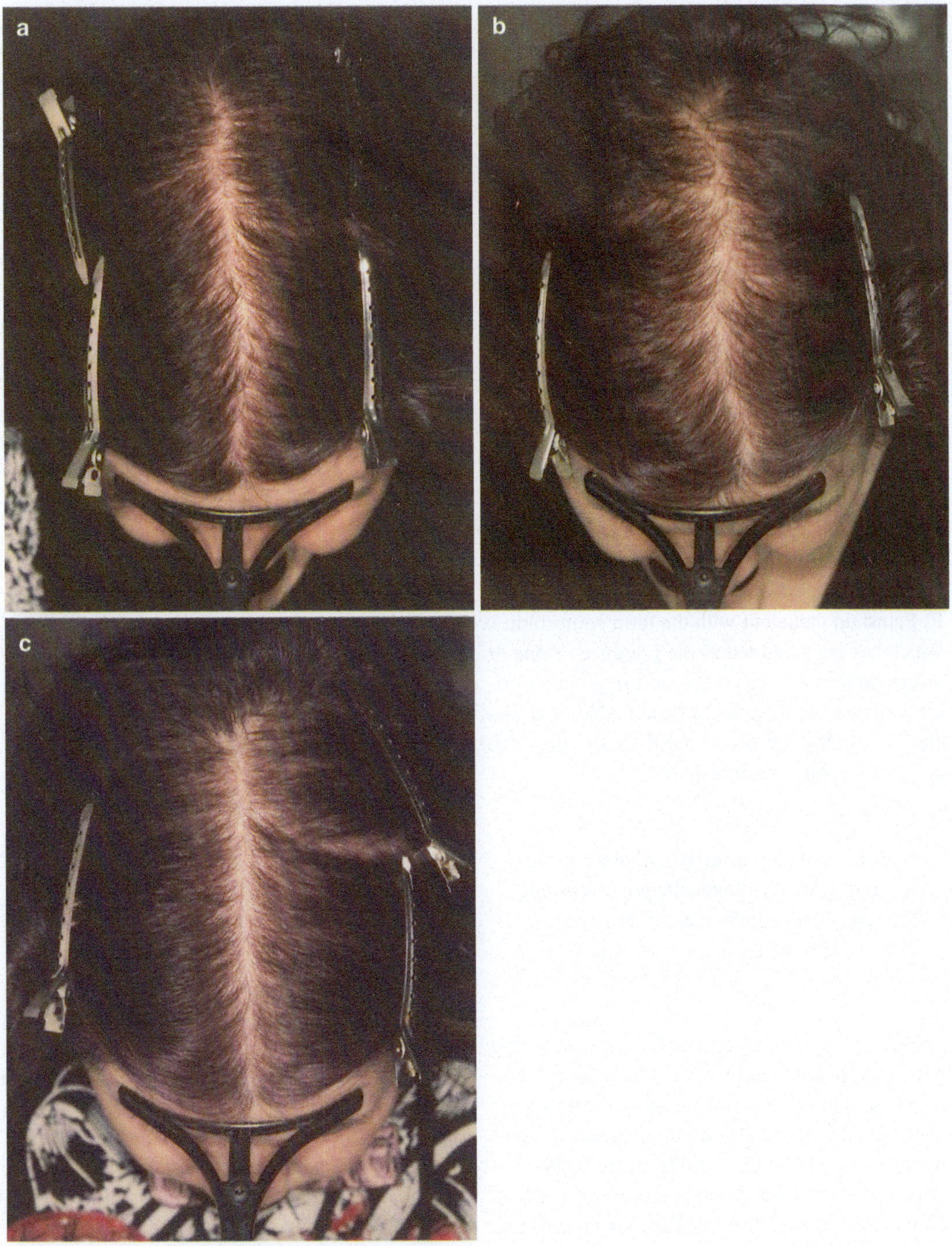

Fig. 8.2 (**a–c**) Subsequent images taken in (**a**) January 2007, (**b**) August 2007, and (**c**) February 2008 (From Kunz M et al. (2009). Seasonality of hair shedding in healthy women complaining of hair loss. *Dermatology* 219:105–110)

problems of comorbidities and multimorbidity in the elderly. The scientific basis for such an approach is given, but there is need for controlled studies to establish increase in efficacy of combination regimens.

8.2.1 Comorbidity

For centuries, physicians propagated the viability of a complex approach in the diagnosis and treatment of disease, while modern medicine, which boasts a wide range of diagnostic methods and variety of therapeutic procedures, stresses specification. This brought up a question: How to wholly evaluate the state of a patient who suffers from a number of diseases simultaneously, where to start from, and which disease(s) requires primary and subsequent treatment? For many years this question stood out unanswered until in 1970 Alvan R. Feinstein came out with the term comorbidity, which has been defined as the presence of one or more additional diseases co-occurring with a primary disease or the effect of such additional diseases, whereby the additional disorder may also be a behavioral or mental disorder.

> The effect of comorbid pathologies on clinical implications, diagnosis, prognosis, and therapy of trichologic conditions is polyhedral and patient specific.

The interrelation of disease, age, and drug pathomorphism greatly affects the clinical presentation and progress of the primary nosology, character, and severity of complications; worsens the patient's life quality; and limits or makes difficult the diagnostic and remedial process. Comorbidity may affect life prognosis and increase the risks of fatality. The presence of comorbidity must be taken into account when selecting the algorithm of diagnosis and treatment plans for any given, including trichologic, disease. Ultimately, the dermatologist participates with the other medical disciplines in the diagnosis and treatment of all types of hair problems as they relate to systemic disease. Selected comorbidities in hair disease are listed in Table 8.2 and illustrated in Fig. 8.3a–u.

8.2.2 Value of Nutritional Therapies

Since an important commercial interest lies in the nutritional value of various vitamin and amino acid supplements, an important question that arises is whether increasing the content of an already adequate diet with specific amino acids, vitamins, and/or trace elements may further promote hair growth. Pharmacy aisles and Internet drugstores are full of nutritional supplements promising full, thick, luscious hair for prices that range from suspiciously cheap to dishearteningly exorbitant.

> It would appear that unless hair loss is due to a specific nutritional deficiency, there's only so much that nutritional therapies can do to enhance hair growth and quality. However, there are internal and external factors, such as aging and oxidative stress, that influence hair health to such a degree that nutritional therapy can boost hair that's suffering from these problems.

Protein is the main component of hair accounting for between 65 and 95 % of the hair by weight. The primary component of the hair fiber is keratin which is made from eighteen amino acids (by alphabetical order: alanine, arginine, aspartic acid, cysteine, glutamic acid, glycine, histidine, isoleucine, leucine, lysine, methionine, phenylalanine, proline, serine, threonine, tryptophane, tyrosine, and valine). The most abundant of these is cysteine which gives the hair fiber much of its strength through the linking of the sulfur in cysteine molecules of adjacent keratin proteins together in disulfide bonds.

Ingesting keratin does not help hair growth, as the protein cannot be broken down and absorbed (in fact, also rhinoceros horn whose use to cure a

Table 8.2 Comorbidities in hair disease

Condition	Comorbidities
Congenital disorders	
Atrichia, hypotrichosis	Mental retardation Epilepsy Immune deficiency Sensorineural deafness Vitamin D-dependent rickets Skeletal anomalies Juvenile macular dystrophy Palmoplantar keratoderma Follicular atrophoderma and basal cell carcinomas (Bazex syndrome) Ectodermal dysplasia
Alopecia	Holocarboxylase synthetase deficiency (inborn error of biotin metabolism) Biotinidase deficiency (inborn error of biotin metabolism) Acrodermatitis enteropathica (zinc deficiency) Progeria
Aplasia cutis congenita	Limb anomalies (Adams–Oliver syndrome) Epidermal or sebaceous nevi (SCALP syndrome) Overlying deeper embryologic malformations with hair collar sign Epidermolysis bullosa Fetus papyraceus, placental infarct Teratogens (intrauterine viral infections, carbimazole exposure) Complex malformation syndromes
Scarring alopecia	Organoid nevi (epidermal, sebaceous) Incontinentia pigmenti (Bloch-Sulzberger syndrome) Epidermolysis bullosa Ichthyosis (alopecia ichthyotica) Ectodermal dysplasia with clefting (AEC and EEC syndrome) Keratosis follicularis (Siemens syndrome)
Hair shaft anomalies:	
Pili torti	Menkes syndrome (inborn error of copper metabolism) Sensorineural deafness (Björnstad syndrome) Hypogonadism (Crandall syndrome)
Twisting dystrophy (pili torti et canaliculi) and corkscrew hairs	Ectodermal dysplasia Clefting (AEC, EEC, and Rapp–Hodgkin syndrome) Ectrodactyly (EEC syndrome)
Uncombable hair (pili trianguli et canaliculi)	Retinal pigmentary dystrophy Brachydactyly
Trichorrhexis invaginata	Congenital erythroderma (Netherton syndrome) Atopic disease Ichthyosis linearis circumflexa
Trichoschisis	Trichothiodystrophy
Congenital trichorrhexis nodosa	Argininosuccinic aciduria Citrullinemia
Woolly hair	Palmoplantar keratoderma Arrhythmogenic cardiomyopathy (Naxos disease) Dilated cardiomyopathy (Carvajal syndrome)
Non-scarring alopecias	
Male androgenetic alopecia	Insulin resistance Metabolic syndrome Coronary heart disease Obesity Smoking status Anterolateral leg alopecia

(continued)

Table 8.2 (continued)

Condition	Comorbidities
Female androgenetic alopecia	Iron deficiency Hypothyroidism Hyperprolactinemia Polycystic ovary syndrome
Senescent alopecia	Nutritional deficiency Endocrine disease Drug related Multimorbidity Dementia
Alopecia areata	Trisomy 21 Atopic disease Autoimmune thyroid disease Pernicious anemia Autoimmune polyendocrinopathy syndrome Celiac disease Iron deficiency Vitamin D deficiency Androgenetic alopecia Trichotillomania
Trichotillomania	Iron deficiency Onychophagia Trichophagia Trichobezoar Rapunzel syndrome
Chemotherapy-induced alopecia	Androgenetic alopecia Anti-estrogen therapy Graft-versus-host disease
Scarring alopecias	
Lupus erythematosus	Systemic disease (see ACR criteria)
Frontal fibrosing alopecia	Androgenetic alopecia Autoimmune thyroid disease Lupus erythematosus Lichen planus (mucous membranes, nails) Anterolateral leg-like alopecia
Folliculitis decalvans	Hypocomplementemia Defective cellular immunity Decreased intracellular killing Hair shaft abnormalities (twisting dystrophy, tufted folliculitis)
Dissecting cellulitis	Acne conglobata Hidradenitis suppurativa Pilonidal sinus
All:	
Psychological comorbidities	Adjustment disorders Personality disorders

variety of ailments is highly praised in the traditional medicine systems in Asia is composed largely of keratin. In other words, there is no evidence to support the plethora of claims about the healing properties of the horns, and one would do just as well chewing on the fingernails or hair). Therefore, constituent amino acids from which the hair follicle can build up the keratin need to be consumed. Cysteine is catabolized in the gastrointestinal tract and blood plasma, while cystine travels safely through the gastrointestinal tract and blood plasma and is promptly reduced to two cysteine molecules upon cell entry. Originally, the role of cystine in the production of wool was investigated

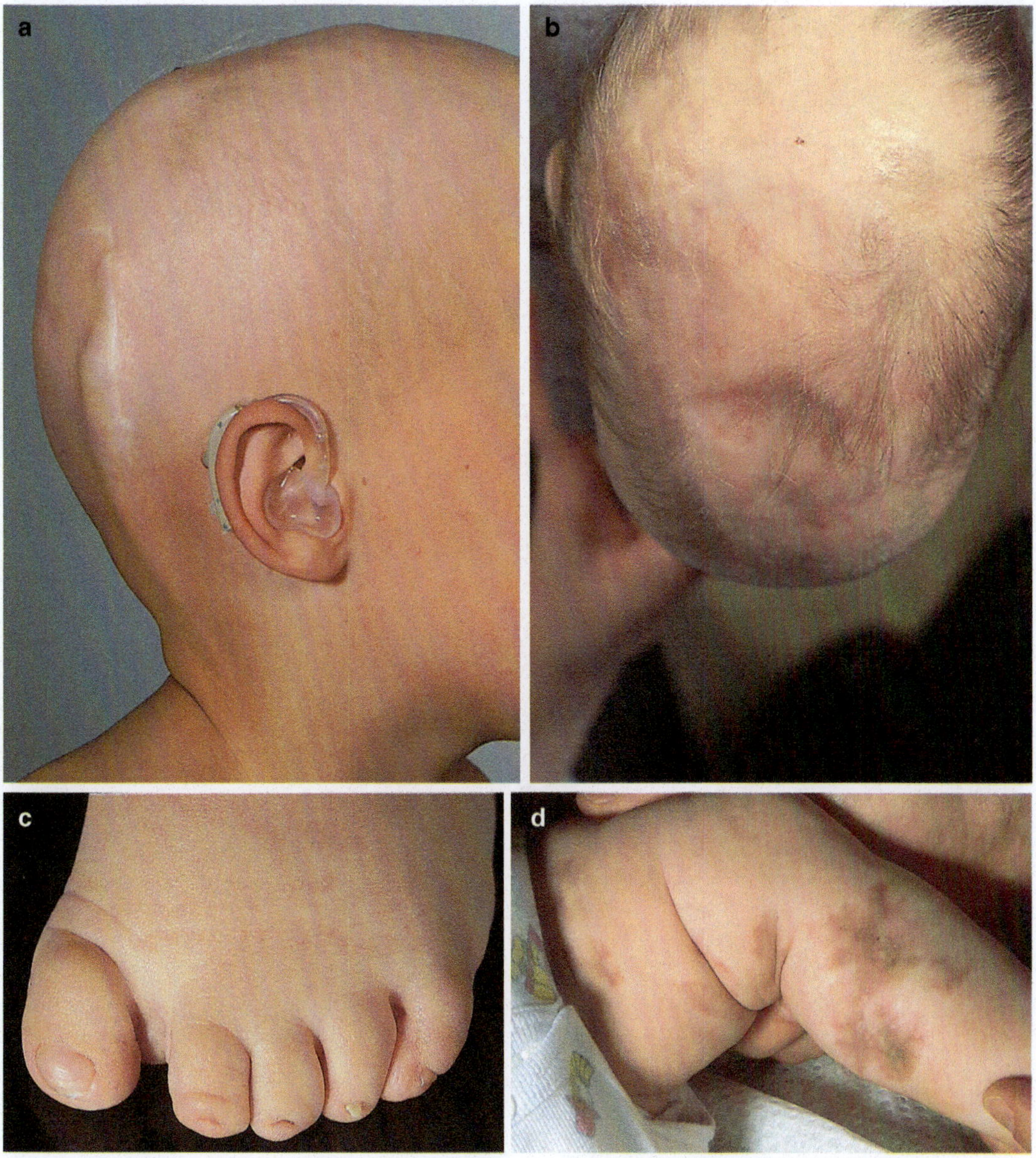

Fig. 8.3 (**a–u**) Comorbidities in congenital and acquired hair disorders. (**a**) Congenital atrichia with sensorineural deafness. (**b–d**) Adams–Oliver syndrome: (**b**) aplasia cutis congenita, (**c**) terminal transverse limb defect, and (**d**) cutis marmorata. (**e–g**) Cranial dysraphism: (**e**) hair collar sign, (**f**) meningocele of the scalp, and (**g**) MRI of underlying neural tube closure defect. (**h–j**) EEC syndrome: (**h**) alopecia with scalp dermatitis, (**i**) ectrodactyly, and (**j**) clefting. (**k, l**) Uncombable hair syndrome with brachydactyly: (**k**) spun-glass hair and (**l**) brachydactyly. (**m, n**) Woolly hair with palmoplantar keratoderma: (**m**) woolly hair and (**n**) palmar keratoderma. (**o**) Anterolateral leg alopecia in androgenetic alopecia. (**p, q**) Polycystic ovary syndrome: (**p**) hirsutism and (**q**) acanthosis nigricans and acrochordons as markers of hyperinsulinemia. (**r**) Alopecia areata in trisomy 21. (**s**) Onychophagia (in trichotillomania). (**t**) Folliculitis decalvans and twisting dystrophy in EEC syndrome. (**u**) Pilonidal sinus in follicular occlusion syndrome

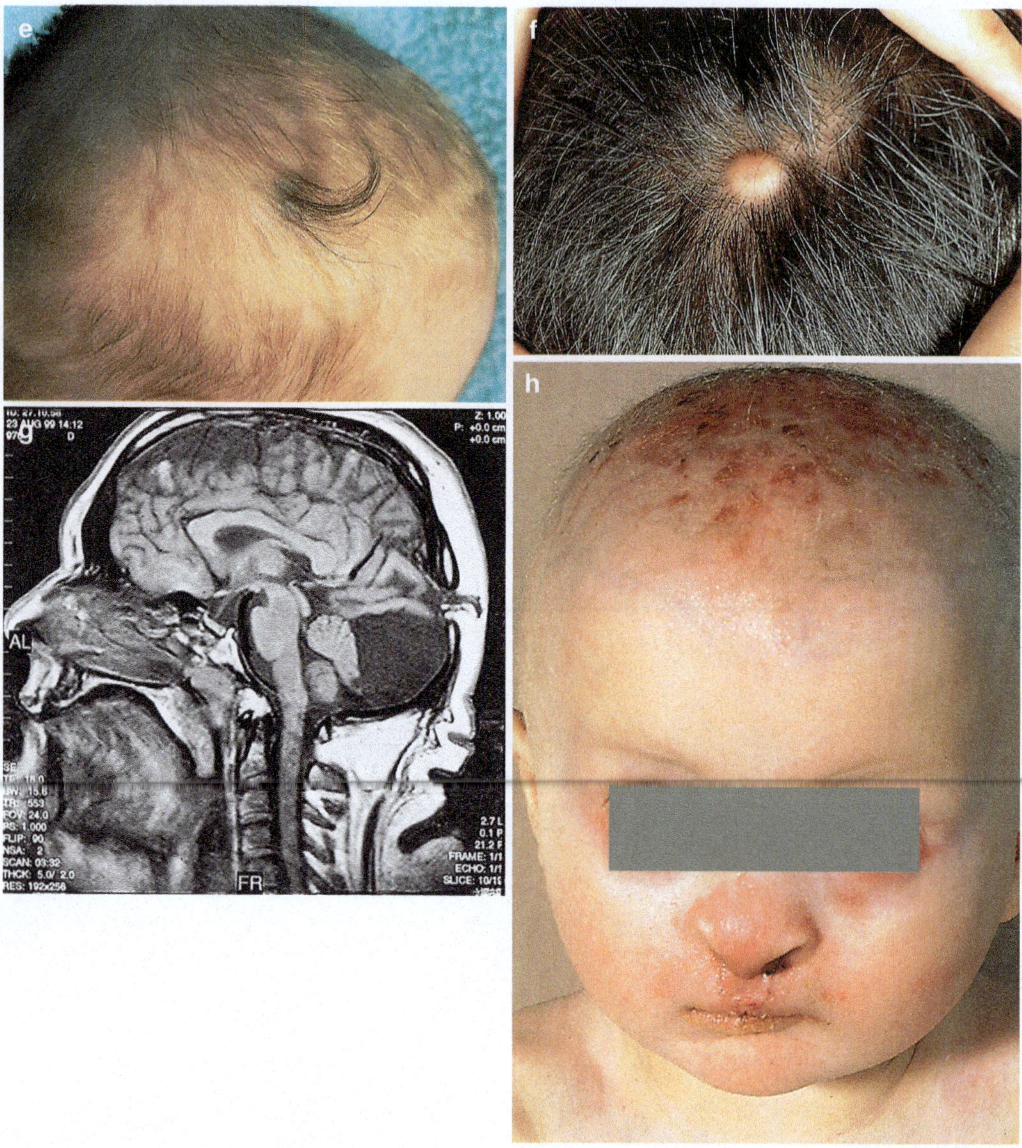

Fig. 8.3 (continued)

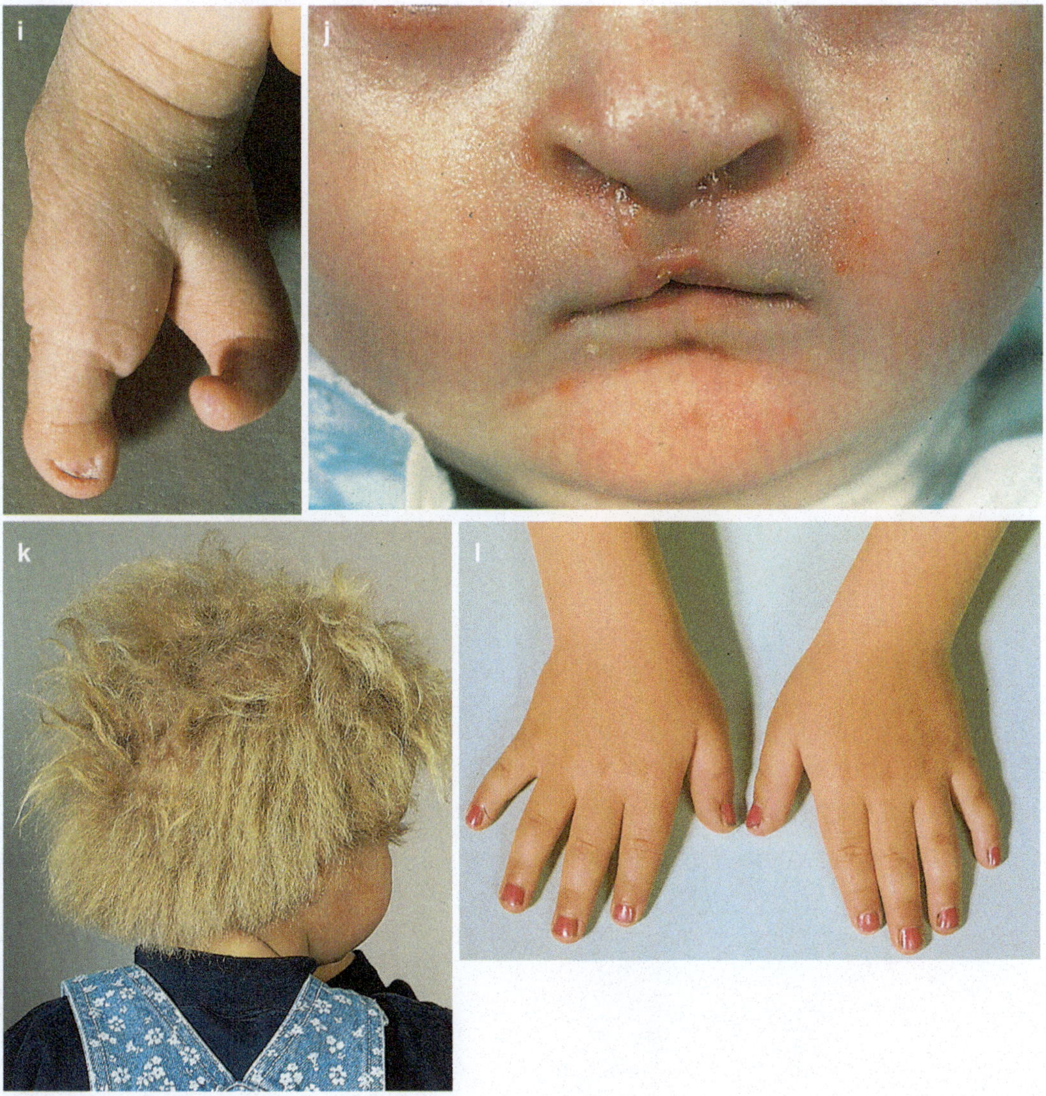

Fig. 8.3 (continued)

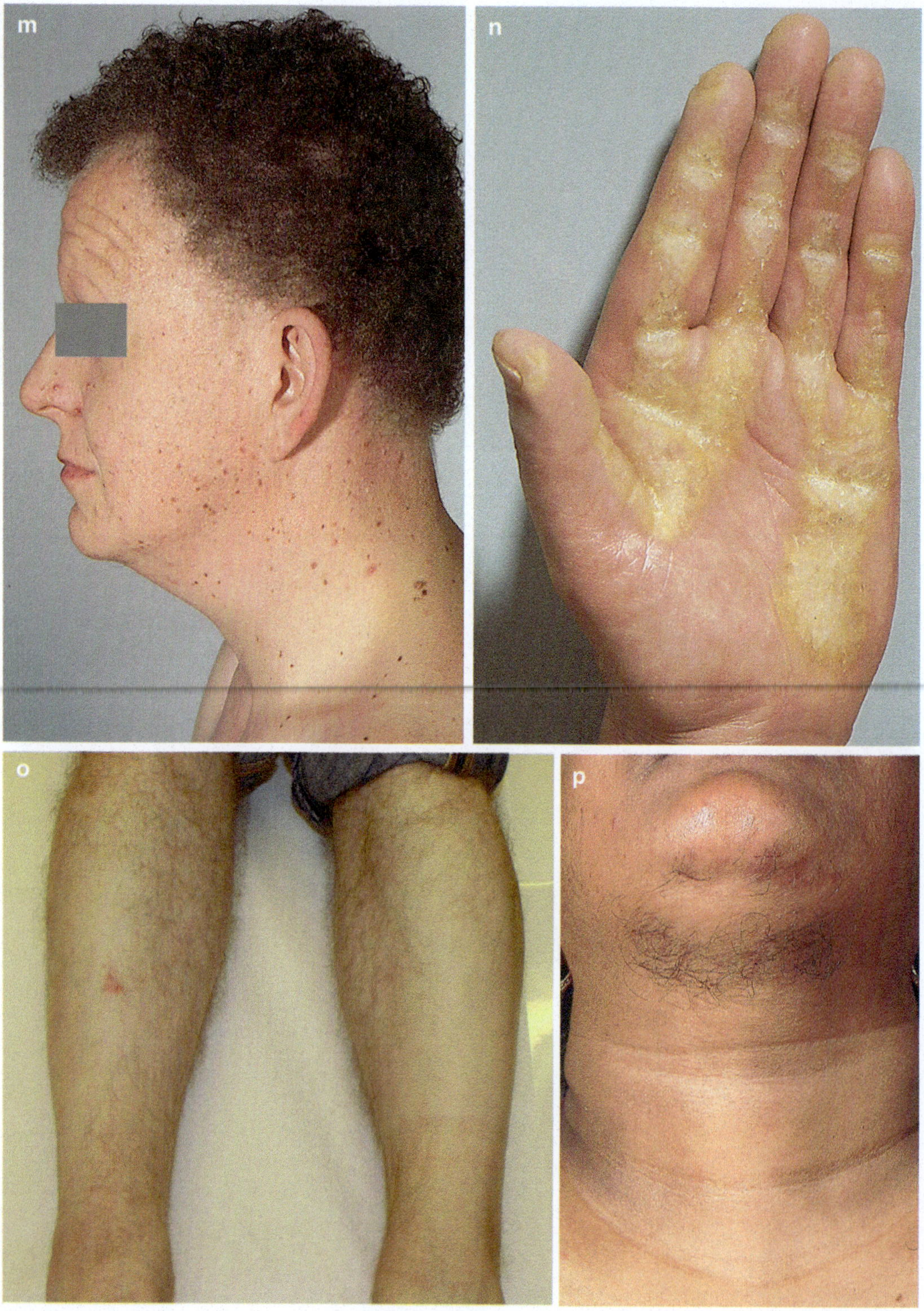

Fig. 8.3 (continued)

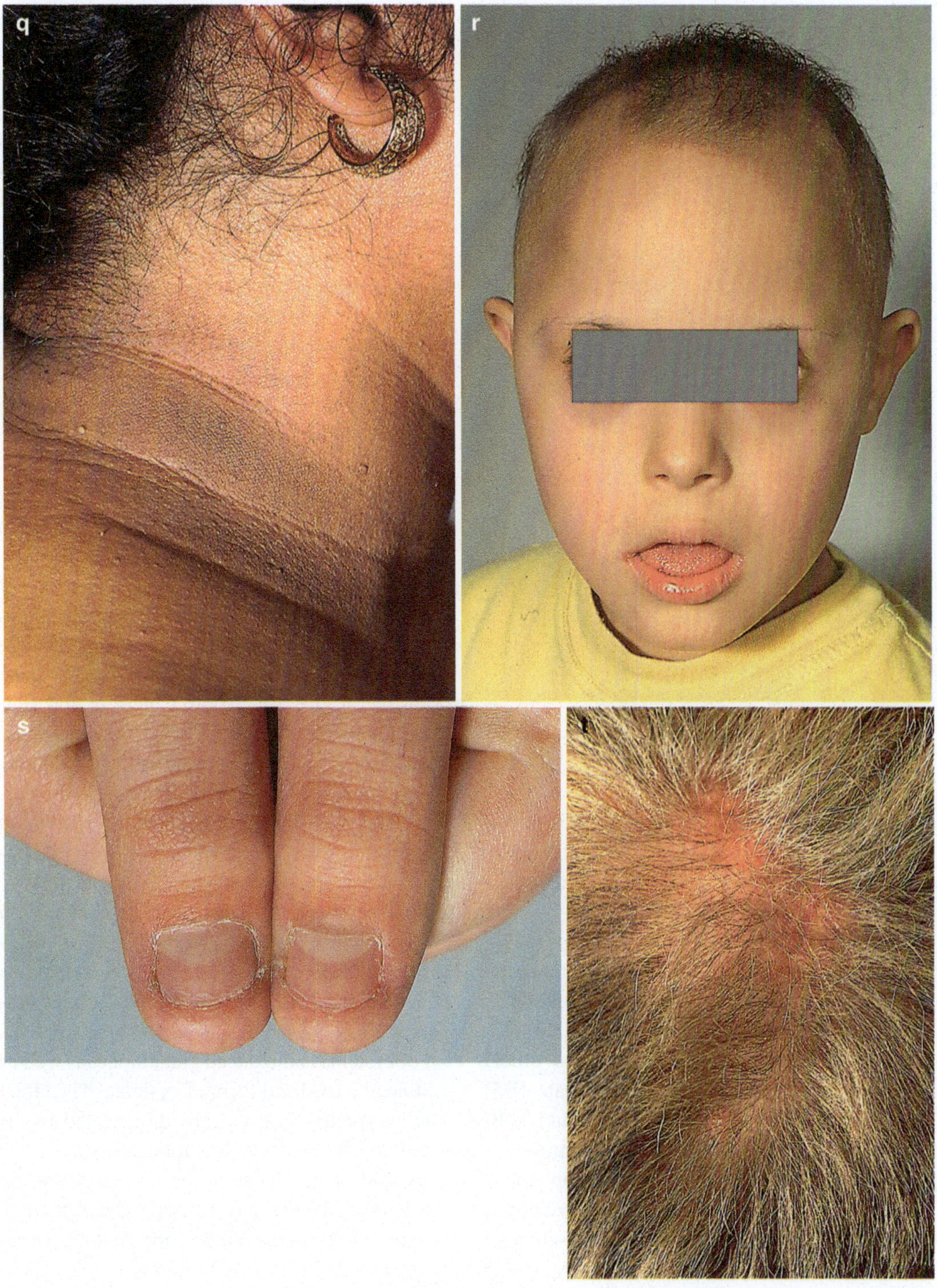

Fig. 8.3 (continued)

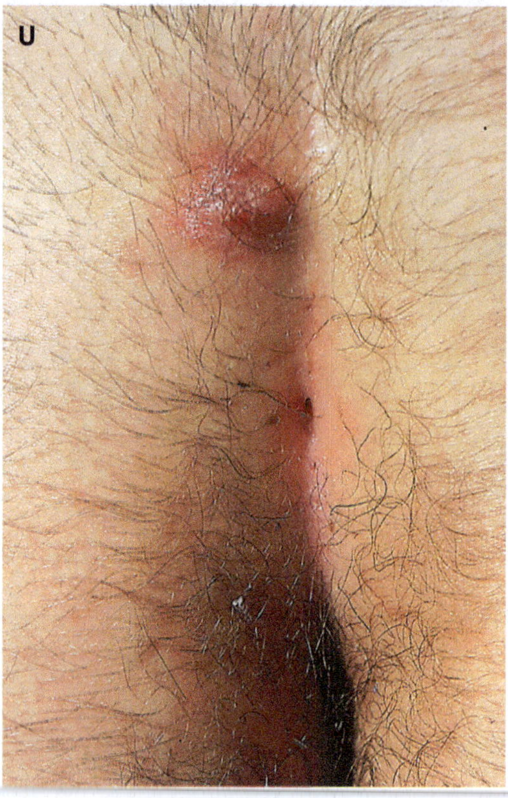

Fig. 8.3 (continued)

in the 1960s, and it was found that enrichment of even what appeared to be a normal diet with the sulfur-containing amino acids cystine and methionine increased wool production in sheep.

The hair follicle exhibits a high rate of metabolism. As a group, B-complex vitamins are important for metabolic functions and therefore required to utilize other nutrients like carbohydrate and amino acids (in alphabetical order): biotin (vitamin H), calcium pantothenate (B5), niacinamide (B3), folic acid, and vitamins B6 (pyridoxal phosphate) and B12 (cobalamin).

When considering which dietary supplements could be used for improving hair growth in humans, cystine in combination with B-complex vitamins or medicinal yeast, a rich natural source of amino acids and B-complex vitamins, was therefore considered. Starting in the early 1990s, studies on the effect of dietary supplements containing cystine, medicinal yeast, and pantothenic acid (CYP-complex) were performed, showing improvements in the trichogram, in hair swelling as a criterion for hair quality, and in the tensile strength of the hair fiber. Eventually, Lengg et al. performed a double-blind, placebo-controlled study in 30 otherwise healthy women suffering from telogen effluvium which demonstrated that a CYP-complex-based dietary supplement increased the anagen hair rate within 6 months of treatment, while placebo did not (Fig. 8.4).

Ultimately, combining with topical minoxidil in the treatment of androgenetic alopecia was speculated to add extra benefit, since it had been shown in whole hair follicle cultures that minoxidil not only increases the incorporation of thymidine as marker of cell division but also leads to increased uptake of cysteine by the hair follicle. This is underlined by the fact that regression analysis in the study performed by Lengg et al. did not show altered treatment efficacy in healthy women with hair loss and concomitant androgenetic alopecia. The proof of concept for superiority of combination treatment with CYP-complex versus minoxidil monotherapy of female androgenetic alopecia was finally presented by Trüeb on the occasion of the 8th World Congress for Hair Research held on May 14–17, 2014 in Jeju Island, Korea: combined therapy resulted in statistically significant higher proportion of patients with normalized percentage of telogen hairs <15 % within 4 months of treatment as compared with minoxidil monotherapy (60 % versus 29 %, $p = 0.03$).

Interestingly, an experiment performed on C57BL/6 mice that developed hair loss when exposed to cigarette smoke demonstrated that this effect could be prevented by the oral administration of N-acetylcysteine, an analogue and precursor of cysteine and reduced glutathione, as well as cystine, the oxidized form of cysteine. The effect was interpreted as to be possibly related to the glutathione-related detoxification system.

A role of the essential amino acid lysine in hair loss has also been suggested to be important. Double-blind data confirmed the findings of an open study in women with increased hair shedding, where a significant proportion responded to combination treatment with lysine and iron.

While nutritional factors affect the hair directly, one should not forget that they also may affect the skin. In the management of subjects with hair loss, evidence of associated scaling problems should

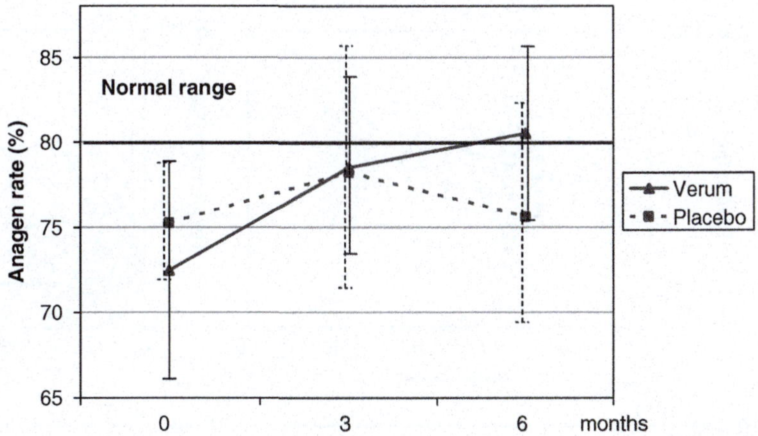

	0	3	6	
Verum	72.5	78.5	80.5	$p = 0.003$
Placebo	75.3	78.2	75.6	$p = 0.85$

Fig 8.4 Double-blinded, placebo-controlled study in healthy women with hair loss using oral combination of cystine, yeast, and pantothenic acid (CYP-complex): active compound led to statistically significant improvement and normalization of mean anagen hair rates within 6 months of treatment (From Lengg N et al. Dietary supplement increases anagen hair rate in women with telogen effluvium: results of a double-blind placebo-controlled trial. *Therapy* 2007;4:59–65)

draw the attention to the possibility of deficiency of vitamin A, biotin, zinc, or essential fatty acids.

Finally, excessive intake of certain nutritional supplements may actually cause hair loss and is not recommended in the absence of a proven deficiency. This applies particularly to vitamin A (>50,000 I.U. daily) and selenium, which in toxic doses cause hair loss.

Also, a caveat should be spoken against uncritical iron supplementations, since there is the possibility that increased iron storage could enhance oxidative injury by inducing the Fenton reaction, with the prospective of increasing the risk of cardiovascular disease and cancer.

Iron deficiency represents the most common nutritional deficiency with the highest prevalence in adolescent girls and women of childbearing age. While the most common causes of iron deficiency are menstrual blood loss, pregnancy, and lactation in premenopausal women, in postmenopausal women and men, they are decreased absorption and gastrointestinal bleeding. Several studies have evaluated the relationship between iron deficiency and hair loss. Almost all of these studies have focused exclusively on women.

Although non-anemic iron deficiency as an etiologic factor for diffuse hair loss in women was first postulated by Hard in 1961, it is not until recently that the significance of iron stores as assessed by serum ferritin levels in women with hair loss has been studied systematically. The various observational studies that evaluated the association between decreased ferritin levels and hair loss have resulted in opposing conclusions. To evaluate the relationship between serum ferritin levels and hair loss activity determined by trichograms, Bregy et al. performed a retrospective case study of 181 women with hair loss who underwent biochemical investigations and trichograms. 61.9 % had a ferritin level >30 μgL^{-1}, 30.4 % between 10 and 30 μgL^{-1}, and 7.7 % $\leq$10 μgL^{-1}, and no correlation was found between ferritin levels >10 μgL^{-1} and telogen rates. The authors only found a correlation between serum ferritin levels and patient age (Fig. 8.5a).

In women with hair loss, the role of tissue iron status within limits regarded as normal has probably been overestimated, since a majority of otherwise healthy women with hair loss had ferritin levels >30 μgL^{-1} (cut-off point with 92 % sensitivity and 98 % specificity for iron deficiency), and no correlation was found between hair loss activity and ferritin levels >10 μgL^{-1} (Fig. 8.5b–d).

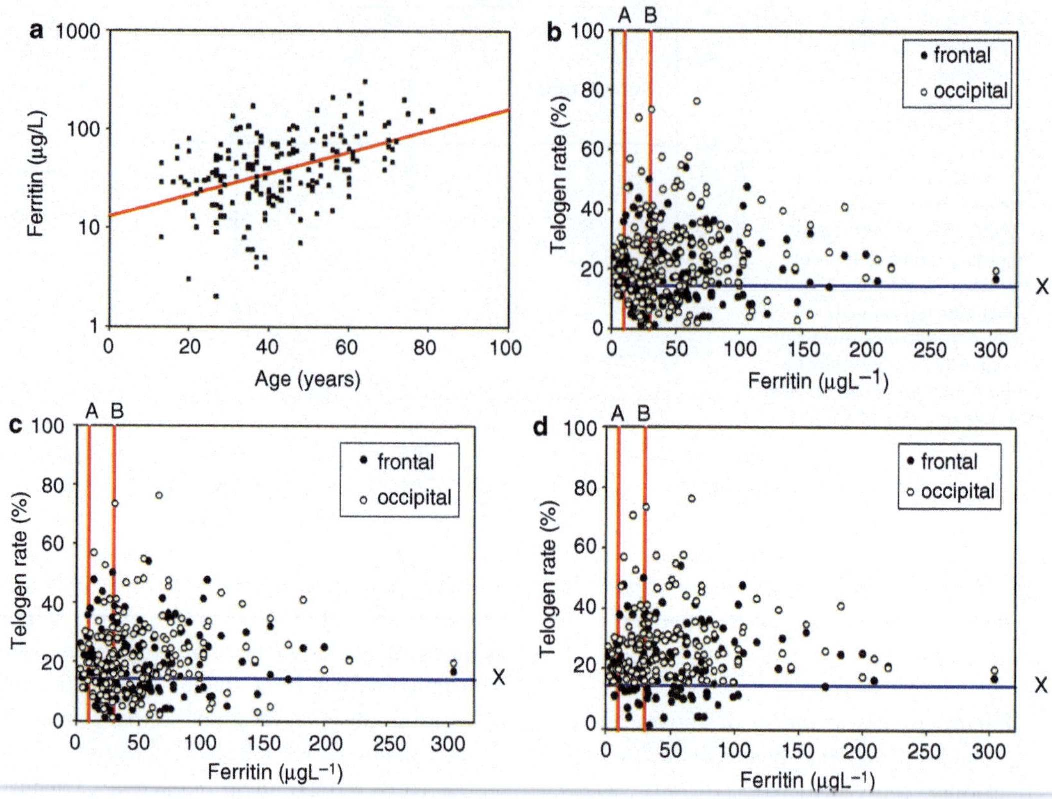

Fig. 8.5 Relationship between serum ferritin levels and hair loss in women. (**a**) Correlation between patient age (years) and serum ferritin values (µg L^{-1}) (From Bregy A, Trüeb RM. No association between serum ferritin levels >10 microg/l and hair loss activity in women. *Dermatology* 2008;217:1–6). (**b–d**) Correlation between telogen rates and ferritin levels in (**b**) all subjects (*n*=181), (**c**) subjects with female androgenetic alopecia (*n*=159), and (**d**) total subjects with telogen effluvium, irrespective of combination with female androgenetic alopecia or not (*n*=135). Diagram shows the ferritin values (µgL^{-1}) and corresponding telogen rates (%) of the frontal and occipital scalp of all patients in a linear scale. Vertical line A represents the lower reference limit of normal with 75 % sensitivity and 98 % specificity for diagnosing iron deficiency in women of childbearing age, and vertical line B represents the cutoff point with sensitivity of 92 % and specificity of 98 % for diagnosing iron deficiency. Horizontal line X represents cutoff point for pathologic telogen rate (>15 %) (From Bregy A, Trüeb RM. No association between serum ferritin levels >10 microg/l and hair loss activity in women. *Dermatology* 2008;217:1–6)

In an attempt to demonstrate the pro-oxidative capacity of oral iron supplementation, King et al. performed a study on women with low iron stores (plasma ferritin < or=20 µg/L) receiving a daily iron supplement for 8 weeks at a level commonly used to treat poor iron status. They measured increased lipid peroxidation by ethane exhalation rates and plasma malondialdehyde. The women served as their own control as pre- and post-supplementation periods were compared. After 6 weeks of iron supplementation, serum ferritin almost doubled and body iron more than doubled, hemoglobin levels increased slightly, and other indicators of iron status became normal. However, plasma malondialdehyde and breath ethane exhalation rates increased by more than 40 % between baseline and 6 weeks of supplementation. These increases correlated significantly with plasma iron and ferritin levels. The authors concluded that the increased indicators of lipid peroxidation with duration of supplementation and as iron status improved suggest that providing daily nearly 100 mg iron may not be a totally innocuous regimen for correcting iron depletion.

Finally, in consideration of the current popularity of intravenous *versus* oral iron therapy, the risk

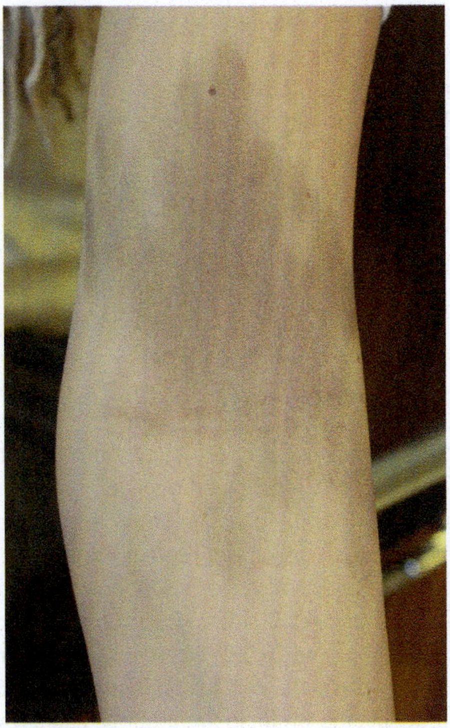

Fig. 8.6 Cutaneous discoloration following paravenous iron infusion

of adverse effects must be taken into account, specifically anaphylactic-like reactions and cutaneous discoloration from paravenous infusion (Fig. 8.6).

8.2.3 Low-Level Laser Therapy

The ability of lasers to induce hair growth was incidentally noted as early as 1967 when Mester et al. used low-level laser therapy (LLLT) to treat cancer in mice with shaved backs. Since then, hypertrichosis has been recognized to be a possible side effect of laser treatment. First described in 2002 with intense pulse light (IPL) therapy, this phenomenon has now been widely acknowledged to occur with an incidence rate ranging from 0.6 to 10 % with low fluences and all laser types. It is thought to be the result of suboptimal fluences that are too low to induce thermolysis, but high enough to stimulate follicular growth.

The hypothesized mechanisms of action of LLLT are increased ATP production, modulation of reactive oxygen species (ROS), and induction of transcription factors. The proposed cellular chromophore responsible for the effect of visible light is cytochrome c oxidase (COX) with absorption peaks in the near infrared, and mitochondria are the likely site for the initial effects. It is believed that LLLT displaces nitric oxide (NO) from COX allowing an influx of oxygen to bond to COX and progress forward in the respiratory process to ATP production and ROS signaling. These effects in turn lead to increased cellular proliferation; modulation in levels of cytokines, growth factors, and inflammatory mediators; and increased tissue oxygenation. While the effects of these biochemical and cellular changes have broadly been studied in both animal models and clinical studies with patients and have shown benefits in diverse conditions, such as increased healing in chronic wounds, improvements in sports injuries and carpal tunnel syndrome, pain reduction in arthritis and neuropathies, and amelioration of damage after heart attacks, stroke, nerve injury, and retinal toxicity, the effects on hair growth stimulation have only recently gained the attention of the scientific community.

Eventually, LLLT has been developed for treatment of androgenetic alopecia. As opposed to other currently marketed systems, the laser comb utilizes hair parting teeth for optimal delivery of laser energy to the exposed scalp. In 2007, the HairMax LaserComb® (Lexington International, LLC) received 510(k) clearance from the FDA for the treatment of androgenetic alopecia for men and 2011 for women. This clearance means that the device is considered a moderate-risk medical device by the FDA and is thereby solely screened for safety. The HairMax LaserComb® has been tested in a company-sponsored study of 110 male patients with the claim of significant increase in mean terminal hair density when compared to a sham device. Avram and Rogers conducted the first independent blinded study of LLLT and hair growth with 7 patients and found that on average, there was a decrease in the number of vellus hairs, an increase in the number of terminal hairs, and an increase in shaft diameter. A consensus written by hair loss experts states that based on anecdotal experience, LLLT, particularly 650–900 nm wavelengths at 5 mW, may be an effective treatment option for patients with androgenetic alopecia.

To evaluate efficacy of the 655 nm HairMax LaserComb® either as monotherapy or concomitant therapy for treatment of male and female androgenetic alopecia, Munck et al. performed a retrospective observational study of global photographic assessments of patients in an office-based setting. Of 32 patients (21 females, 11 males), 11 showed significant, 17 moderate, and 4 no improvement. Improvement was seen both with monotherapy and concomitant therapy. Improvement was observed as early as 3 months and was sustained up to a maximum observation time of 24 months.

The technology appears to work better for some than for others, and predictive factors which will most benefit from LLLT are to be determined. It seems though that patients with intermediate alopecia (Hamilton–Norwood III and IV and Ludwig I and II, resp.) respond best, since effective photobiostimulation depends on a minimum of hair for effective photobiostimulation and on a maximum of hair for the laser beam to reach the scalp without absorption or interference from existing hairs.

> From these observations, the authors concluded LLLT represents a safe and potentially effective treatment option for patients with androgenetic alopecia who do not respond or are not tolerant to standard treatment of androgenetic alopecia. Moreover, combining LLLT with topical minoxidil and oral finasteride may act synergistic to enhance hair growth. Due to the known beneficial effect on wound healing, it is conceivable that LLLT as an adjunctive therapy in hair transplant surgery may also reduce postoperative shedding, reduce healing time, and increase graft patency.

8.2.4 Value of Cosmetic Treatments

Hair care, color, and style play an important role in people's physical appearance and self-perception. Hair defines an individual's gender, age, sexual attitude, and social status. There are no significant differences in the number of hair follicles between men and women or between different races.

> Differences in the appearance of hair are due to the type of hair produced by a follicle and to the type of hair care and cosmetics practiced by the individual.

Treatments for age-dependent thinning of hair in the course of either androgenetic alopecia or senescent alopecia focus on improving scalp hair density and on preventing further damage to the hair fiber. For the former, prescription drugs such as topical minoxidil solution and oral finasteride are available and for the latter over-the-counter cosmetic products. While medicinal treatments aim at specific problems relating to hair growth and shedding or the superficial condition of the scalp, such as dandruff, redness, and itchiness, cosmetic hair treatments aim at cleansing the hair, conditioning hair, styling hair, changing hair color, and perming hair. Table 8.3 lists the main types of hair cosmetics.

Shampoos are the most commonly used treatment for hair and scalp conditions. Today, shampoos are expected to be more than mere cleansing agents. They are expected to not dry out the hair, to produce lather in hard and soft water and when applied to oily hair, to be non-irritating to skin and mucous membranes, to be chemically and

Table 8.3 Hair cosmetics

Hair shampoos: to remove sebum and environmental dirt without decreasing cosmetic appearance of hair
Hair conditioners: to improve hair manageability, decrease hair static electricity, add luster, and enhance styling ease
Hairstyling aids: to maintain hair in fashionable arrangement while improving the quality of hair fibers
Hair dyes: to lighten or darken hair color while covering gray hair
Permanent hair waving/straightening: to reposition hair keratin disulfide bonds in a new curly or straight position

physically stable, to possess conditioning benefits, to be biodegradable, and to be affordable.

Shampoos are expected to improve the hair cosmetically, while being tailored to the needs of various hair types as well as age and individual habits.

The aim of conditioning agents in a shampoo and of hair conditioners is to maintain the natural condition of newly grown hairs for as long as possible. Sebum is the ideal hair conditioner. Excessive removal of sebum in the course of washing the hair and scalp created the need for synthetic sebum-like substances that attempt to supply hair with the positive attributes of sebum while avoiding the greasy appearance of excessive sebum and dirty hair. Virtually all standard shampoos used today contain conditioning agents. Damaged hair can, of course, not be restored to the condition of healthy, newly growing hair, and more than a reparative effect cannot be expected.

Nonetheless, it is possible to increase shine and make hair more manageable and easier to comb by using a shampoo with a high proportion of conditioning agents or a hair conditioner.

Hair conditioners aim at imparting softness, increasing luster and gloss, reducing flyaway, enhancing disentangling facility, and alleviating defects related to certain types of hair and hair treatments. Table 8.4 lists the hair conditioner categories with their primary ingredients, main advantages, and hair grooming benefits.

Finally, hairstyling aids are intended to maintain hair in fashionable arrangement while improving the quality of hair fibers. They aim at maintaining hair in desired position, adding increased hold to hair, creating illusion of fullness, creating a wet "spiky" look, straightening, conditioning, moisturizing, and adding shine to kinky hair. They are available as hair spray, hairstyling gel, hair sculpting gel, hair wax, hair mousse, and ethnic styling aids, such as pomade, brilliantine, oil sheen spray, and curl activator. Table 8.5 lists available styling products and their formulation, aim, and application.

Since hair fiber diameter has been recognized to represent a key contributor to age-related hair thinning, a novel leave-on technology has been developed at Procter & Gamble that combines caffeine, niacinamide, panthenol, dimethicone, and an acrylate polymer (CNPDA) to affect the diameter and behavior of individual scalp hair fibers as an approach to improve decreasing fiber diameter. Utilizing laser scan micrometer for assessment of fiber diameter measures and tensile break stress and torsion pendulum testing for

Table 8.4 Hair conditioning agents

Hair conditioner category	Primary ingredient	Main advantage	Hair grooming benefit
Fatty ingredients	Fatty alcohols, lanolin derivatives, oils, waxes, lecithins	Increase hair shine, increase hair manageability	Improve appearance of dry hair
Cationic detergents and film formers	Quaternary ammonium compounds (quats)	Smooth cuticle, decrease static electricity	Excellent to restore damaged, chemically processed hair
	Polymers (polyquaternium)	Fill hair shaft defects, decrease static electricity, improve shine	Improve appearance of dry hair, improve grooming of coarse, kinky hair
Protein containing	Hydrolyzed proteins (keratin, collagen, silk, wheat, soya)	Penetrate hair shaft to minimally increase strength	Temporarily mend splits
Silicones	Dimethicone, cyclomethicone, amodimethicone	Thin coating placed on hair shaft	Decrease static electricity, decrease combing friction, add shine

Table 8.5 Hairstyling aids

Styling product	Formulation	Aim	Application
Hair spray	Aerosolized spray polymer (PVP, VA, MEA)	Maintain hair in desired position	Sprayed on finished hairstyle
Hairstyling gel, hair sculpturing gel	Clear gel polymer	Hold hair away from scalp for fullness or "spiky look"	Rubbed with hands on towel-dried hair
Hair wax	Soft opaque formable wax	Add increased hold to hair	Massaged into dry hair after softening in palm
Hair mousse	Aerosolized polymer foam	Hold hair away from scalp for fullness or "spiky look"	Squirted onto hand and dabbed through towel-dried hair
Ethnic styling aids			
Pomade	Ointment of petrolatum	Straighten, condition, moisturize, add shine to kinky hair	Combed with hands through hair
Brilliantine	Liquid oil	Allow ease of styling and proved shine	Massaged with hands through hair
Oil sheen spray	Aerosolized oil	For shine and moisturization	Sprayed onto hair
Curl activator	Clear glycerin gel	For ringlet hairstyles	Massaged with hands through hair

From: Draelos ZD (2005) Hair grooming cosmetics. In: Draelos ZD (ed) Hair Care. An Illustrated Dermatologic Handbook. Taylor & Francis, London /New York, p. 75

assessment of behavioral properties, it was found that CNPDA significantly increased the diameter of individual terminal scalp hair fibers by 2–5 μm, which yields an increase in the cross-sectional area of approximately 10 %. Beyond the increase in hair fiber diameter, the CNPDA-thickened fibers demonstrated enhanced mechanical properties characteristic of thicker fibers, such as increased suppleness/pliability and better ability to withstand force without breaking.

Ultimately, cosmetic products represent a key integral part of management of hair loss and thinning, since they may significantly improve the condition of the hair fiber with more immediate effects, while pharmacologic agents take their time.

8.2.5 Targeting the Inflammatory Component in Androgenetic Alopecia

The limited success rate of treatment of androgenetic alopecia with topical minoxidil or oral finasteride means that further pathogenic pathways may be taken into account. Clinical and investigative advances have helped us to understand some of the pathogenic steps leading to androgenetic alopecia: besides androgens and genetic imbalance, additional pathogenic factors are suspected, such as microbial flora, endogenous and exogenous stress, microinflammation, and others. While further suspects are likely to be exposed, individual diversity of causal agents, as well as of the sequence of events, or combined factors, must be kept in mind, when addressing the biological conditions contributing to androgenetic alopecia. Ultimately, dissecting the molecular controls of immune-mediated hair follicle degeneration by apoptosis-mediated organ deletion could provide insights into how progression to permanent hair loss due to follicular inflammatory phenomena and fibrosis might be halted.

So far, the inflammatory component has not been included in treatment protocols for androgenetic alopecia.

In an early study, Piérard-Franchimont et al. hypothesized on a microbial-driven inflammatory reaction abutting on the hair follicles and conducted a study to compare the effect of 2 % ketoconazole shampoo to that of an unmedicated shampoo used in combination with or without 2 % minoxidil therapy. They found that hair density and size and proportion of anagen follicles were improved almost similarly by both ketoconazole and minoxidil regimens and concluded that there may be a significant action of ketoconazole upon the course of androgenetic alopecia and that *Malassezia* spp. may play a role in the inflammatory reaction. Later, Berger et al. performed a 6-month, randomized, investigator-blinded, parallel-group clinical study with healthy men between the ages of 18 and 49 years exhibiting Hamilton–Norwood type III vertex or type IV baldness to assess the hair growth benefits of a 1 % pyrithione zinc shampoo. The efficacy of a 1 % pyrithione zinc shampoo (used daily) was compared with that of 5 % minoxidil topical solution (applied twice daily), a placebo shampoo, and a combination of the 1 % pyrithione zinc shampoo and the 5 % minoxidil topical solution. Hair count results showed a significant net increase in total visible hair counts for the 1 % pyrithione zinc shampoo, the 5 % minoxidil topical solution, and the combination treatment groups relative to the placebo shampoo after 9 weeks of treatment. The relative increase in hair count for the 1 % pyrithione zinc shampoo was slightly less than half that for the minoxidil topical solution. However, no advantage was seen in using both the 5 % minoxidil topical solution and the 1 % pyrithione zinc shampoo.

Surprisingly, the use or addition of topical corticosteroids or of systemic anti-inflammatory agents such as oral hydroxychloroquine or oral doxycycline in the treatment plan of androgenetic alopecia (with microinflammation and fibrosis) has so far not been systematically studied. For now, we can only deduce a putative added benefit by analogy from their preliminary (successful) use in cicatricial pattern hair loss or in central centrifugal cicatricial alopecia.

Proposed pathogenic mechanisms in androgenetic alopecia and respective therapeutic strategies are summarized in Fig. 8.7.

CG210® is a novel topical botanical hair growth-promoting agent based on *Allium cepa* (onion), *Citrus medica limonum* (lemon), *Theobroma cacao* (cocoa), and *Paullinia cupana* (guaraná) with a proposed three-level mechanism of action including (1) regulation of the intracellular anti-apoptotic Bcl-2 protein, (2) reduction of microinflammation, and (3) increase of collagen content and collagen remodeling. Safety and efficacy of the compound have been tested in more than 400 male and female volunteers with male and female androgenetic alopecia, respectively. Phototrichogram evaluations revealed the efficacy of the product in normalizing the proportion of hair in telogen, which is understood to be the consequence of premature follicular cell apoptosis in androgenetic alopecia.

8.3 Off-Label Use of Drugs

When a drug is used for unapproved indications, it is termed off-label use. Off-label use of drugs is legal, but the promotion of drugs toward unapproved indications is illegal.

> The prescribing physician should be aware that the off-label prescription of drugs occurs at the discretion of the prescriber.

More than 2,000 different diseases are treated in dermatology, and for many there is no explicitly approved medication. Additional limitations in the approval status are related to patient age (children), pregnancy, and comorbidities. Therefore, for medical and ethical reasons in many treatment situations, prescription of medications off label is necessary. There are no standardized regulations on off-label use for dermatological indications.

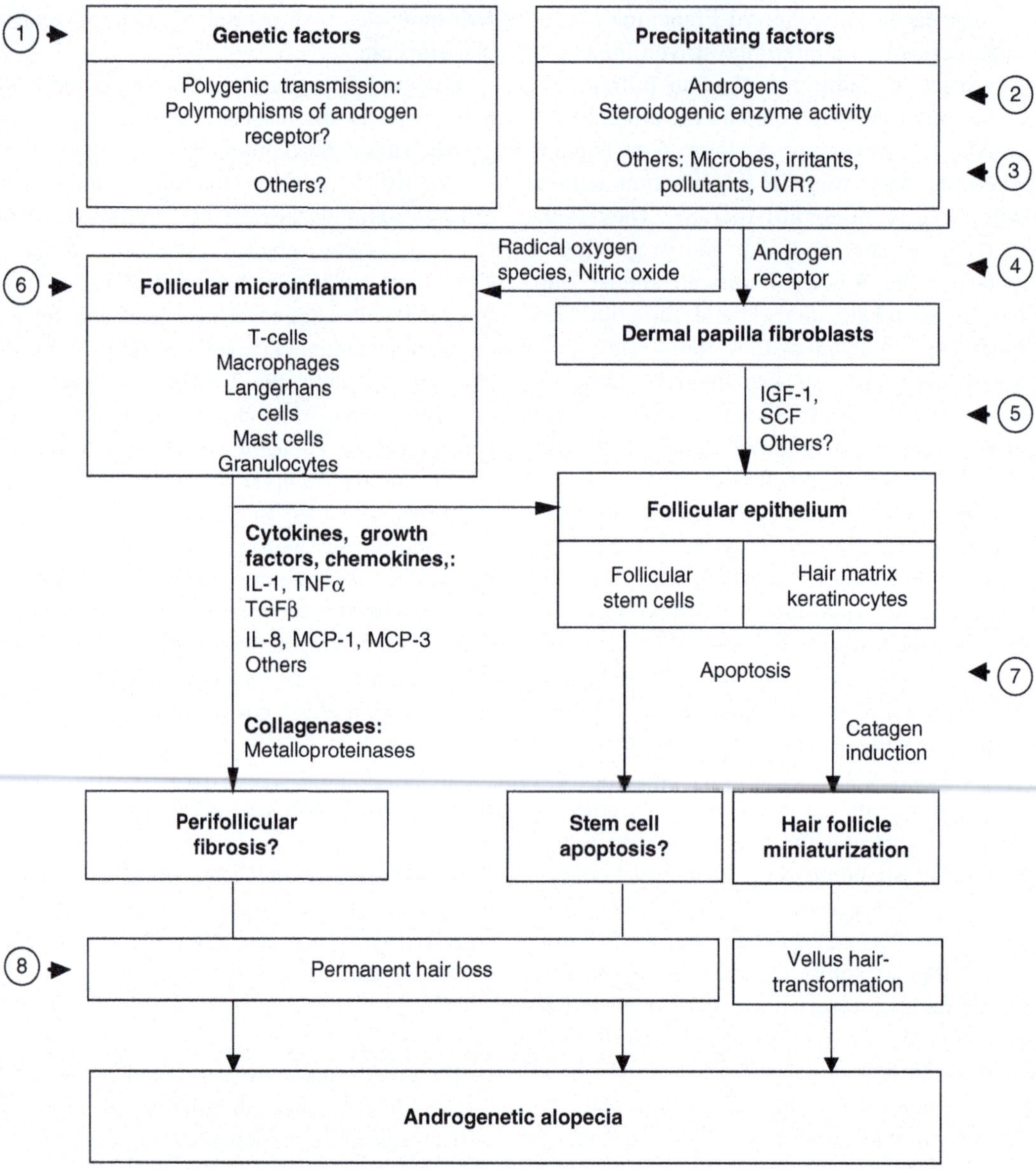

Therapeutic strategies:

1. Gene therapy? (currently not available)
2. Modifiers of androgen metabolism: finasteride (available for men)
3. Antimicrobial shampoos?
4. Antiandrogens: cyproterone acetate (available for women)
5. Hair growth promoters: minoxidil (available for men and for women)
6. Antiinflammatory agents?
7. Apoptosis modulating agents? (currently not available)
8. Hair transplantation (available), implantation of dermal papilla cells or cells of follicle dermal-sheath (impending)

Fig. 8.7 Androgenetic alopecia: pathogenic mechanisms and therapeutic strategies (From Trüeb RM (2002). Molecular mechanisms of androgenetic alopecia. *Exp Gerontol* 37:981–990)

As a general rule, off-label use can be justified in exceptional cases and from the socio-legal perspective can even be demanded by patients, if the existing indications represent a serious life-threatening disease or one which permanently reduces the quality of life, a suitable therapy under approved conditions is not available, and there is a well-founded prospect of successful treatment.

For appropriate prescription in off-label use, it is necessary to carry out an appropriate and thorough evaluation and documentation of previous treatment and of the degree of suffering on the side of the patient and to have knowledge of the international literature on studies involving the selected substance. Off-label use is involved in approximately 5–15 % of necessary pharmaceutical prescriptions in dermatology and affects some 30 drugs and several hundred indications in routine treatment. Examples in the treatment of hair diseases are the use of oral finasteride for treatment of female androgenetic alopecia and the use of oral tetracyclines, hydroxychloroquine, mycophenolate mofetil, cyclosporine A, or pioglitazone in the treatment of lichen planopilaris and related conditions.

The case of the oral antidiabetic pioglitazone that has been proposed for treatment of lichen planopilaris sheds light on the risks of liability issues: on June 9, 2011, the French Agency for the Safety of Health Products decided to withdraw pioglitazone in regard to high risk of bladder cancer; on June 10, 2011, Germany's Federal Institute for Drugs and Medical Devices advised doctors not to prescribe the medication until further investigation of the cancer risk had been conducted; and ultimately, on June 15, 2011, the USFDA announced that pioglitazone use for more than 1 year may be associated with an increased risk of bladder cancer and that the information about this risk will be added to the warnings and precautions section of the label for pioglitazone-containing medicines. On April 7, 2014, a jury in Lafayette, Louisiana, awarded a plaintiff over $1.475 million in compensatory damages and $9 billion in punitive in a suit against Takeda Pharmaceutical Company and Eli Lilly and Company, manufacturers of the diabetes medication Actos® (pioglitazone). The suit alleged that defendants downplayed the risk of cancer in producing and marketing the diabetes drug.

Nevertheless, prescriptions for off-label use are an integral component of qualified dermatologic treatment. Despite regulatory and legal hurdles, off-label use can be implemented with knowledge of the juridical and formal conditions.

Further Reading

Impact of Seasonality on Hair Growth and Shedding

Courtois M, Loussouarn G, Hourseau S, Grollier JF (1996) Periodicity in the growth and shedding of hair. Br J Dermatol 134:47–54

Hotzenköcherle Trüeb B (2015) Impact of seasonality of hair growth and shedding on clinical trials with hair growth promoting agents. Inaugural Dissertation, University of Zurich

Kunz M, Seifert B, Trüeb RM (2009) Seasonality of hair shedding in healthy women complaining of hair loss. Dermatology 219:105–110

Orentreich N (1969) Scalp replacement in man. In: Montagna W, Bobson RL (eds) Advances in biology of skin. Vol IX: Hair growth. Pewrgamon, Oxford, pp 99–108

Randall VA, Ebling FJG (1991) Seasonal changes in human hair growth. Br J Dermatol 124:146–151

Concept of Multitargeted Treatment

Rajput RJ (2010) Controversy: is there a role for adjuvants in the management of male pattern hair loss? J Cutan Aesthet Surg 3(2):82–86

Concept of Multitargeted Treatment: Comorbidity

Feinstein AR (1970) The pre-therapeutic classification of co-morbidity in chronic disease. J Chronic Dis 23(7):455–468

Jakovljević M, Ostojić L (2013) Comorbidity and multimorbidity in medicine today: challenges and opportunities for bringing separated branches of medicine

closer to each other. Psychiatr Danub 25(Suppl 1):18–28
Mangin D, Heath I, Jamoulle M (2012) Beyond diagnosis: rising to the multimorbidity challenge. BMJ 344, e3526
Valderas JM, Starfield B, Sibbald B, Salisbury C, Roland M (2009) Defining comorbidity: implications for understanding health and health services. Ann Fam Med 7(4):357–363
Weel V, Chris S, François G (2006) Comorbidity and guidelines: conflicting interests. Lancet 367(9510):550–551

Concept of Multitargeted Treatment: Value of Nutritional Therapies

Ahrens J (1994) Systemische Behandlung des diffusen Haarausfalls. Therapiewoche Schweiz 10:551–554
Aldosary BM, Sutter ME, Schwartz M, Morgan BW (2012) Case series of selenium toxicity from a nutritional supplement. Clin Toxicol (Phila) 50:57–64
Aydingoz I, Ferhanoglu B, Guney O (1999) Does tissue iron status have a role in female alopecia? J Eur Acad Dermatol Venereol 13:65–67
Bregy A, Trueb RM (2008) No association between serum ferritin levels >10 microg/l and hair loss activity in women. Dermatology 217:1–6
Budde J, Tronnier H, Rahlfs VW, Frei-Kleiner S (1993) Systemische Therapie von diffusem Effluvium und Haarstrukturschäden. Hautarzt 144:380–384
Buhl AE, Waldon DJ, Kawabe TT, Holland JM (1989) Minoxidil stimulates mouse vibrissae follicles in organ culture. J Invest Dermatol 92:315–320
D'Agostini F, Balansky R, Pesce C et al (2000) Induction of alopecia in mice exposed to cigarette smoking. Toxicol Lett 114:117–123
D'Agostini F, Fiallo P, Pennisi TM, De Flora S (2007) Chemoprevention of smoke-induced alopecia in mice by oral administration of L-cystine and vitamin B6. J Dermatol Sci 46:189–198
Finner AM (2013) Nutrition and hair: deficiencies and supplements. Dermatol Clin 31:167–172
Frenkel MJ, Gillepsie JM, Reis PJ (1974) Factors influencing the biosynthesis of the tyrosine-rich proteins of wool. Aust J Biol Sci 27:31–38
Garneata L (2008) Intravenous iron, inflammation, and oxidative stress: is iron a friend or an enemy of uremic patients? J Ren Nutr 18:40–45
Gillespie JM, Reis PJ (1966) Dietary regulated biosynthesis of high-sulfur wool proteins. Biochem J 98:669–677
Gummer CL (1985) Diet and hair loss. Semin Dermatol 4:35–39
Hard S (1963) Non-anemic iron deficiency as an etiologic factor in diffuse loss of hair of the scalp in women. Acta Derm Venereol 43:562–569
Kantor J, Kessler LJ, Brooks DG, Cotsarelis G (2003) Decreased serum ferritin is associated with alopecia in women. J Invest Dermatol 121:985–988
King SM, Donangelo CM, Knutson MD, Walter PB, Ames BN, Viteri FE, King JC (2008) Daily supplementation with iron increases lipid peroxidation in young women with low iron stores. Exp Biol Med 233:701–707
Lopez RE, Knable AL Jr, Burruss JB (2010) Ingestion of a dietary supplement resulting in selenium toxicity. J Am Acad Dermatol 63:168–169
Petri H, Perchalla P, Tronnier H (1990) Die Wirksamkeit einer medikamentösen Therapie bei Haarstrukturschäden und diffusen Effluvien – vergleichende Doppelblindstudie. Schweiz Rundsch Med Prax 79:1457–1462
Reis PJ, Tunks DA, Sharry LF (1973) Plasma amino acid patterns in sheep receiving abomasal infusions of methionine and cystine. Aust J Biol Sci 26:635–644
Rushton DH (2002) Nutritional factors and hair loss. Clin Exp Dermatol 27:396–404
Rushton DH, Dover R, Sainsbury AW et al (2002) Iron deficiency is neglected in women's health. Br Med J 325:1176
Rushton DH, Ramsay ID (1992) The importance of adequate serum ferritin levels during oral cyproterone acetate and ethinyl oestradiol treatment of diffuse androgen-dependent alopecia in women. Clin Endocrinol (Oxf) 36:421–427
Rushton DH, Ramsay ID, James KC et al (1990) Biochemical and trichological characterization of diffuse alopecia in women. Br J Dermatol 123:187–197
Schümann K, Ettle T, Szegner B, Elsenhans B, Solomons NW (2007) On risks and benefits of iron supplementation recommendations for iron intake revisited. J Trace Elem Med Biol 21:147–168
Senol E, Ersoy A, Erdinc S, Sarandol E, Yurtkuran M (2008) Oxidative stress and ferritin levels in haemodialysis patients. Nephrol Dial Transplant 23:665–672
Sinclair R (2002) There is no clear association between low serum ferritin and chronic diffuse telogen hair loss. Br J Dermatol 147:982–984
Trost LB, Bergfeld WF, Calogeras E (2006) The diagnosis and treatment of iron deficiency and its potential relationship to hair loss. J Am Acad Dermatol 54:824–844
Vinceti M, Wei ET, Malagoli C, Bergomi M, Vivoli G (2001) Adverse health effects of selenium in humans. Rev Environ Health 16:233–251
Waalen J, Felitti V, Beutler E (2002) Haemoglobin and ferritin concentrations in men and women: cross sectional study. BMJ 325:137
Yoshimura K, Nakano H, Yokoyama K, Nakayama M (2005) High iron storage levels are associated with increased DNA oxidative injury in patients on regular hemodialysis. Clin Exp Nephrol 9:158–163

Concept of Multitargeted Treatment: Low Level Laser Therapy

Avci P, Gupta GK, Clark J, Wikonkal N, Hamblin MR (2014) Low-level laser (light) therapy (LLLT) for treatment of hair loss. Lasers Surg Med 46(2):144–151
Avram MR, Leonard RT Jr, Epstein ES, Williams JL, Bauman AJ (2007) The current role of laser/light sources in the treatment of male and female pattern hair loss. J Cosmet Laser Ther 9(1):27–28

Avram MR, Rogers NE (2009) The use of low-level light for hair growth: part I. J Cosmet Laser Ther 11(2):110–117
Bernstein EF (2005) Hair growth induced by diode laser treatment. Dermatol Surg 31(5):584–586
Chung H, Dai T, Sharma SK, Huang YY, Carroll JD, Hamblin MR (2012) The nuts and bolts of low-level laser (light) therapy. Ann Biomed Eng 40(2):516–533
Ghanaat M (2010) Types of hair loss and treatment options, including the novel low-level light therapy and its proposed mechanism. South Med J 103(9):917–921
Gupta AK, Daigle D (2014) The use of low-level light therapy in the treatment of androgenetic alopecia and female pattern hair loss. J Dermatolog Treat 25(2):162–163
Jimenez JJ, Wikramanayake TC, Bergfeld W, Hordinsky M, Hickman JG, Hamblin MR, Schachner LA (2014) Efficacy and safety of a low-level laser device in the treatment of male and female pattern hair loss: a multicenter, randomized, sham device-controlled, double-blind study. Am J Clin Dermatol 15(2):115–127
Lanzafame RJ, Blanche RR, Bodian AB, Chiacchierini RP, Fernandez-Obregon A, Kazmirek ER (2013) The growth of human scalp hair mediated by visible red light laser and LED sources in males. Lasers Surg Med 45(8):487–495
Lanzafame RJ, Blanche RR, Chiacchierini RP, Kazmirek ER, Sklar J (2014) The growth of human scalp hair in females using visible red light laser and LED sources. Lasers Surg Med 46(8):601–607
Leavitt M, Charles G, Heyman E, Michaels D (2009) HairMax LaserComb laser phototherapy device in the treatment of male androgenetic alopecia: a randomized, double-blind, sham device-controlled, multicentre trial. Clin Drug Investig 29(5):283–292
Mester E, Szende B, Gärtner P (1968) [The effect of laser beams on the growth of hair in mice]. [Article in German]. Radiobiol Radiother (Berl) 9(5):621–626
Munck A, Gavazzoni MF, Trüeb RM (2014) Use of low-level laser therapy as monotherapy or concomitant therapy for male and female androgenetic alopecia. Int J Trichol 6(2):45–49
Moreno-Arias G, Castelo-Branco C, Ferrando J (2002) Paradoxical effect after IPL photoepilation. Dermatol Surg 28(11):1013–1016
Satino JL, Markou M (2003) Hair regrowth and increased hair tensile strength using HairMax LaserComb for low-level laser therapy. Int J Cosmet Surg Aesthet Dermatol 5(2):113–117
Tin SS, Wiwanitkit V (2014) Low-level laser therapy for androgenic alopecia. Int J Trichol 6(4):189

Concept of Multitargeted Treatment: Value of Cosmetic Treatments

Bouillon C (1996) Shampoos. Clin Dermatol 14:113–121
Davis MG, Thomas JH, van de Velde S, Boissy Y, Dawson TL Jr, Iveson R, Sutton K (2011) A novel cosmetic approach to treat thinning hair. Br J Dermatol 165(Suppl 3):24–30
Dawber R (1996) Hair: its structure and response to cosmetic preparations. Clin Dermatol 14:105–112
Draelos ZD (2005) Hair grooming cosmetics. In: Draelos ZD (ed) Hair care. An illustrated dermatologic handbook. Taylor & Francis, London/New York
Draelos ZD (2010) Care of aging hair and photoprotection. In: Trüeb RM, Tobin DJ (eds) Aging hair. Springer, Berlin Heidelberg, pp 183–191
Rushton H, Gummer CL, Flasch H (1994) 2-in-1 shampoo technology: state of the art shampoo and conditioner in one. Skin Pharmacol 7:78–83
Trüeb RM (2007) Shampoos: ingredients, efficacy and adverse effects. J Dtsch Dermatol Ges 5:356–365
Trüeb RM (2005) Dermocosmetic aspects of hair and scalp. J Investig Dermatol Symp Proc 10:289–292
Urbano CC (1995) 50 years of hair care development. Cosmet Toiletries 110:85–104

Concept of Multitargeted Treatment: Targeting the Inflammatory Component in Androgenetic Alopecia

Berger RS, Fu JL, Smiles KA, Turner CB, Schnell BM, Werchowski KM, Lammers KM (2003) The effects of minoxidil, 1% pyrithione zinc and a combination of both on hair density: a randomized controlled trial. Br J Dermatol 149:354–362
Cucé L, Consuelo JR, Régia CRP (2011) Celium® GC: evaluation of a new natural active ingredient in 210 mg/ml topical solution, through scalp biopsy. Surg Cosmet Dermatol 3:123–128
Piérard-Franchimont C, De Doncker P, Cauwenbergh G, Piérard GE (1998) Ketoconazole shampoo: effect of long-term use in androgenic alopecia. Dermatology 196:474–477
Trüeb RM (2002) Molecular mechanisms of androgenetic alopecia. Exp Gerontol 37:981–990

Off-Label Use of Drugs

Augustin M (2013) Appropriate off-label prescription in practice. Hautarzt 64(10):728–735
Brucklacher U, Brockmeyer NH, Riedel C (2013) Off-label use and G-BA. Legal framework for off-label use. Hautarzt 64(10):736–742
Brunne V, Mertins G, Reimann G, Brockmeyer NH (2004) Off-label use in dermatological practice. The conflict between professional duty and legal requirements. Hautarzt 55(8):727–734
Picard D, Carvalho P, Bonnavia C, Louin L, Josset V, Lauret P, Joly P, Ensemble des Consultants de la Clinique Dermatologique du CHU de Rouen (2003) Assessment off-label prescribing in dermatology. Ann Dermatol Venereol 130(5):507–510

9 Exemplary Case Studies of Successful Treatments

The art of medicine was to be properly learned only from its practice and its exercise.
Thomas Sydenham (1624–1689)

In every art, there are many techniques, but few principles. The only way to achieve success is to have a firm foundation of principles to build upon and the right attitude about achieving one's goals. In the chapters of this book, the basic principles of clinical trichology as well as the attitudes to effectively translate these principles into live practice are discussed.

In the first three chapters, the prerequisites for successful management of hair loss are reviewed—basically, making a diagnosis and understanding the patient and his or her problem. In the following two chapters, guidance is provided to the management of difficult dermatologic conditions and of the psychopathological disorders associated with the complaint of hair loss. Finally, important aspects of follow-up are covered, specifically the problems of adverse effects, patient noncompliance, and their management, before concluding with the ultimate goal of optimizing therapy beyond evidence-based medicine.

The following set of clinical case studies of successful management of alopecia and related conditions aims at encouraging physicians to apply with confidence what is learned from the former chapters with the certainty of success and of reward.

9.1 Acquiring the Skills for Effective Treatment of Alopecia and Related Conditions

From experience, the patient complaining of hair loss takes a low position in the scale of popularity in dermatologic practice. Few dermatologic problems carry as much emotional overtones as the care of hair loss, both on the part of patients and of the attending physicians. This attitude on the part of physicians is related to lack of comprehension of the psychological impact of hair loss or fear of hair loss on patients and to a general lack of confidence in successful treatment of alopecia.

Is there any reason why treatment of hair loss should not be as straightforward and rewarding as that of acne or of eczema? This book provides the principles to achieve success in management of alopecia and related conditions. In order to get the most out of this book, the same four *guideposts* proposed by Dale Carnegie (1888–1955, American author and lecturer on self-improvement, public speaking, and interpersonal skills) for effective speaking

R.M. Trüeb, *The Difficult Hair Loss Patient: Guide to Successful Management of Alopecia and Related Conditions*, DOI 10.1007/978-3-319-19701-2_9

in public will prove to be useful for effective treatment of hair loss:

- Taking heart from the experience of others
- Keeping your goal before you
- Predetermining your mind to success
- Seizing every opportunity to practice

Taking heart from the experience of others. Despite what sophisticated publications would suggest us to believe, effective trichological practice is not a closed art to be mastered only after years of perfecting and struggling with the mysteries of hair growth and shedding. I have spent much of my teaching career proving to fellow physicians that it is easy to effectively treat hair loss, provided you follow a few simple, but important, rules. I have assured them, on the basis of my experiences with young trainees in clinical trichology at my practice, that there is no doubt in my mind that anyone can succeed. Positive testimonials from the trainees provide the evidence.

Keeping your goal before you. "Whoever strives with all his might, that man we can redeem" is a maxim of Johann Wolfgang von Goethe (German writer and statesman, 1749–1832). In almost any subject, your passion for the subject will save you. If you care enough for a result, you will most certainly achieve it. Project yourself into the future and then work toward bringing that projection into reality. If you wish to be learned, you will be learned. If you wish to be good, you will be good. Only then you must really wish these things and wish them with exclusiveness and not wish 100 other incompatible things just as strongly. Think of the satisfaction and pleasure that will be yours when you succeed in effectively treating hair loss and alopecia. You will get a sense of strength and a feeling of power. At the same time, try your best to develop the ability to let your patients feel into your head and heart. You will find, as you progress in your efforts, that you are making an impression and impact on your patients such as you never made before. You will obtain a double benefit from this approach, since your self-confidence will strengthen with your success and your whole personality will grow warmer and better.

Predetermining your mind to success. Once you have set your mind on the goal of increased confidence and more effective trichological practice, you must keep thinking positively about your chances to succeed. Always keep in mind the great importance of what you think, for your own thoughts make you what you are. To succeed, you need the qualities that are essential in any endeavor: desire amounting to enthusiasm, persistence to overcome all obstacles, and the self-assurance to believe you will succeed.

Seizing every opportunity to practice. You could read every textbook available on hair growth and disorders and still not be able to treat hair loss effectively. This book is a thorough guide going beyond the technical aspects of trichology and evidence-based medicine. But you must put its suggestions into practice. "I know all about that" you may argue, "but I hesitate to face the ordeal of trichological practice." What ordeal? You must think of practicing in the right spirit, the spirit of adventure on the path to success while unfolding your personality in the practice of clinical trichology. As you follow this book in putting its principles into practice, you too will be heading into adventure.

9.2 Androgenetic Alopecia

Case 9.1 A 35-year-old male with androgenetic alopecia. He had been transplanted twice, 6 and 7 years earlier, respectively. He was not advised to follow with a pharmacological treatment and progressed with hair loss over the next 6 years. He was successfully treated with 1 mg oral finasteride: (**a**) before, (**b**) after 3 months, and (**c**) after 12 months of treatment

Comment Autologous hair transplantation remains the only treatment option for advanced patterned baldness. With the advent of micrografting, hair restoration surgery has in general become satisfying. Modern techniques use the visual qualities of hair and varying design patterns to create the optical illusion of more hair

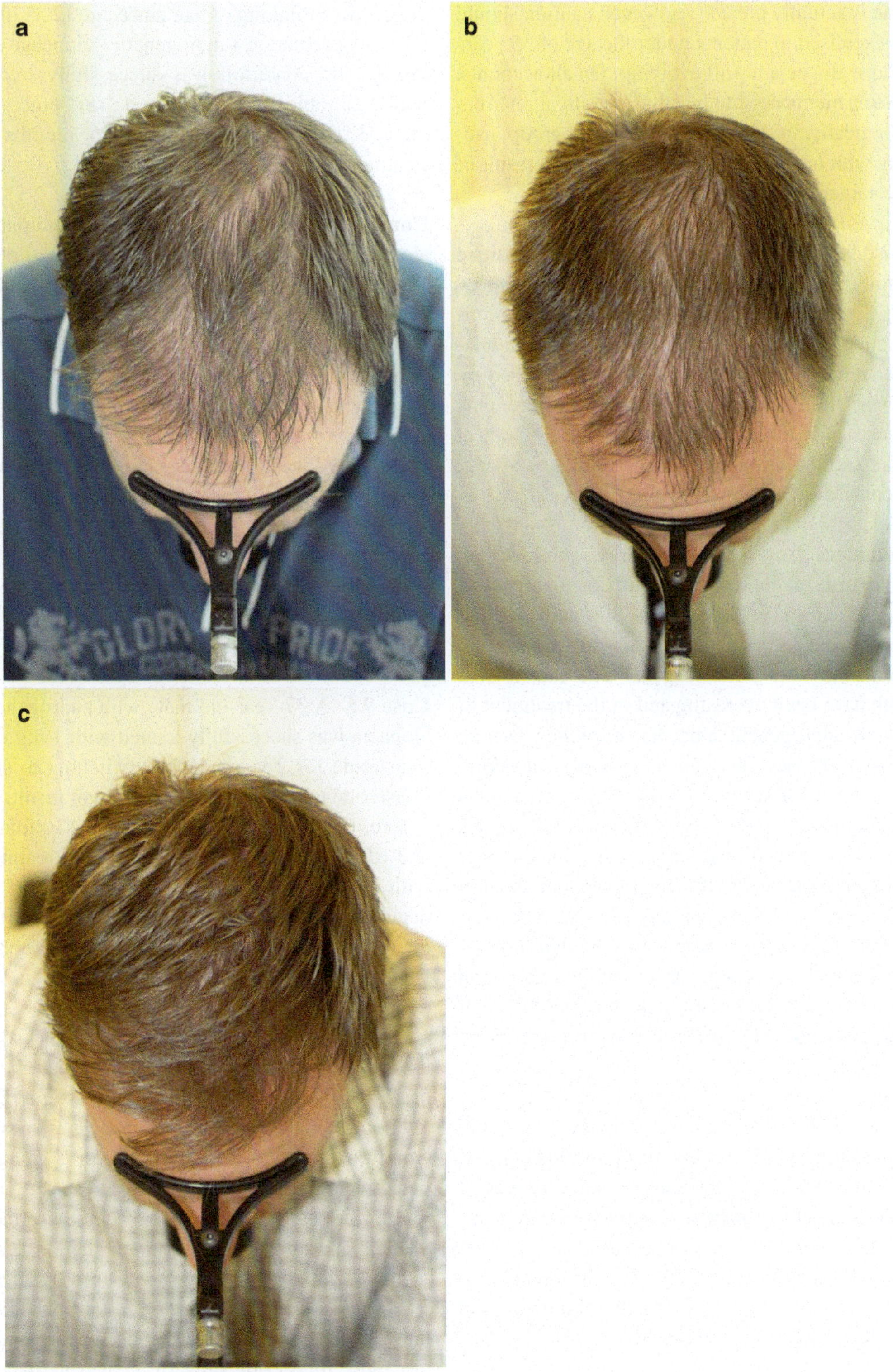

Fig. 9.1 (a–c)

than is actually present. However, caution should be exercised in patients under the age of 35 years whose alopecia is still evolving. On all accounts, these patients need to be advised to treat pharmacologically, in the 18 to 40 years age group, usually with oral finasteride for a sustained result of the surgery.

Case 9.2 A 30-year-old female, with a positive family history for alopecia and a personal history of 10-year hair loss progression, despite previous treatment with topical alfatradiol, iron supplementations, and an oral contraceptive based on 20 µg ethinylestradiol and 3 mg drospirenone. She was successfully treated with 5 % topical minoxidil solution b.i.d.: (**a**) before, (**b**) after 9 months, and (**c**) after 15 months of treatment

Comment This is an exemplary example for the superiority of topical minoxidil for treatment of female androgenetic alopecia. Traditionally, hair loss in women has been treated with iron supplementation and antiandrogens. The fact is that both have been overestimated in the treatment of female androgenetic alopecia, since they have no proven efficacy in women with normal serum androgen and ferritin levels. Minoxidil causes hair follicles at rest to grow, promotes hair growth through increasing anagen duration, and enlarges suboptimal follicles. Its effect may start as early as 8 weeks and is typically recognizable at 6 months. This case is noteworthy, in that minoxidil treatment increased hair growth even between months 9 and 15, underlining the importance of long-term patient adherence to treatment for best results.

Case 9.3 A 10-year-old otherwise healthy girl of Indian origin with a positive family history and 2-year personal history of progressive thinning of hair in the crown area. A diagnosis of premature (androgenetic) alopecia was made. The condition was successfully treated with 2 % topical minoxidil once daily: (**a**) before, (**b**) after 3 months, and (**c**) after 6 months of treatment

Case 9.4 A 15-year-old otherwise healthy boy with a positive family history of alopecia noticed progressive thinning of hair since age 12. A diagnosis of premature (androgenetic) alopecia was made. The condition was successfully treated with 2 % topical minoxidil b.i.d.: (**a**) before, (**b**) after 3 months, and (**c**) after 6 months of treatment

Comment The first case series of premature alopecia in children was reported by Tosti et al. There usually is a strong family history of androgenetic alopecia, the children are otherwise healthy, and the hair loss shows a characteristic female pattern distribution (also in males). Efficacy and safety data for topical minoxidil solution are not available before the age of 18 years. Moreover, systemic side effects of topical minoxidil (hypertrichosis and cardiovascular) are observed more frequently in children. Nevertheless, treatment with topical 2 % minoxidil solution, before the age of 12 once daily, thereafter twice daily, is usually safe and very effective.

Case 9.5 A 37-year-old male with androgenetic alopecia was successfully treated with 1 mg oral finasteride for 2 years, before switching to split finasteride tablets with deterioration of result: (**a**) before, (**b**) after 6 months, (**c**) after 12 months, and (**d**) after 24 months of successful treatment with 1 mg oral finasteride (Propecia®) and (**e**) deterioration within 9 months after switching to a quarter tablet daily of a 5 mg oral finasteride generic

Comment In an effort to save money, some users buy 5 mg finasteride tablets instead of the original 1 mg pill and split them into several parts to approximate the 1 mg dosage. Navarro Guerrero et al. performed a galenic-pharmaceutical study of pieces of Proscar® (5 mg finasteride) tablets and Propecia® in the treatment of male androgenetic alopecia and demonstrated a high variability in the dosage of pieces of tablets ranging from 0.49 to 1.81 mg of finasteride, only 10 % being within the dosage range. Finally, the 1 mg finasteride pills are coated to prevent contact with the active ingredient during handling, and dust or crumbs from broken 5 mg fin-

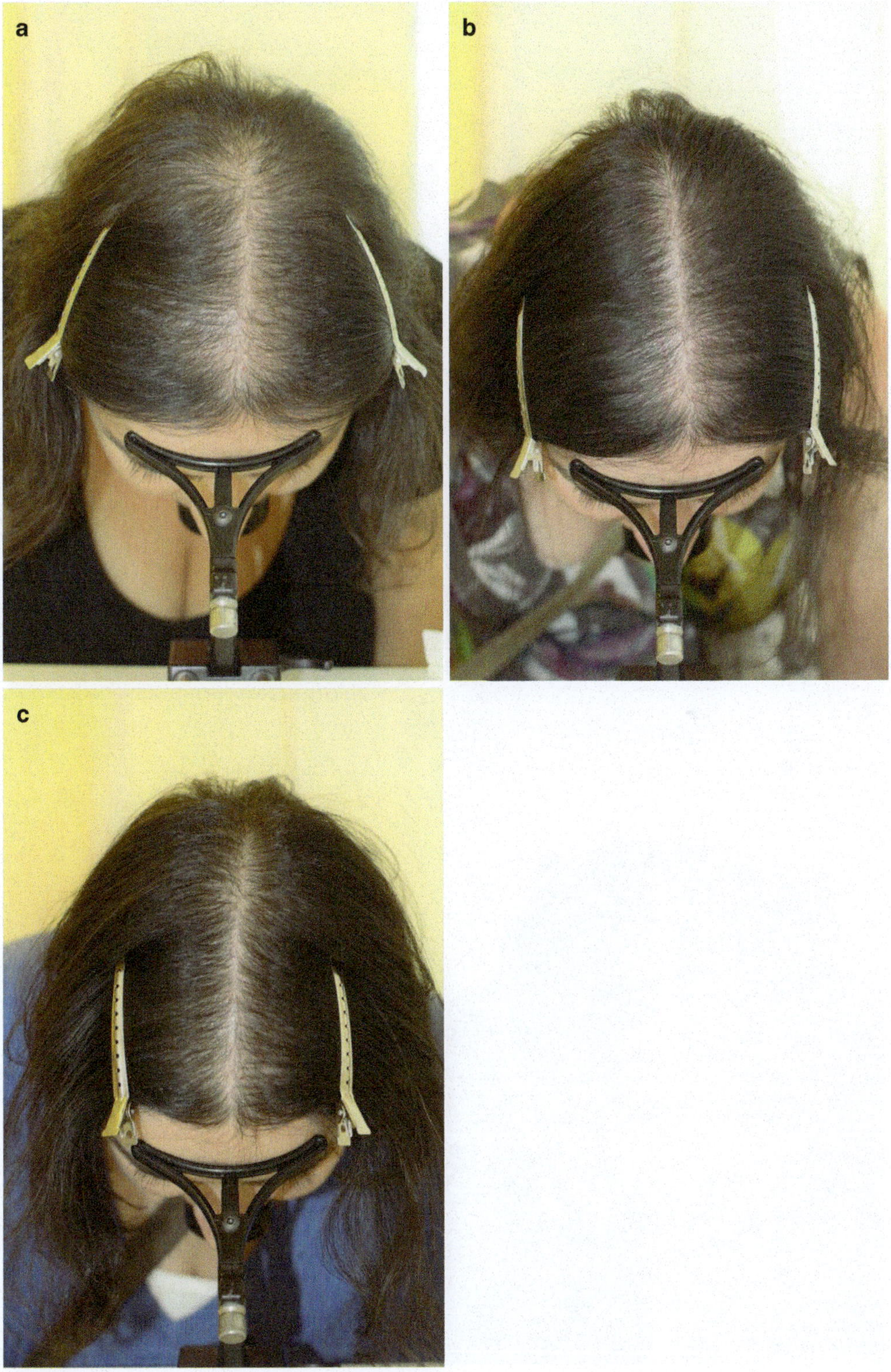

Fig. 9.2 (a–c)

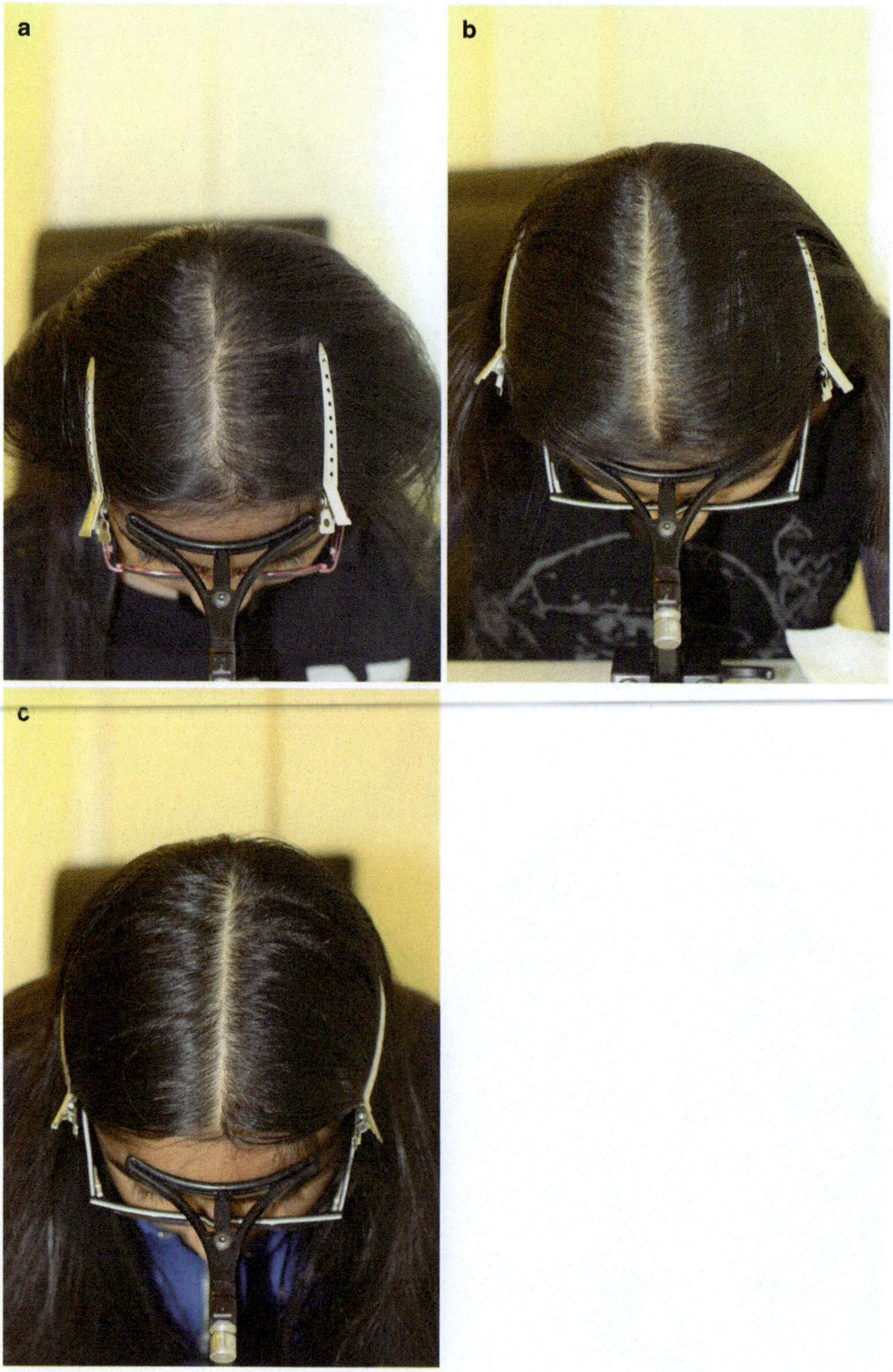

Fig. 9.3 (a–c)

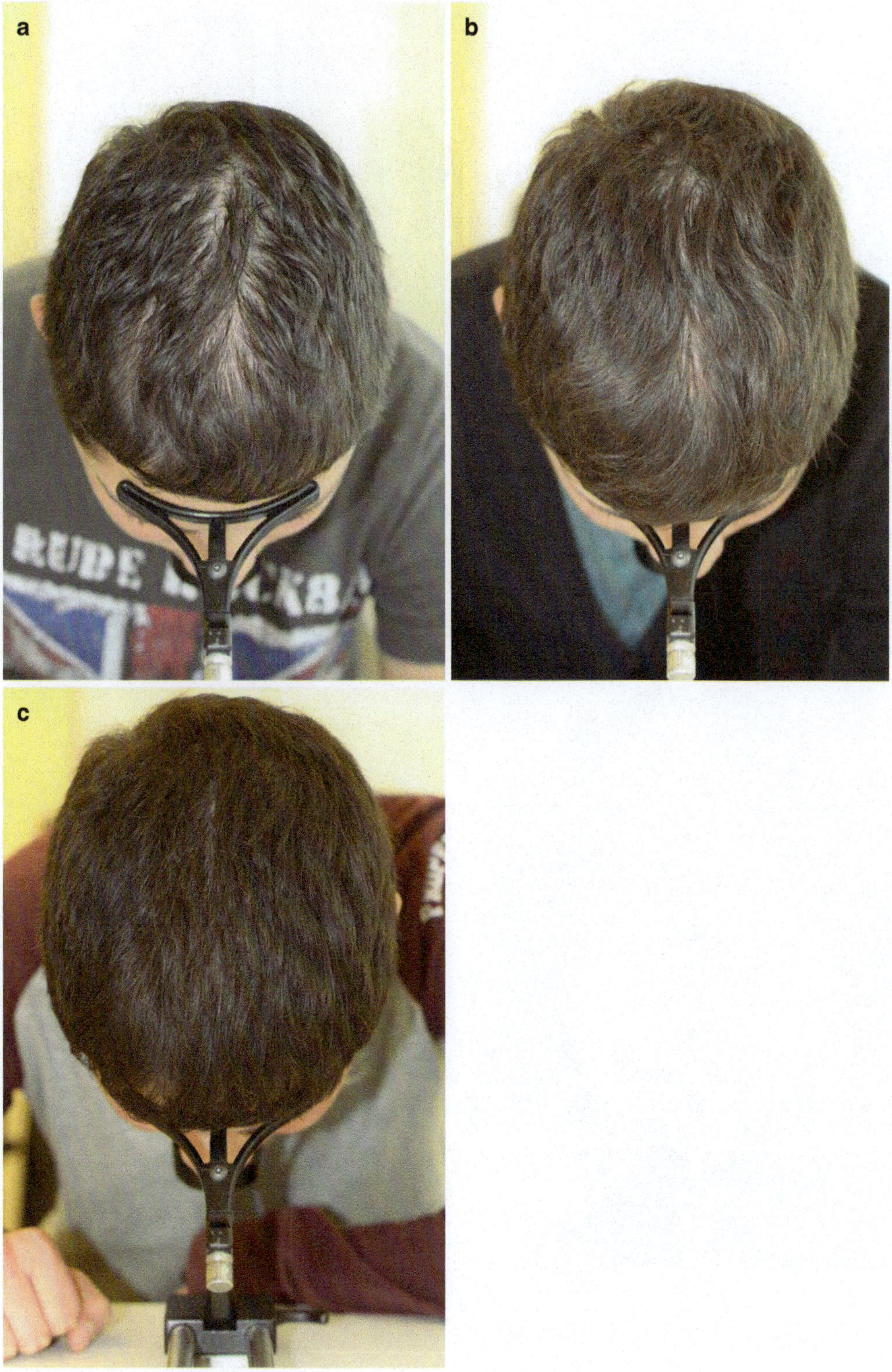

Fig. 9.4 (a–c)

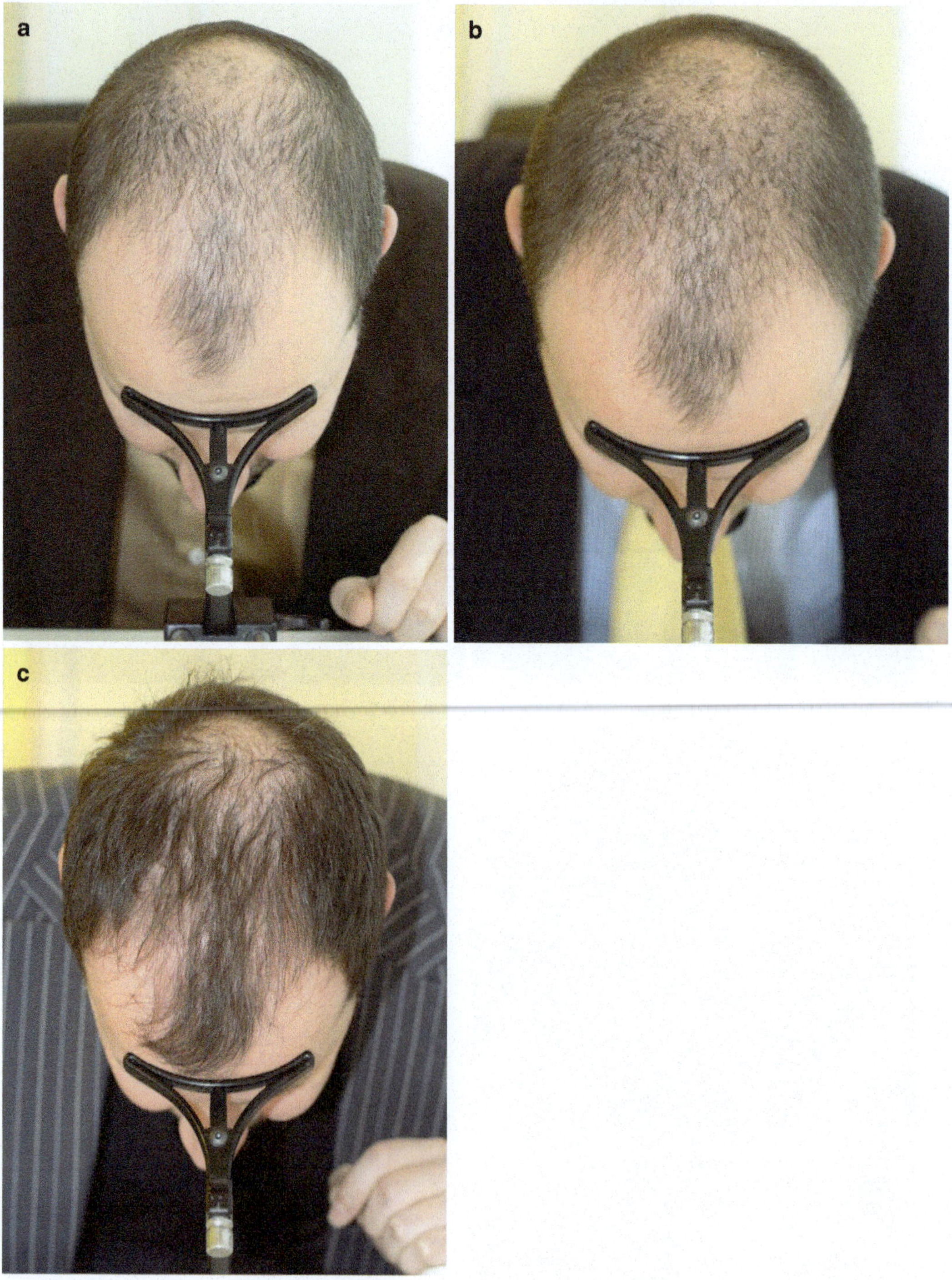

Fig. 9.5 (a–e)

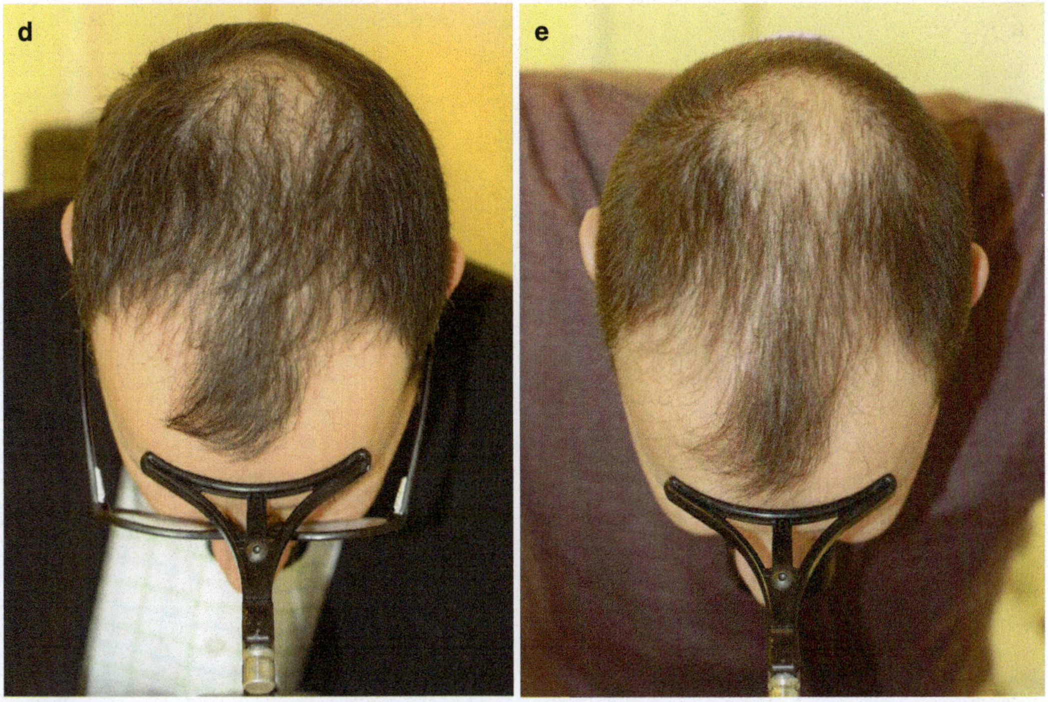

Fig. 9.5 (continued)

asteride tablets should be kept away from pregnant women or women who may become pregnant due to teratogenicity. Splitting 5 mg finasteride tablets to treat androgenetic alopecia is therefore an inappropriate practice from the point of view of dosage variability and safety.

Case 9.6 A 28-year-old male with androgenetic alopecia successfully treated with 1 mg oral finasteride over 12 months was successfully switched to 0.5 mg oral dutasteride for further improvement: (**a**) before, (**b**) after 6 months, and (**c**) after 12 months of 1 mg oral finasteride treatment and (**d**) further improvement within 3 months after switching to 0.5 mg oral dutasteride

Comment Gubelin Harcha et al. recently demonstrated efficacy and safety of 0.5 mg dutasteride in increasing hair growth and restoration in male androgenetic alopecia while being well tolerated. In another study performed by Jung et al., 0.5 mg dutasteride/day also proved to be effective in men with androgenetic alopecia recalcitrant to finasteride. As opposed to finasteride, which is a selective 5-alpha reductase isotype I-inhibitor, dutasteride is a dual inhibitor of 5-alpha reductase isotypes I and II, therefore further lowering circulating plasma levels of dihydrotestosterone. A point to be made is that the plasma half-life time of dutasteride (3–5 weeks) is significantly longer than that of finasteride (age-dependent, from 5 to 8 h).

Case 9.7 A 60-year-old female with androgenetic alopecia allergic to minoxidil successfully treated with 5 mg oral finasteride: (**a**) before, (**b**) after 6 months, and (**c**) after 12 months of treatment

Comment Thai and Sinclair originally reported successful oral finasteride treatment of female androgenetic alopecia in a postmenopausal woman. Trüeb et al. later reported successful treatment with 2.5 or 5 mg/d oral finasteride in 5 normoandrogenic, postmenopausal women. In the so far largest series of 37 premenopausal women treated for 1 year with finasteride in doses

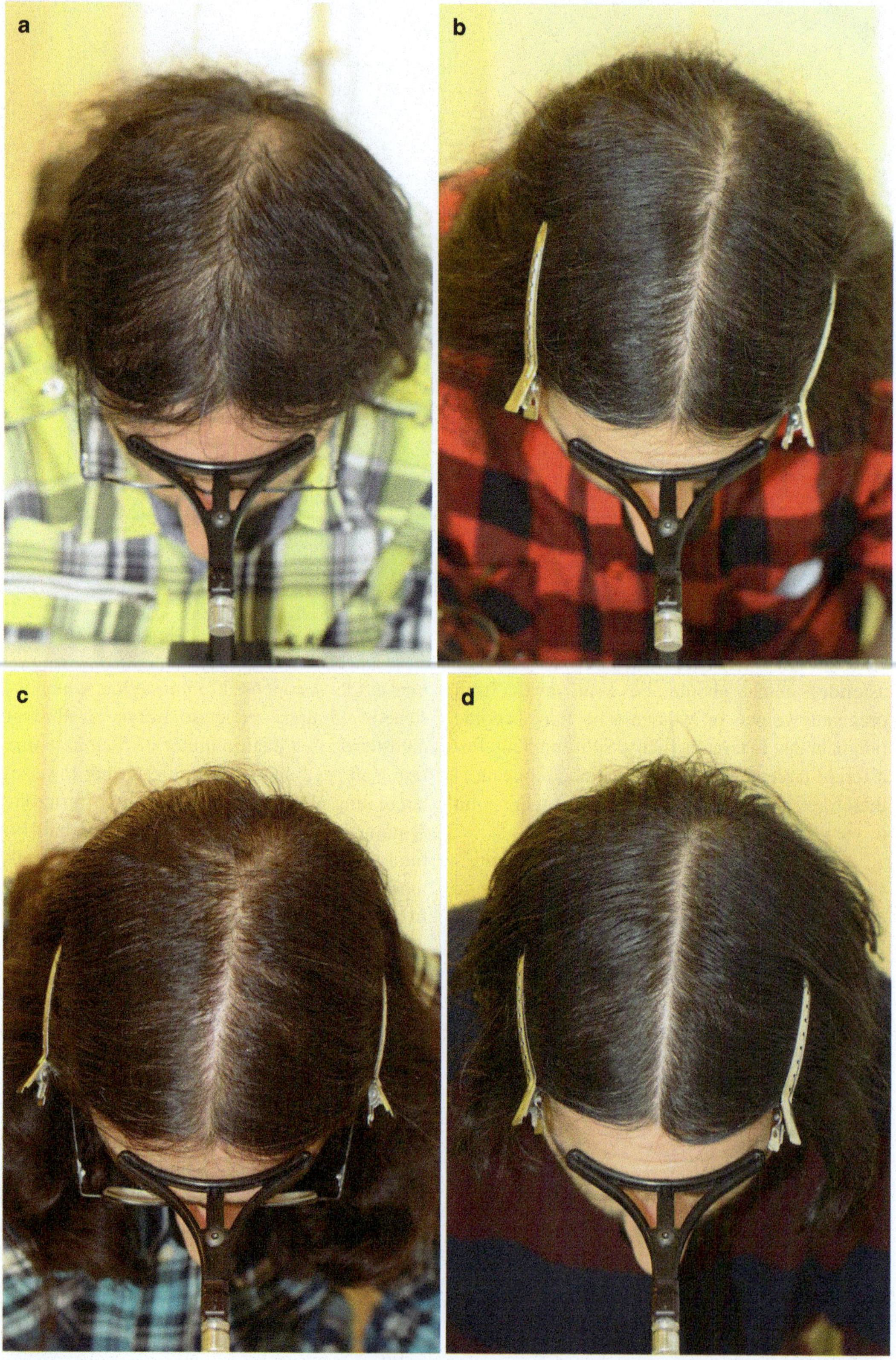

Fig. 9.6 (a–d)

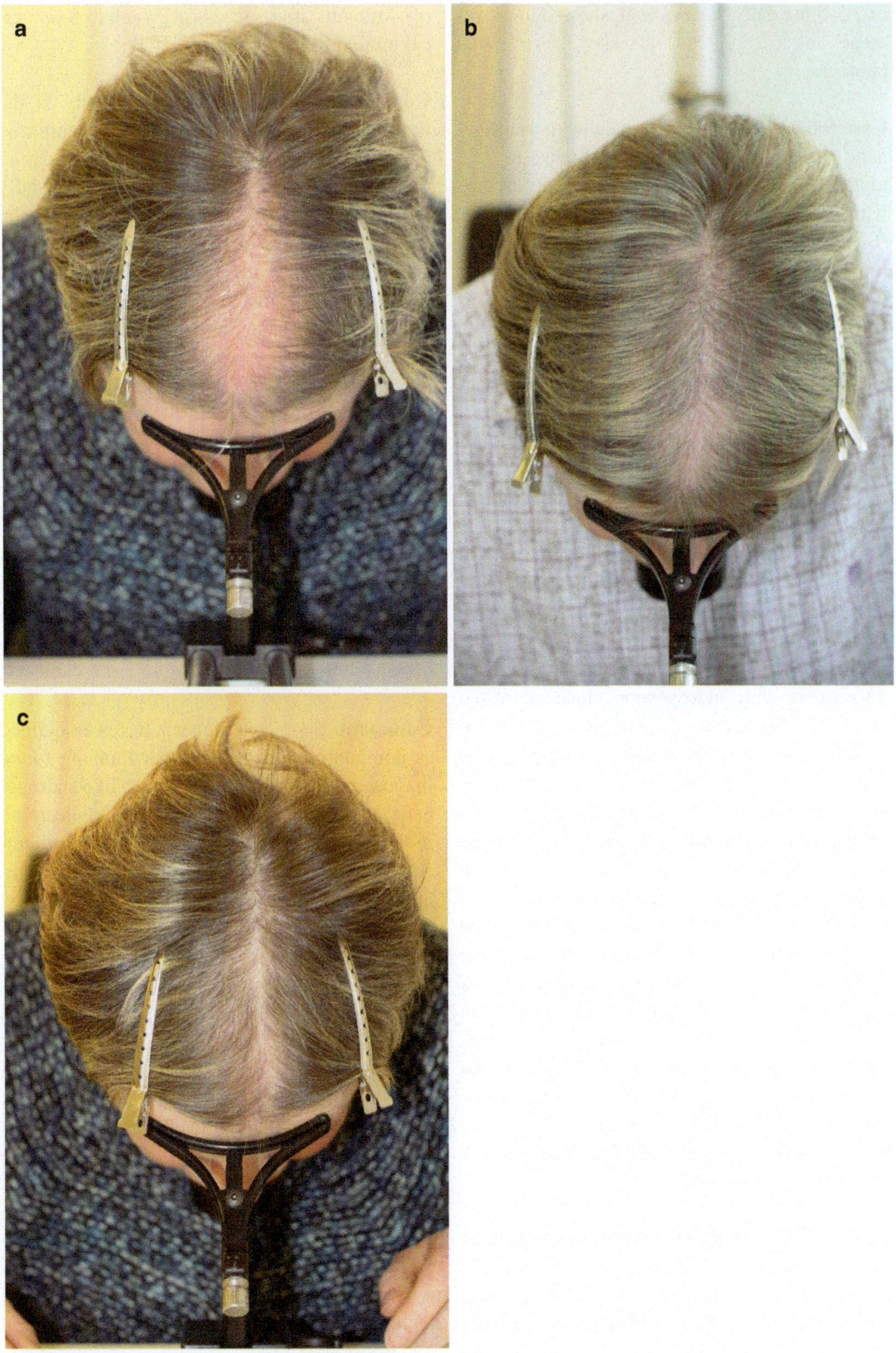

Fig. 9.7 (a–c)

of 2.5–5 mg daily, Iorizzo et al. showed improvement in 62 % as assessed by global photography.

Case 9.8 A 34-year-old female with androgenetic alopecia and inadequate response to 5 % topical minoxidil b.i.d. was successfully treated with low-level laser therapy (LLLT): (**a**) before, (**b**) after 1 year of 5 % topical minoxidil b.i.d, and (**c**) after 6 months adding on LLLT

Comment Currently, topical minoxidil solution and 1 mg oral finasteride are the treatments with the highest levels of medical evidence for treatment of female and male androgenetic alopecia, respectively, but patients who exhibit intolerance or poor response to these treatments are in need of additional treatment modalities. Although low-level energy laser treatments (LLLT) have been therapeutically used in medicine for photobiostimulation in a variety of indications more than 30 years, it has only recently found the attention of the scientific community for the treatment of androgenetic alopecia. In a study of 32 patients with androgenetic alopecia treated with LLT, Munck et al. demonstrated clinical efficacy of the device both as monotherapy and as concomitant therapy, in terms of clinically relevant improvement of appearance of hair. Of the patients, 25 % showed significant improvement, and 62.5 % showed moderate improvement in global photographic assessments. The effect was observed as early as 3 months of treatment and was sustained up to a maximum observation time of 24 months. The technology appears to work better for some than for others, and it seems that patients with intermediate alopecia respond best, since effective photobiostimulation depends on a minimum of hair for effective photobiostimulation and on a maximum of hair for the laser beam to reach the scalp without absorption or interference from existing hairs.

Case 9.9 A 37-year-old male with androgenetic alopecia was successfully treated with 1 mg oral finasteride for 15 months and wished to switch to 5 % topical minoxidil b.i.d.: (**a**) before, (**b**) after 15 months of 1 mg oral finasteride treatment, and (**c**) 4 months after successful switch to 5 % topical minoxidil b.i.d

Comment 1 mg oral finasteride daily is the first-line agent for improvement or prevention of progression of male androgenetic alopecia in male patients aged 1–40 years. Finasteride daily has also proven to be effective in aging male, though with a lesser degree of efficacy and a higher frequency of sexual adverse effects. Therefore, in men aged 35 years or more, a successful switch from oral finasteride to topical minoxidil may be considered in anticipation of age-related more frequent sexual function-related problems

9.3 Senescent Alopecia

Case 9.10 A 70-year-old otherwise healthy male complaining of age-related thinning of hair was successfully treated with 5 % topical minoxidil b.i.d.: (**a**) before, (**b**) after 3 months, and (**c**) 6 months of treatment

Comment Senescent alopecia has been defined as non-androgen-dependent hair thinning found in those over 60 years of age. Much like androgenetic alopecia, it involves a progressive decrease in the number of anagen follicles and hair diameter. It frequently occurs together with androgenetic alopecia, further complicating its delineation from the latter. Nevertheless, recent data comparing androgenetic and senescent alopecia using microarray analysis have demonstrated significant differences in the gene expression patterns suggesting they represent different entities. Moreover, topical minoxidil has not been studied in the specific perspective of aging and senescent alopecia. Nevertheless, clear treatment benefits of topical minoxidil solution are noted in the older age group that has retained some hair.

Case 9.11 A 83-year-old otherwise healthy female with age-related thinning of hair was successfully treated with 2 % topical minoxidil b.i.d.: (**a**) before, (**b**) after 3 months, and (**c**) 6 months of treatment

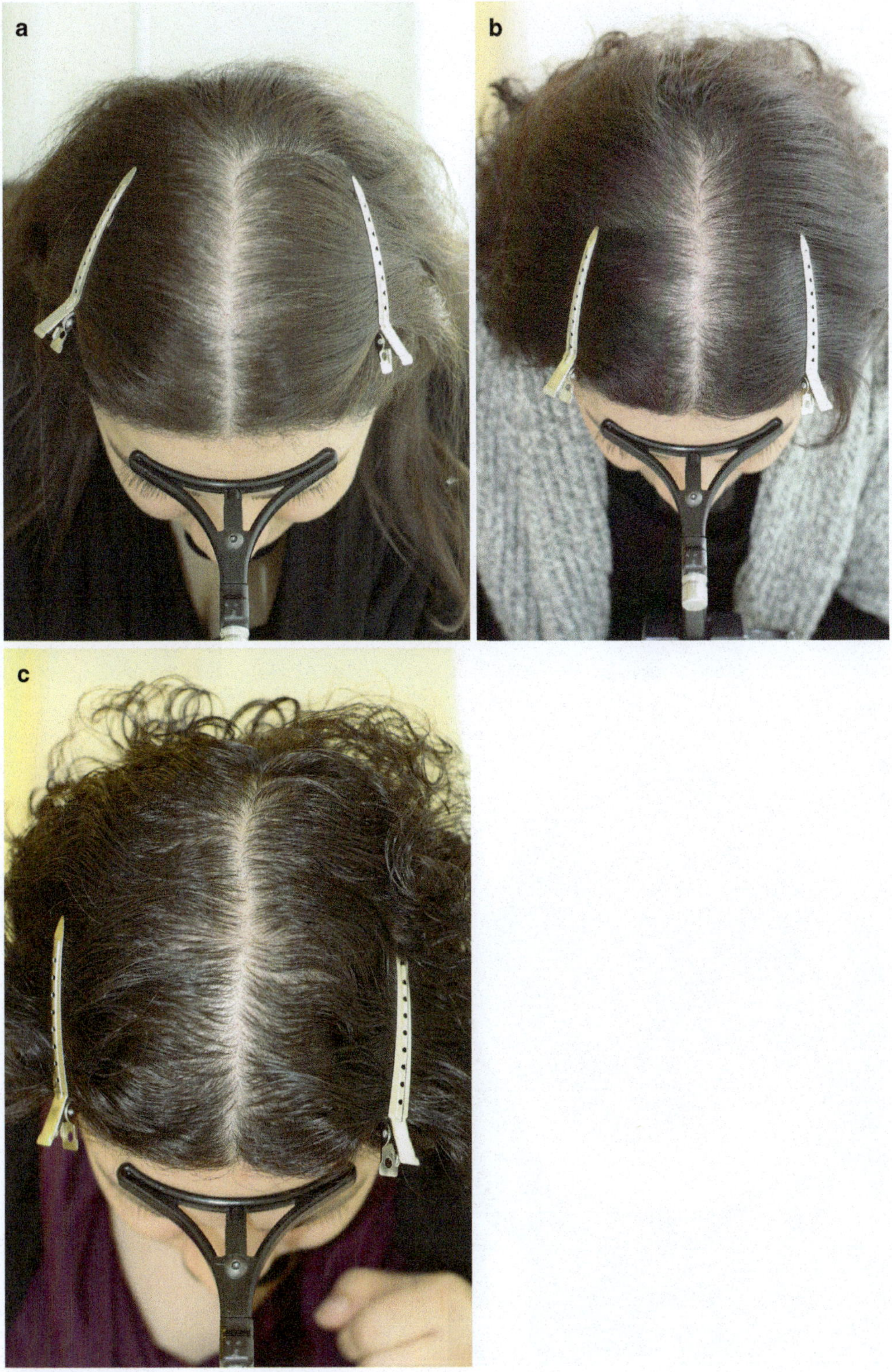

Fig. 9.8 (a–c)

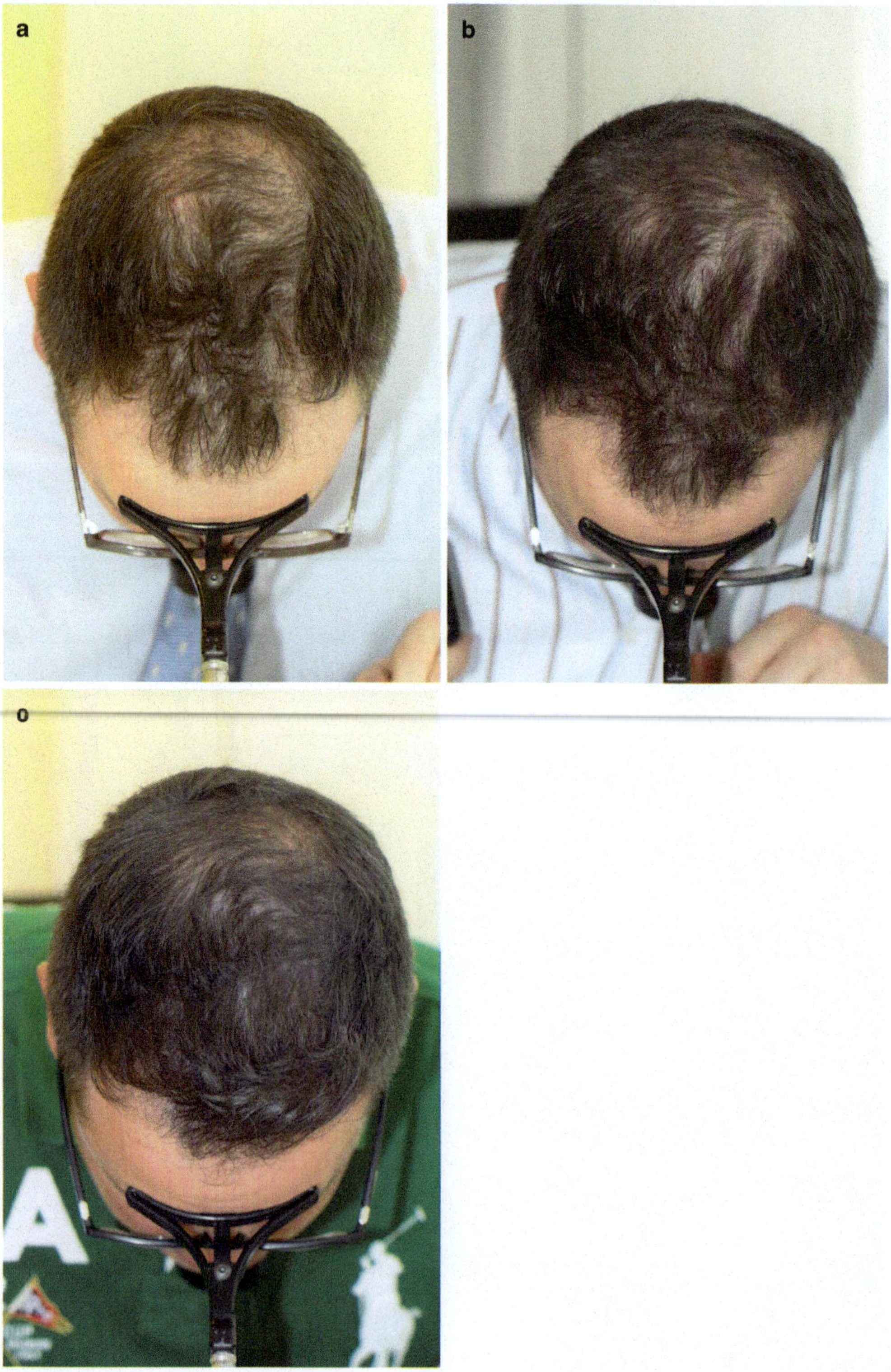

Fig. 9.9 (a–c)

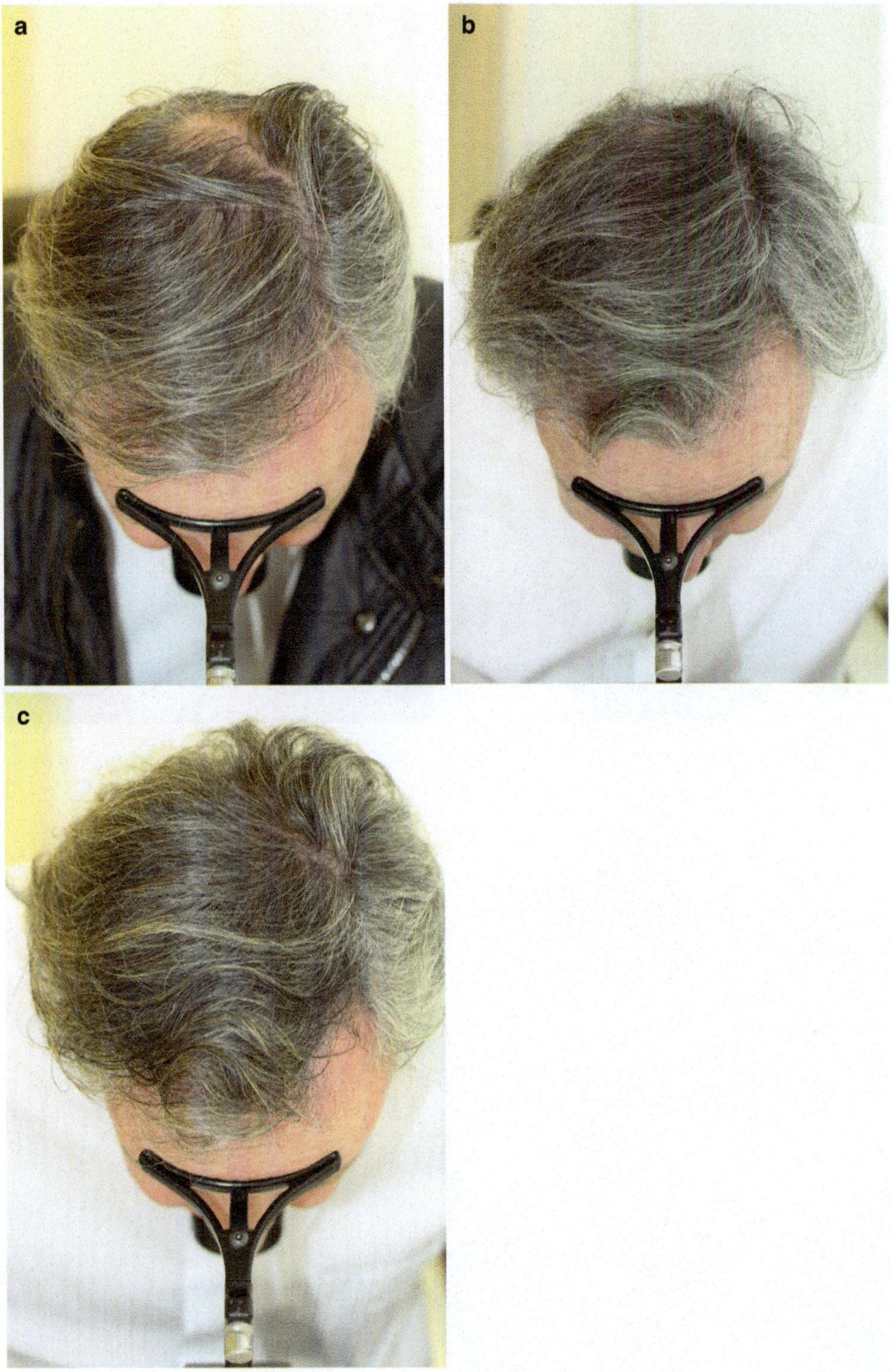

Fig. 9.10 (a–c)

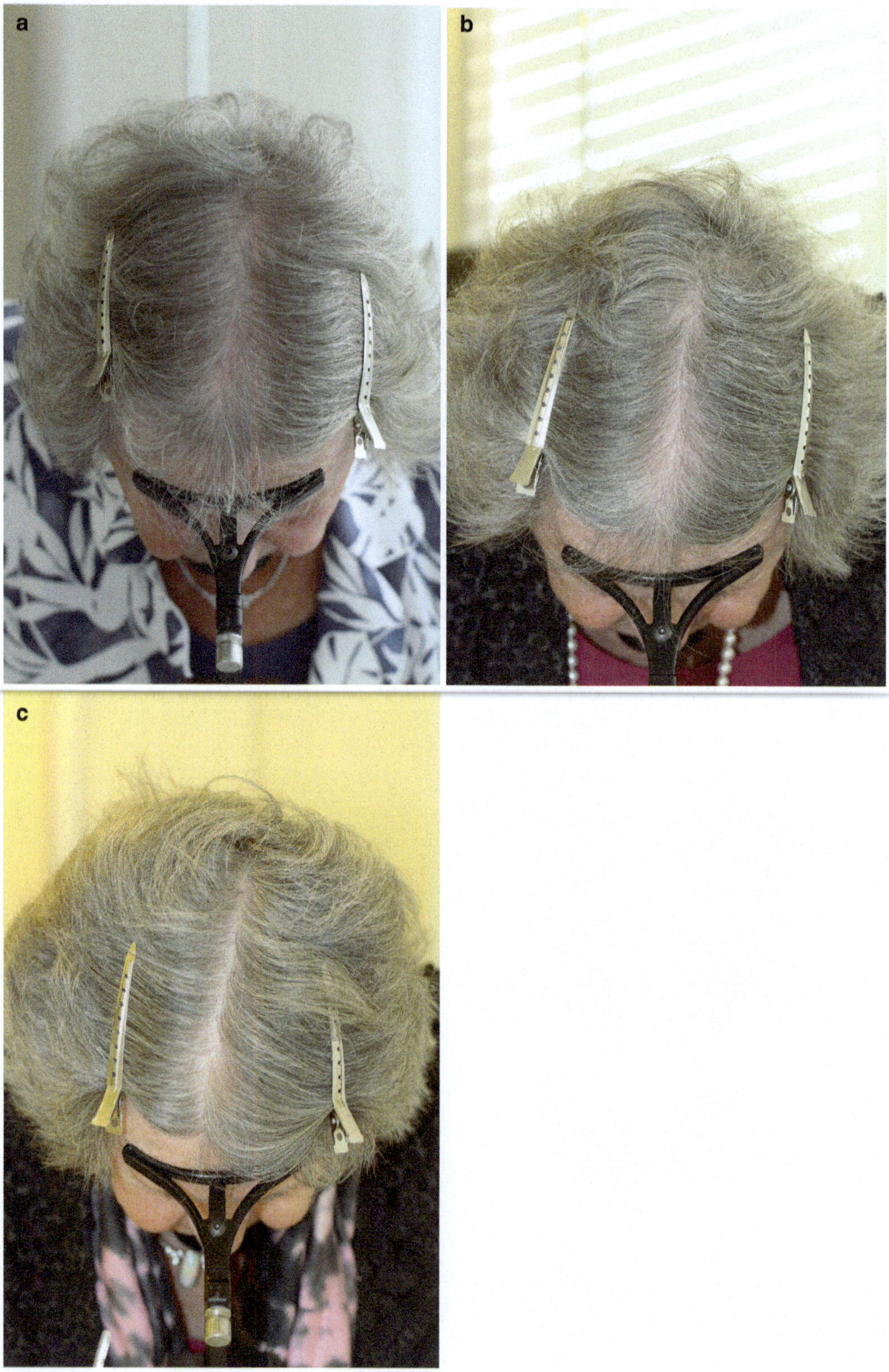

Fig. 9.11 (a–c)

Comment Hair length, color, and cosmetic properties play an important role in people's physical appearance and self-perception. Our preoccupation with the condition of our hair is heightened as today's increasing life expectancy fuels the desire to preserve youthfulness. For the time being, the current available treatment for age-related hair loss is topical minoxidil, though with some limitations: Specifically, older patients often suffer from a variety of conditions that may also affect the condition of the hair—nutritional deficiency, endocrine disorders, psychological problems, and drug-related adverse effects. Therefore, one must remain suspicious of the possibility of a more general problem underlying the patient's complaint in taking care of the elderly with hair problems. Finally, nocebo reactions are observed more frequently in women of the older age group. Symptoms have a high level of psychosomatic background and include nausea, headaches, and drowsiness. Frequently observed objective findings are increased pulse frequency and blood pressure. The influence of the prescribing physician should be kept in mind, since inspiring confidence versus skepticism and fear clearly impacts the outcome of treatment.

Case 9.12 A 74-year-old otherwise healthy female suffering of hair loss was prescribed 5 % topical minoxidil once daily without success after 6 months of treatment. It was found that she was not supplied with an appropriate pipette and therefore underdosed her medication. After a switch to the appropriate 1 mL pipette, her hair growth increased within 3 months: (**a**) before treatment, (**b**) after 6 months of inadequate treatment, and (**c**) 3 months after switching to the appropriate 1 mL pipette. (**d**) At the left is the wrong pipette, and at the right the correct 1 mL pipette for application of 5 % minoxidil solution

Comment Even with a correct diagnosis of a hair condition and appropriate treatment for that specific condition, a proportion of patients do not get better. When it comes to topical treatments, poor adherence is the most likely reason for non-response. In this case, the patient was provided with a wrong pipette and therefore unknowingly underdosed her topical minoxidil. In the treatment of hair loss, one must always remain open-minded for the possibility of a multitude of cause-relationships underlying hair loss and treatment failures.

9.4 Alopecia Areata

Case 9.13 A 16-year-old female with alopecia areata >30 % of scalp surface and >6 months' duration and evidence of female pattern hair loss as a comorbid condition. She was successfully treated with a combination treatment of repeated intralesional triamcinolone acetonide 10 mg/ml and a compound of topical 5 % minoxidil and 0.2 % triamcinolone acetonide: (**a, b**) before, (**c, d**) after 3 months, and (**e, f**) after 6 months of treatment

Comment A recent meta-analysis of published trials on treatment of alopecia areata states that only few treatments have been well evaluated in randomized trials. The authors found no randomized controlled trials on the use of diphenylcyclopropenone (DCP), or intralesional corticosteroids, and although topical steroids and minoxidil are widely prescribed, the authors found no convincing evidence that they are beneficial. Therefore, they concluded that considering the possibility of spontaneous remission, especially for those in early stages of the disease, the options of not being treated therapeutically or, depending on individual preference, of wearing a wig may be alternative ways of dealing with this condition. Nevertheless, depending on patient age, surface area, and disease duration, a treatment algorithm for successful treatment of alopecia areata can be designed.

Case 9.14 A 25-year-old female with diffuse alopecia areata of <3 months' duration. Successful i.v. methylprednisolone pulse therapy (500 mg on 3 consecutive days, repeated after 1 and 2 months): (**a**) before, (**b**) after 4 months, and (**c**) after 8 months of treatment

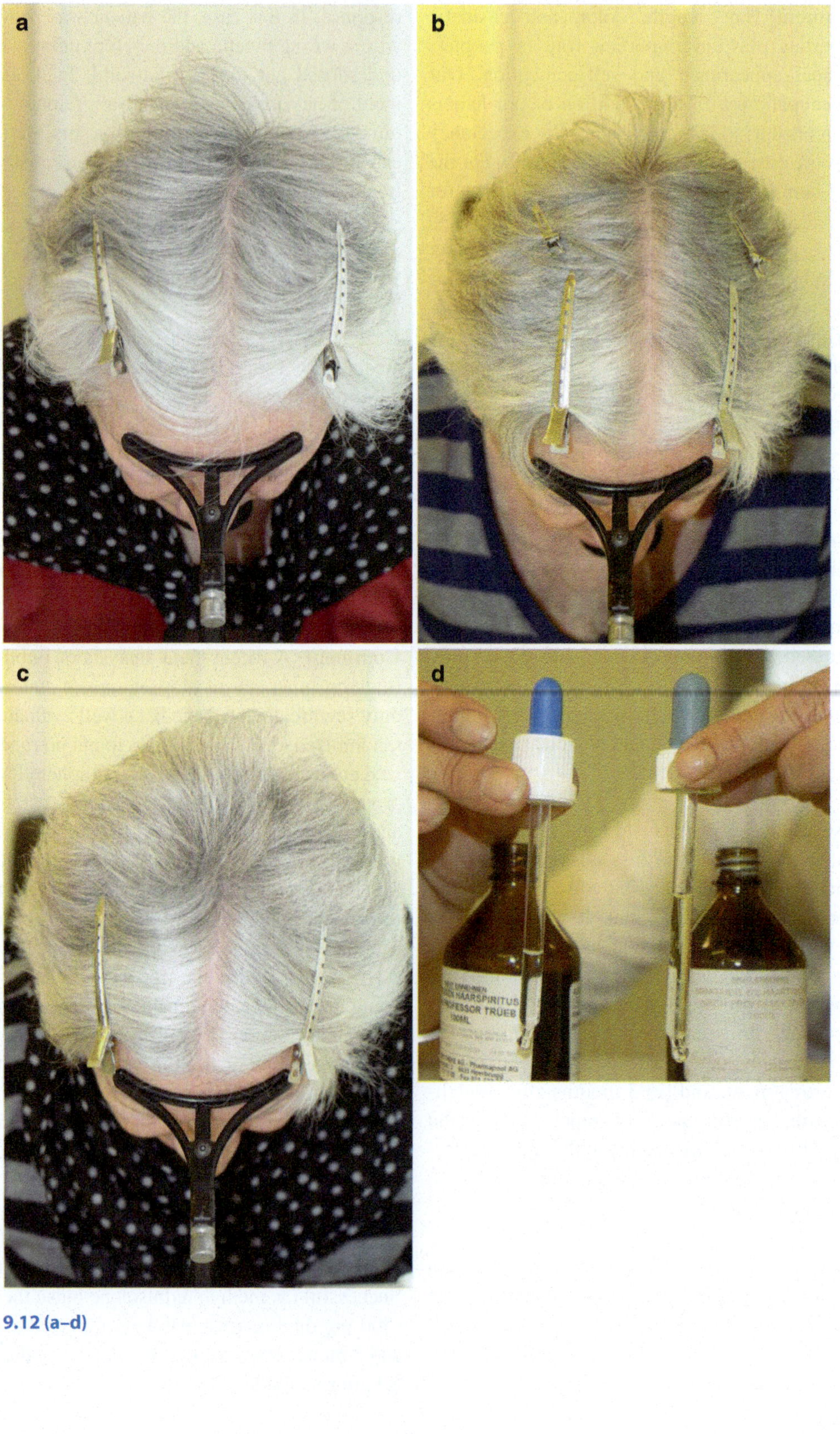

Fig. 9.12 (a–d)

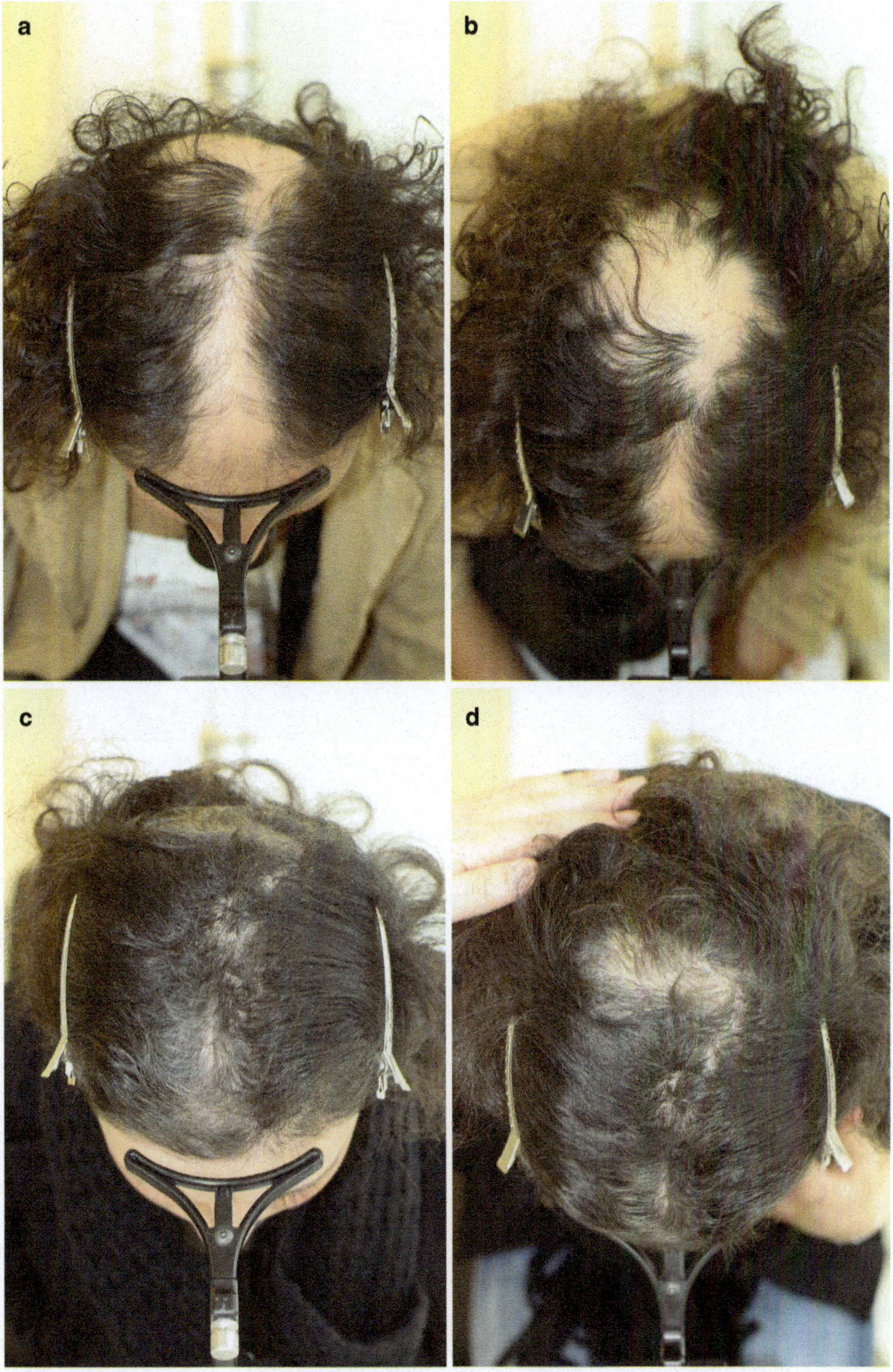

Fig. 9.13 (a–f)

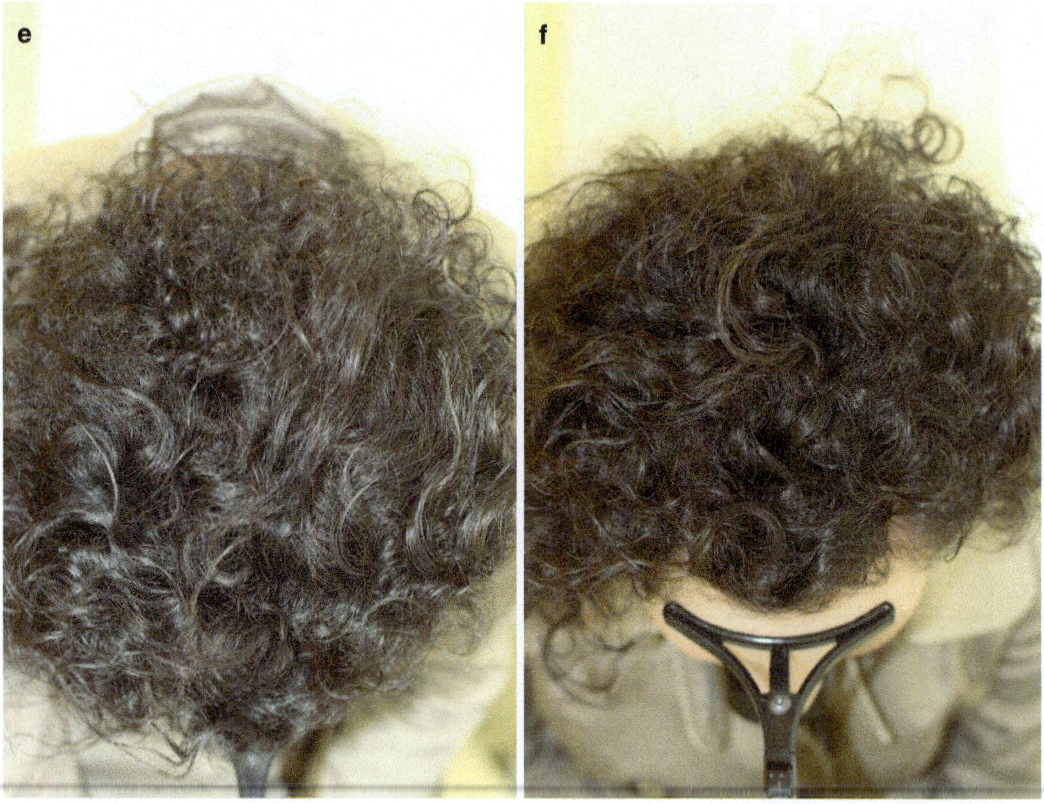

Fig. 9.13 (continued)

Case 9.15 A 55-year-old female with diffuse alopecia areata of <3 months' duration. Successful i.v. methylprednisolone pulse therapy (500 mg on 3 consecutive days, repeated after 1 and 2 months) followed by a compound of topical 5 % minoxidil and 0.02 % triamcinolone acetonide b.i.d: (**a**) before, (**b**) after 6 months, (**c**) after 9 months, (**d**) after 12 months, and (**e**) after 15 months of successful treatment, including repigmentation of initial regrowth of white hair

Comment The art of using corticosteroids for treatment of alopecia is maximizing efficacy and minimizing toxicity. Friedli et al. originally reported effectiveness of intravenous methylprednisolone pulse therapy for alopecia areata with rapid and extensive hair loss much in the same way as for treatment of other autoimmune diseases. Subsequently, Nakajima confirmed efficacy of intravenous methylprednisolone pulse therapy and found remission rates 88 % for multilocular disease with surface area <50 %, 59.4 % with surface area >50 %, and 21.4 % in alopecia totalis/universalis. After 6 months of disease onset, the remission rate was 15.8 %. Finally, Im et al. identified disease duration before treatment in relation to the type of alopecia areata to be of prognostic relevance, with good response obtained for all types of alopecia areata with a duration of <3 months before treatment and for the multifocal type of alopecia areata with a duration of <6 months.

Case 9.16 A 50-year-old otherwise healthy male with sudden graying of hair (**a**) before, (**b**) after 6 months, and (**c**) after 9 months of successful treatment with a compound of topical 3 % minoxidil and 0.2 % triamcinolone acetonide b.i.d

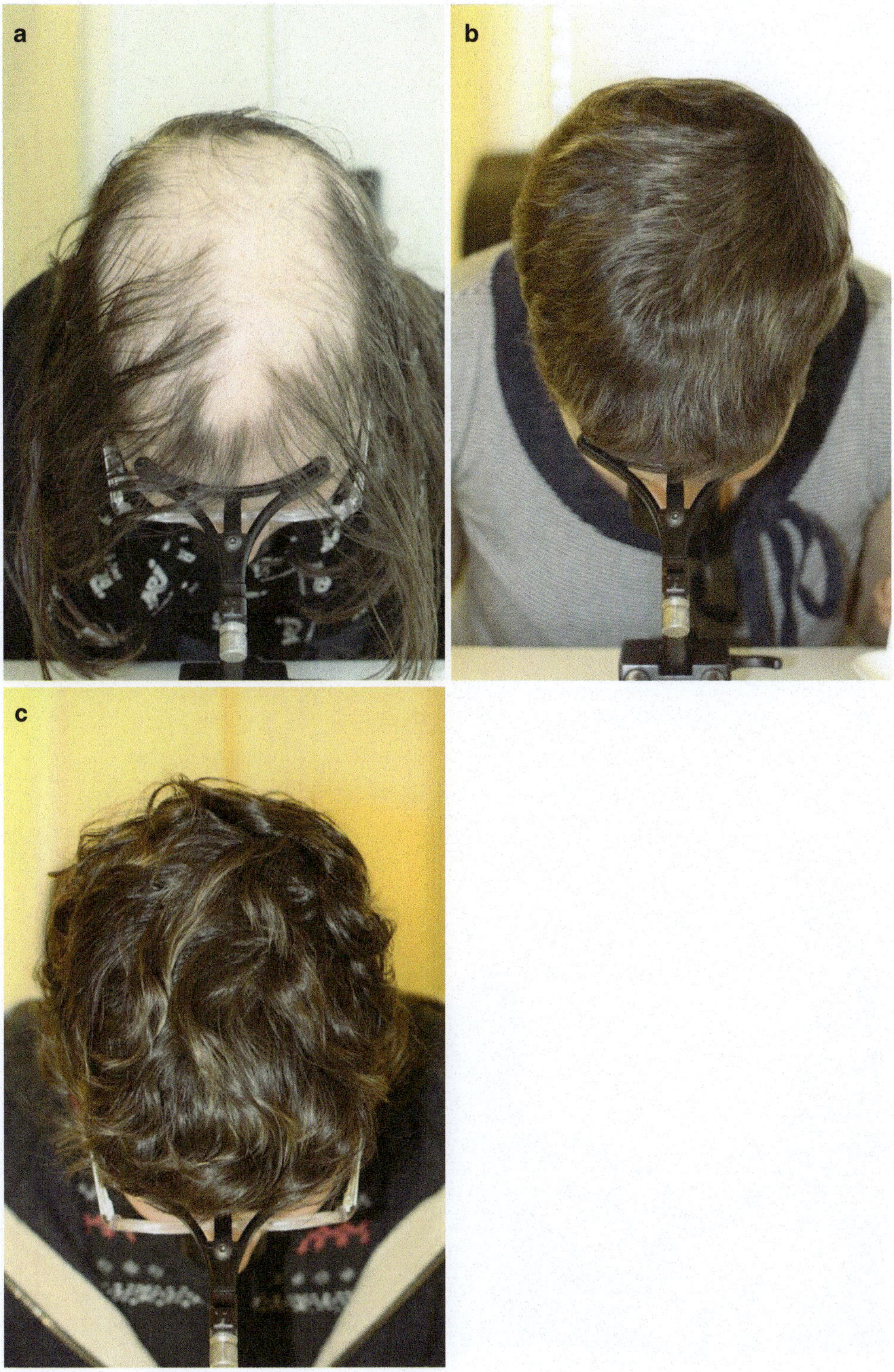

Fig. 9.14 (a–c)

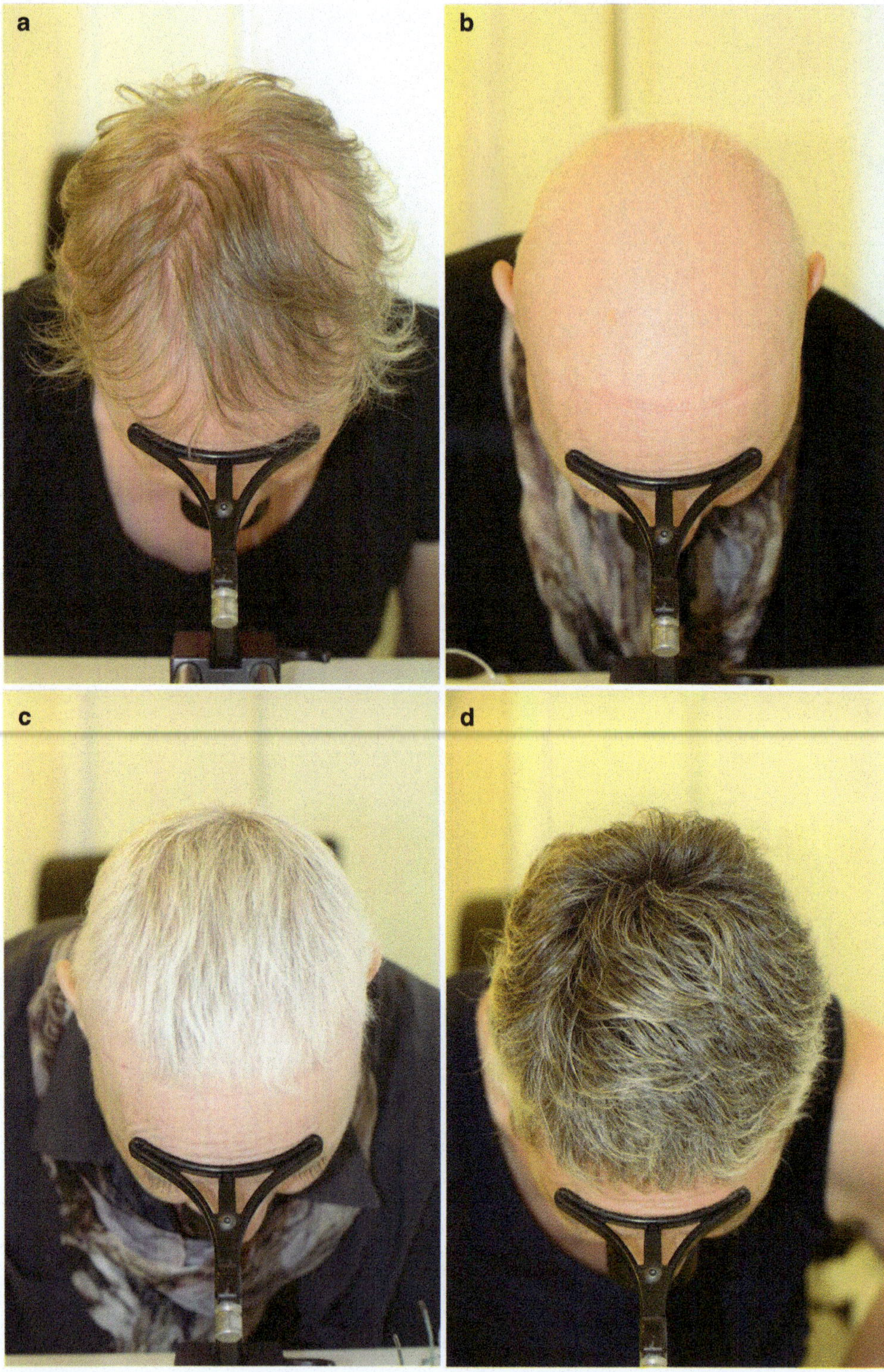

Fig. 9.15 (a–e)

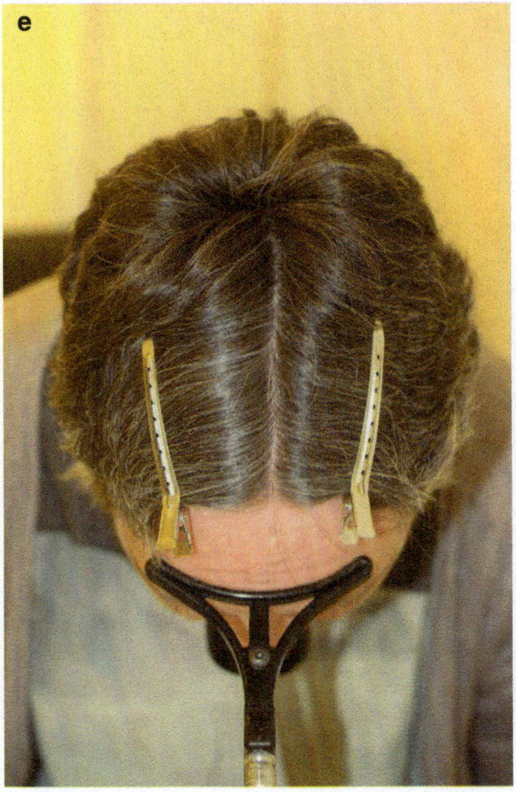

Fig. 9.15 (continued)

Comment

The condition of sudden graying or whitening of scalp hair has most recently been designated Thomas More syndrome, alluding to the English martyr Thomas More, whose hair allegedly turned white overnight in the Tower of London before his execution. Although the actual incidence is rare, this stigmatizing phenomenon has captured storytellers' imagination like few other afflictions as a sign of grave sorrow. History also records that the hair of the ill-fated French Queen Marie Antoinette turned white the night before her walk to the guillotine during the French Revolution, hence the original term Marie Antoinette syndrome for the same condition. Although Marie Antoinette has originally been chosen as eponym for the syndrome, presumably out of dermatological gallantry, Thomas More, whose hair turned white in 1535, ought to have the right of seniority over Marie Antoinette who succumbed to the same fate in 1793. Since there seems to be no other particular reason for favoring Marie Antoinette over Thomas More, out of fairness, it seems appropriate to use the term 'Marie Antoinette syndrome' for the condition afflicting women and 'Thomas More syndrome' in men. Today, the syndrome is interpreted as an acute episode of diffuse alopecia areata in which the 'overnight' whitening of hair is caused by the preferential loss of pigmented hairs in a supposedly immune-mediated disorder. Ultimately, these observations have led authorities to speculate that the autoimmune target in alopecia areata may be related to the hair follicle melanin pigment system. Treatment is the same as of alopecia areata with the potential of repigmentation.

Case 9.17 A 40-year-old male with a 20-year history of recurring alopecia areata and total alopecia for 1 year. A trial with homeopathic treatment did not have any effect. Successful treatment with clobetasol propionate 0.05 % ointment under occlusion with Saran wrap on 6 consecutive nights per week: (**a**) before, (**b**) after 4 months, and (**c**) after 6 months of treatment. Small residual patches were thereafter injected with 10 mg/ml triamcinolone acetonide

Case 9.18 A 48-year-old male with a 2-year history of reticular alopecia areata was formerly unsuccessfully treated with topical minoxidil. Successful treatment with clobetasol propionate 0.05 % foam applied twice daily on 5 consecutive days per week during 6 months: (**a**) before, (**b**) after 3 months, and (**c**) after 9 months of treatment. Small residual patches were thereafter injected with 10 mg/ml triamcinolone acetonide

Case 9.19 A 75-year-old female with diffuse alopecia areata of 5 weeks' duration. After 6 months of unsuccessful treatment with clobetasol foam, the patient was successfully switched to clobetasol ointment under occlusion followed by topical 5 % minoxidil b.i.d.: (**a**) before, (**b**) after 6 months of clobetasol foam treatment, and (**c**) after 3 months and (**d**) 6 months of clobetasol ointment treatment, followed by (**e**) 6 months of topical minoxidil for comorbid patterned hair loss

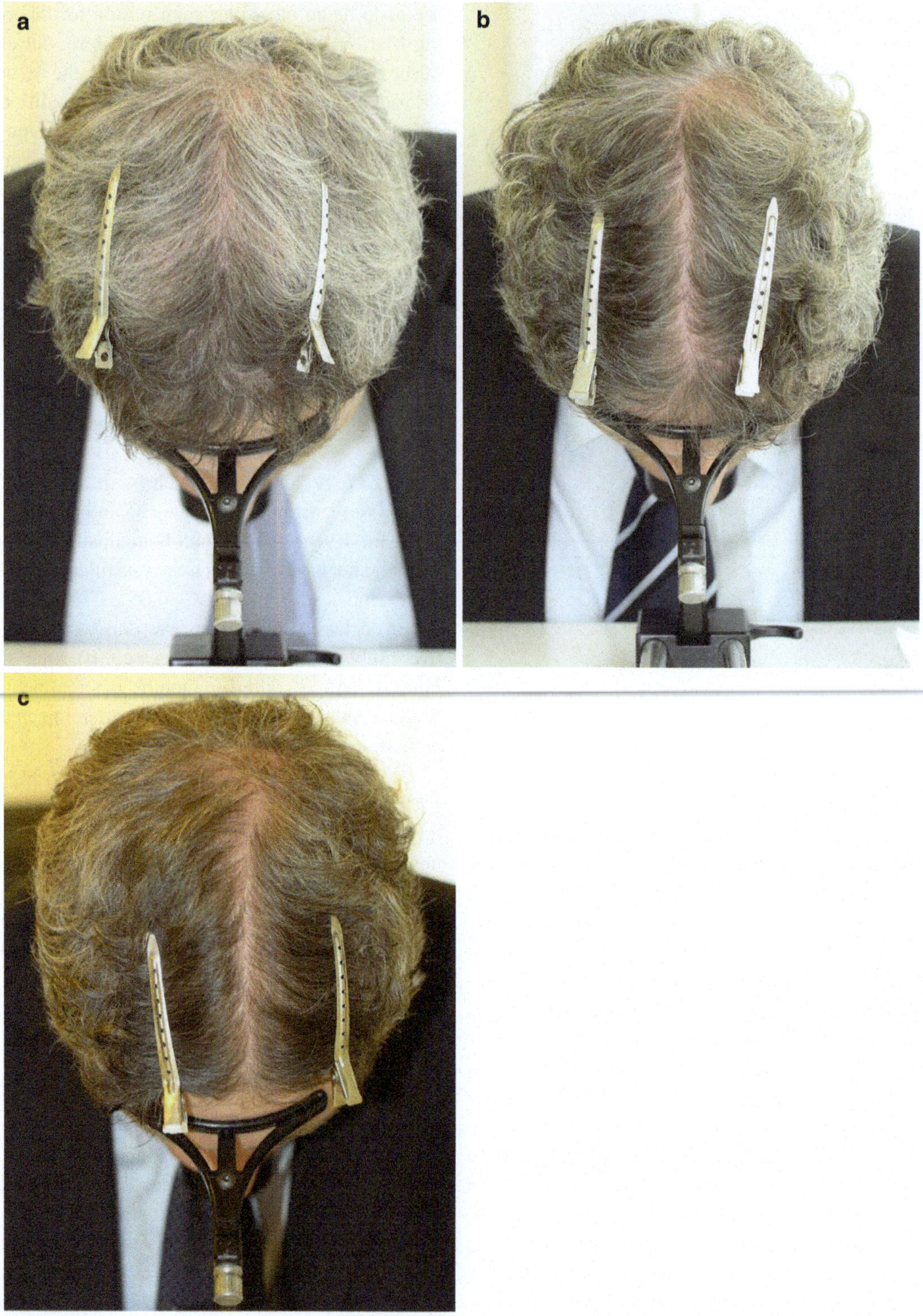

Fig. 9.16 (a–c)

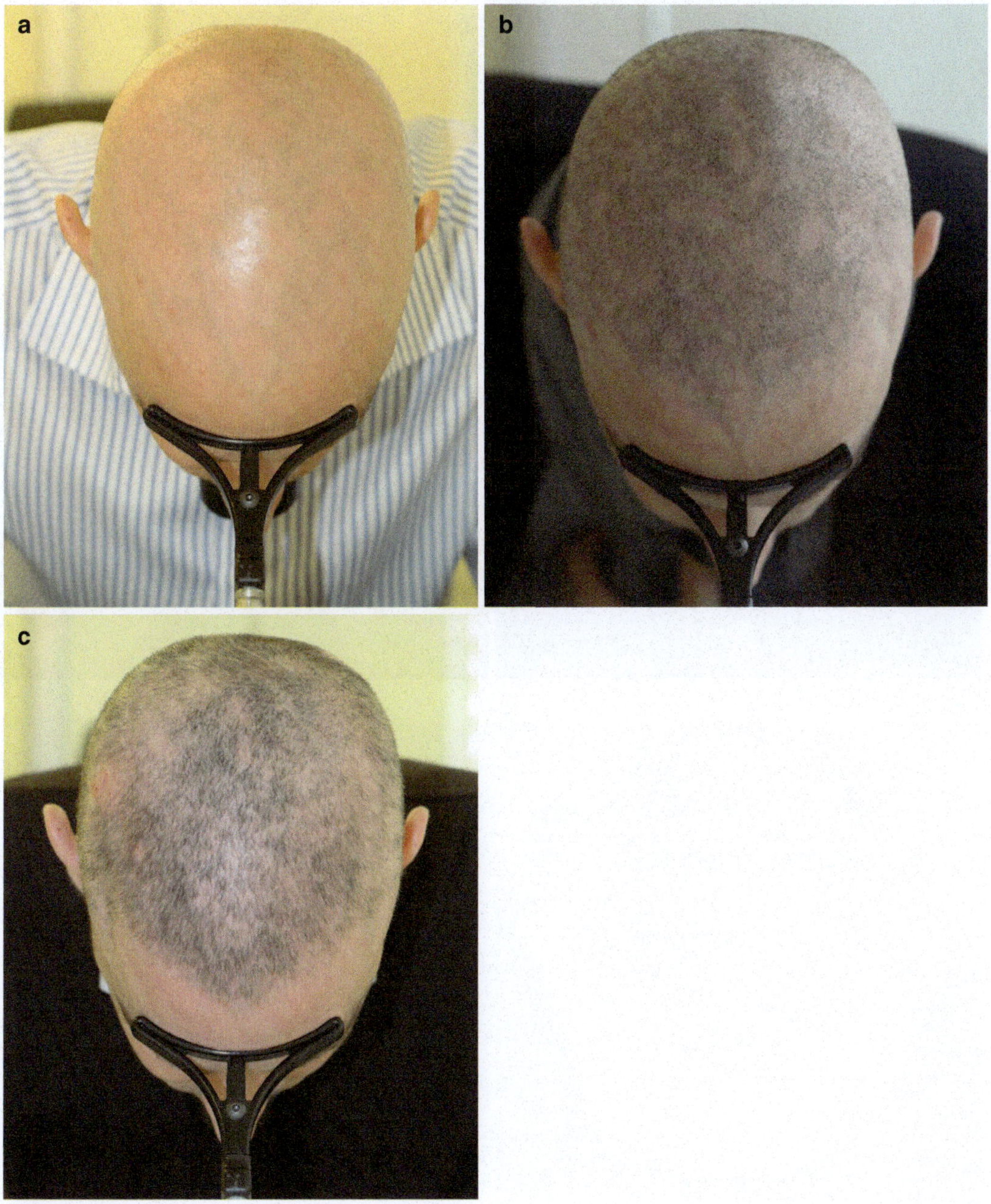

Fig. 9.17 (a–c)

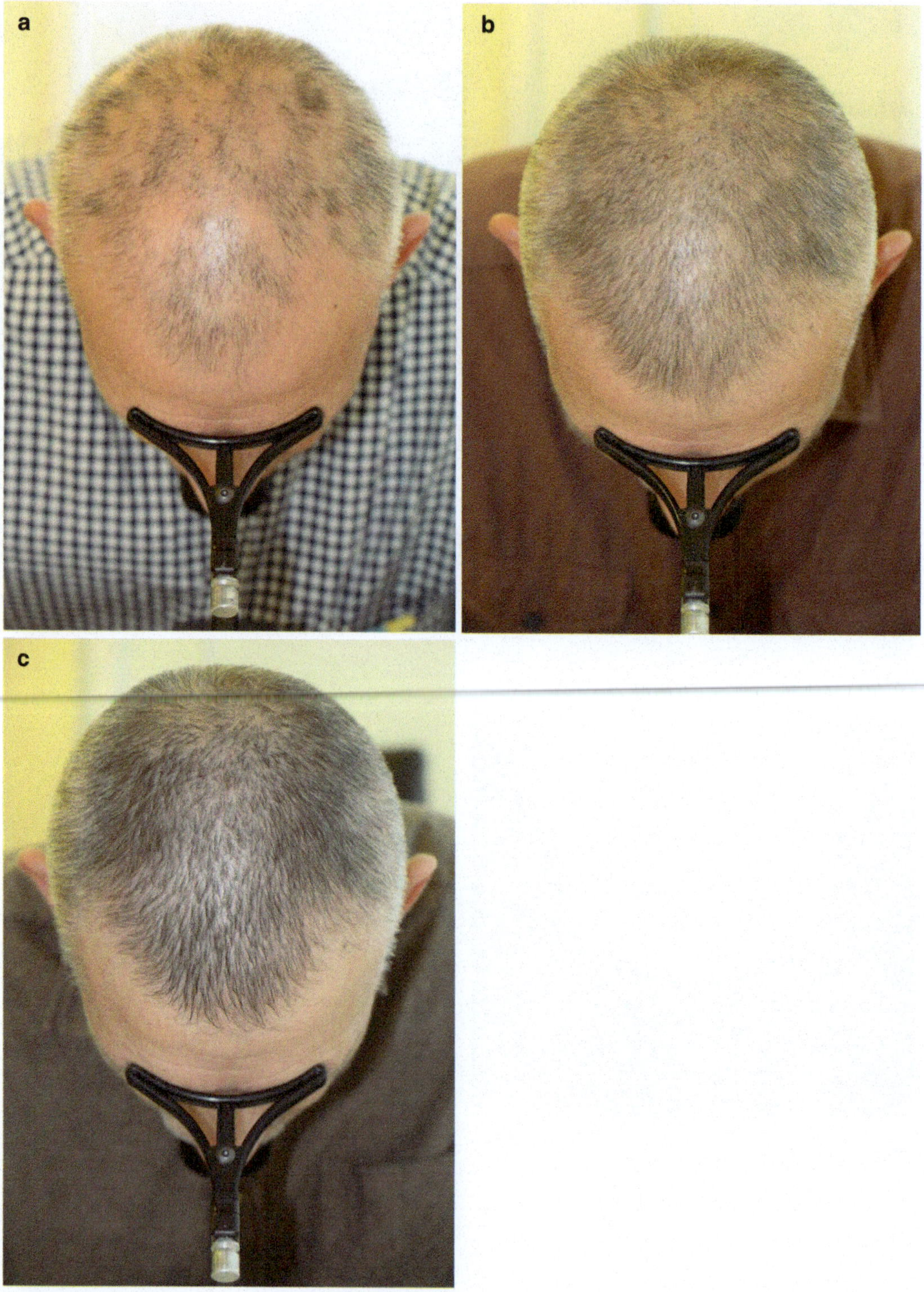

Fig. 9.18 (a–c)

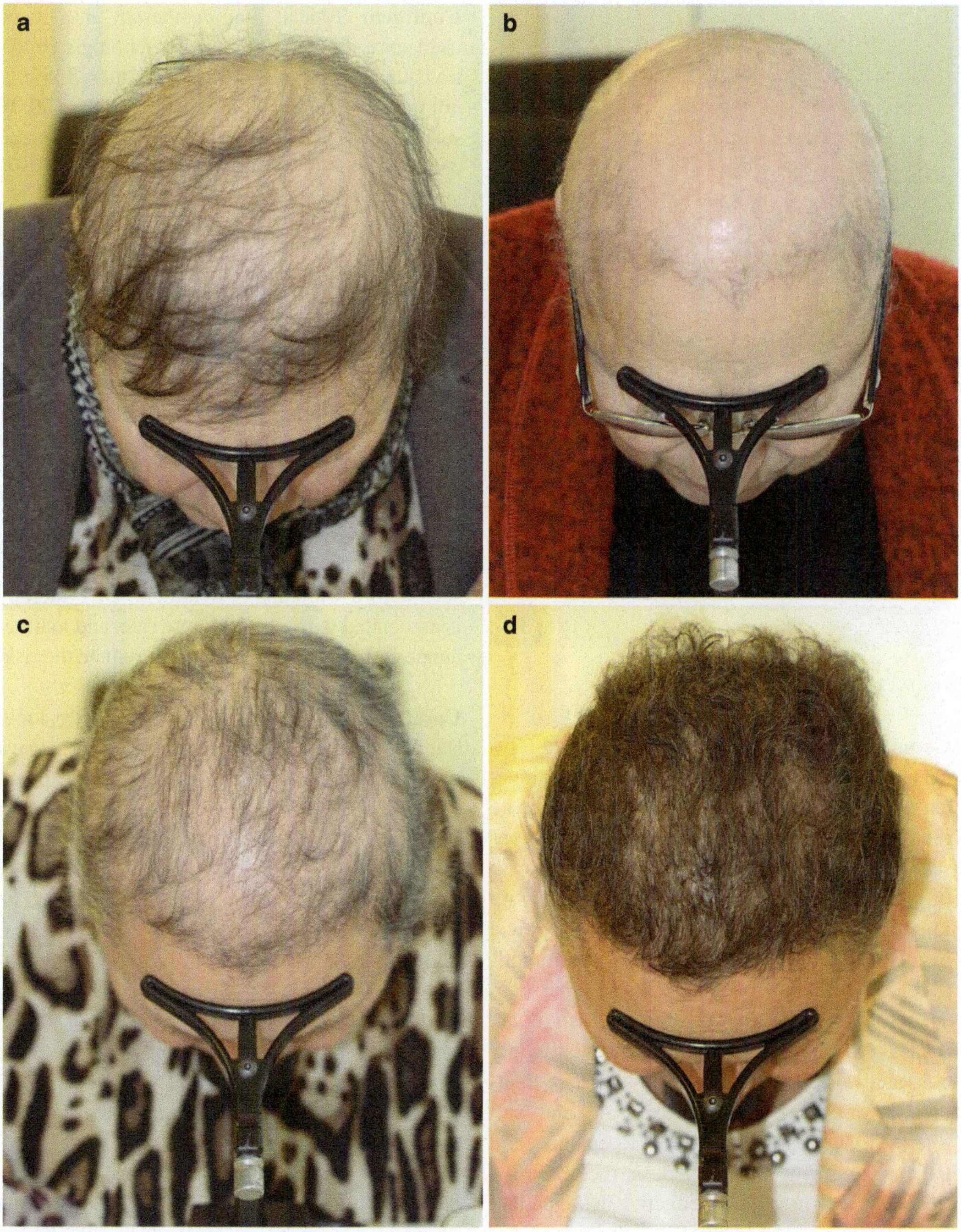

Fig. 9.19 (a–e)

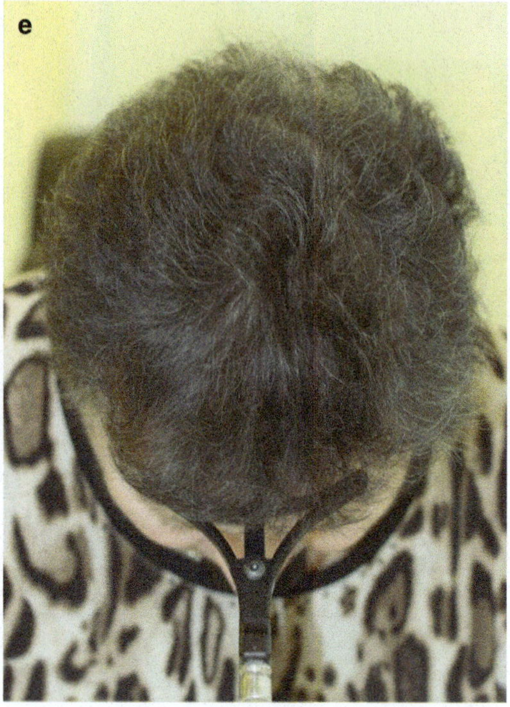

Fig. 9.19 (continued)

Comment Tosti et al. originally evaluated topical clobetasol for treatment of widespread alopecia areata. With 0.05 % clobetasol propionate ointment under occlusion (Saran wrap) on 6 consecutive nights per week, over 6 months' regrowth of hair was achieved in 17.8 % of patients with long-standing disease. Despite positive clinical results, this approach has a low patient compliance, especially in patients with residual hair. Therefore, in a subsequent study, Tosti et al. applied 0.05 % clobetasol foam twice daily on 5 consecutive days per week. The alternative treatment proved to also be effective, safe, and well tolerated, with good cosmetic acceptance and patient compliance. Nevertheless, the occlusive treatment may prove to be effective in the patient who fails to respond to clobetasol foam.

Case 9.20 A 12-year-old girl with a 3-year history of widespread alopecia areata and unsuccessful therapy with topical dithranol. Successful topical immunotherapy with diphenylcyclopropenone (DCP): (**a**) before, (**b**) after 4 months, and (**c**) 8 months of treatment

Comment Topical immunotherapy has been used since the 1970s to treat dermatologic conditions understood to result from an altered immunological state, including widespread (>30 % surface area) and long-standing (>6 months) alopecia areata. The extent of hair loss before therapy is the main predictor for therapeutic success, and a long period of therapy is needed to increase the percentage of responders. In a retrospective study of patients with severe alopecia areata treated with topical DCP, Pericin and Trüeb found an overall response rate of 30.9 % complete remission: complete remission rates for multilocular alopecia areata was 43.8 %, for subtotal alopecia areata and ophiasis 33.3 %, and for alopecia totalis or universalis 21.4 %, irrespective of disease duration. Treatment should be tried for at least 8 months, before regarding it as ineffective, and regrowth of hair is usually not seen before 4 months of treatment. DCP therapy is associated with a high relapse rate, and maintenance therapy is recommended to reduce the risk.

Case 9.21 A 43-year-old female with long-standing widespread alopecia areata nonresponsive to topical immunotherapy. Successful treatment with initially 30 mg s.c. methotrexate (MTX) in combination with 20 mg oral prednisone until total remission. Thereafter, prednisone was tapered to 10 mg oral prednisone e.o.d. and 15 mg s.c. MTX: (**a**) before, (**b**) after 3 months, (**c**) after 6 months, (**d**) after 9 months, and (**e**) after 12 months of treatment. (**f**) Recurrence occurred when the patient inadvertently switched from subcutaneous to oral MTX at 15 mg weekly dose. (**g**) Regrowth of hair after reinstitution of s.c. MTX treatment and 10 mg intralesional triamcinolone acetonide

Comment Joly originally proposed the use of MTX for treatment of recalcitrant alopecia areata. Best results are achieved with subcutaneous MTX in the maximal dosage of 30 mg weekly in combination with 20 mg oral prednisone daily with regrowth of hair beginning within 2–4 months of therapy. Lasting improvement requires continuous treatment at lower dosages. Drug toxicities are to be carefully weighed out against treatment benefit, and therapeutic drug

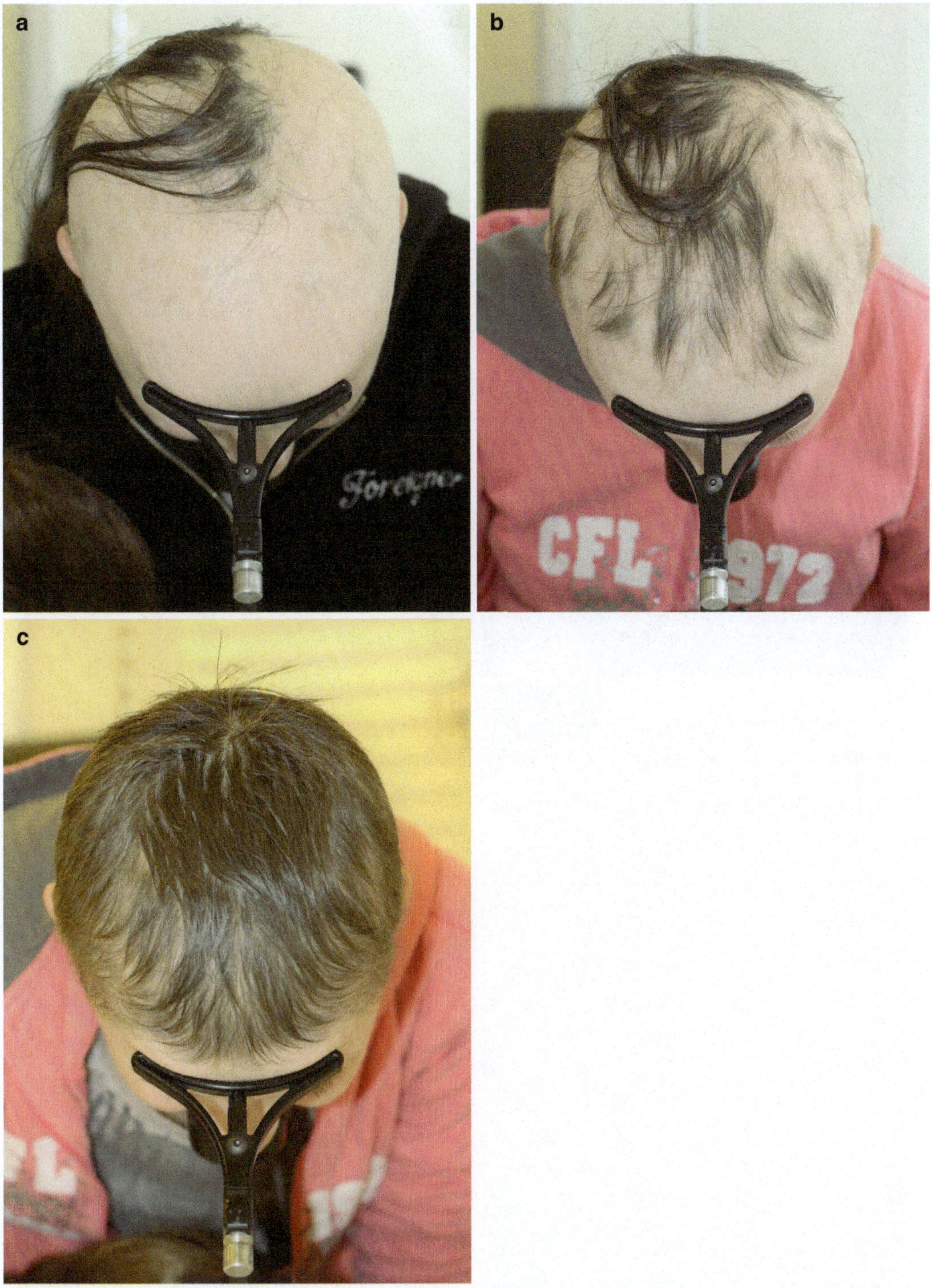

Fig. 9.20 (a–c)

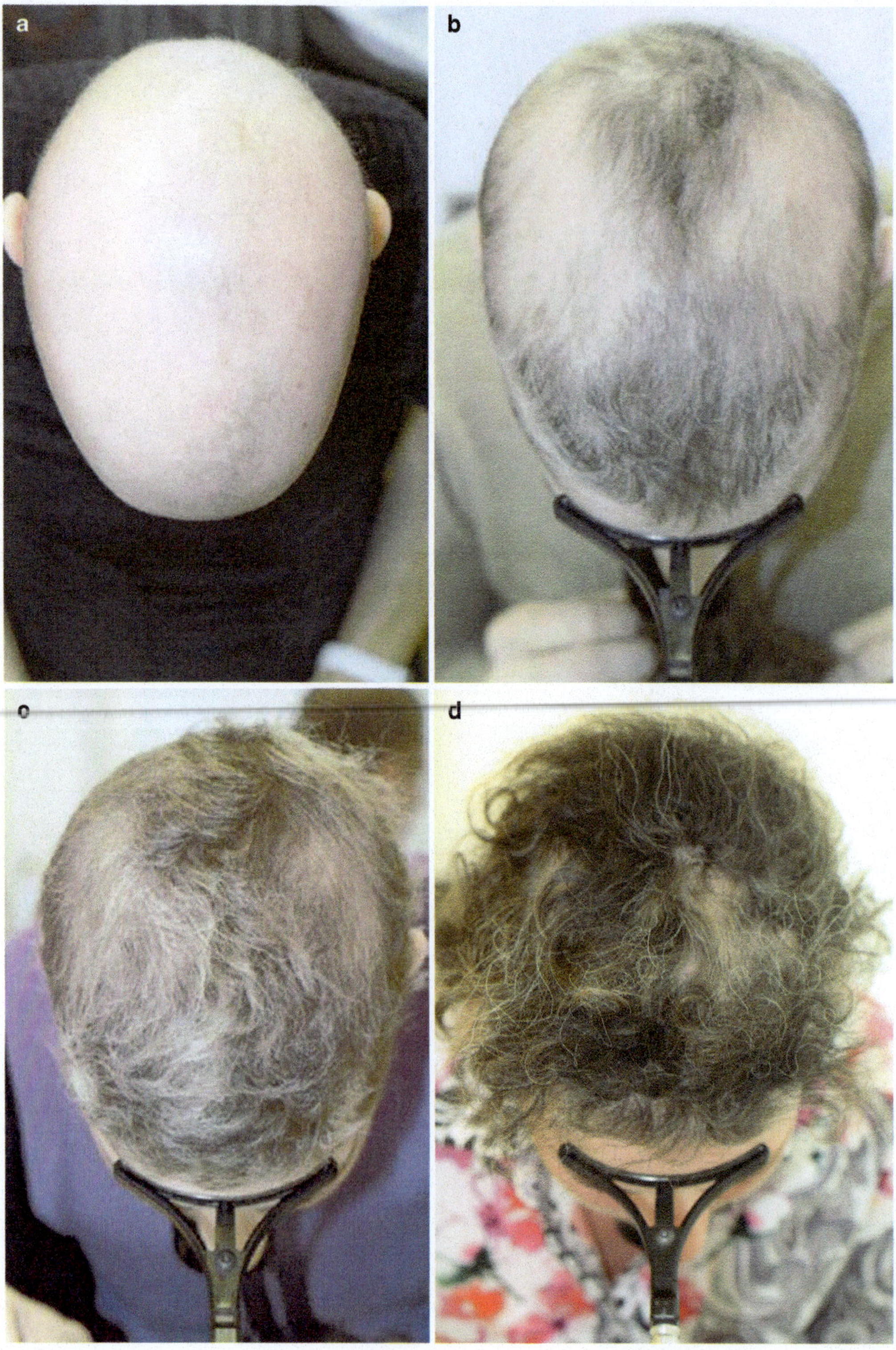

Fig. 9.21 (a–g)

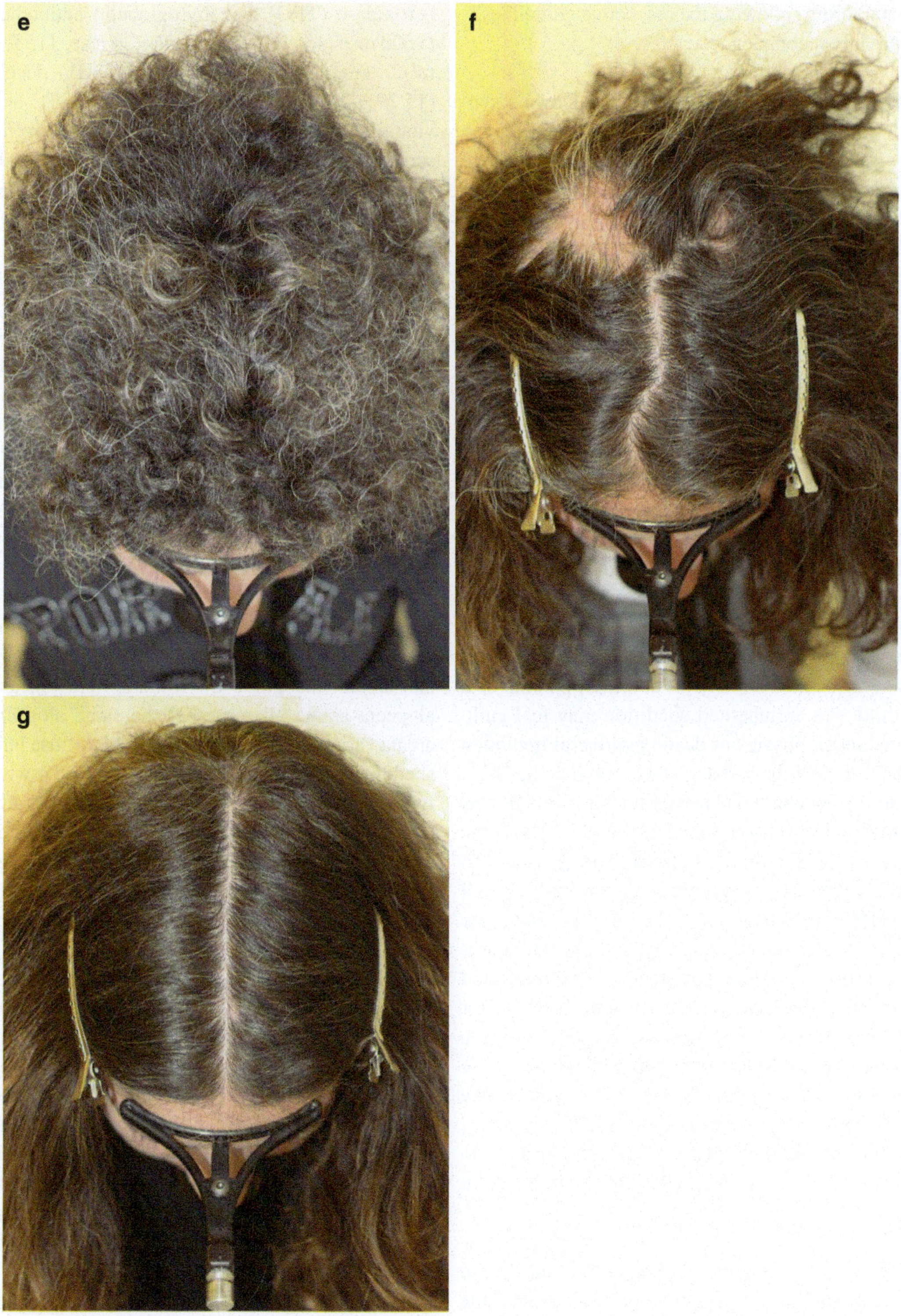

Fig. 9.21 (continued)

monitoring following the respective guidelines is strongly recommended.

Case 9.22 A 9-year-old boy with Down's syndrome and long-standing (3 years), widespread (>30 % surface area) alopecia areata. Successful treatment with topical 0.1 % mometasone furoate twice daily on 5 consecutive days per week: (**a**) before, (**b**) after 6 months, and (**c**) after 15 months of treatment. The lotion was used for widespread disease and later the cream for residual patches

Case 9.23 A 10-year-old boy with diffuse alopecia areata of <6 months' duration. Successful i.v. methylprednisolone pulse therapy (500 mg on 3 consecutive days, repeated after 1 month): (**a**) before and (**b**) after 5 months of treatment

Comment Alopecia in childhood is a source of high concern, frustration, and anxiety. The younger children usually lack self-awareness, and it may be the parents who, projecting their own concerns onto the child, most acutely feel any associated anxiety. In addition, parents of a child with an inherited condition may feel guilt. In a sense, physicians dealing with children often have to treat the parents rather than just the child. In treating childhood alopecia areata, it is imperative to avoid doing harm. Such variables as the ability of the child to absorb, metabolize, and excrete medications must be considered, as well as the expected action of the drug, possible side effects, and potential toxicity. 1 % topical hydrocortisone, 0.1 % mometasone or anthralin, and oral zinc gluconate are usually unproblematic for use in the pediatric age group with alopecia areata. Intravenous methylprednisolone pulse therapy much in the same way as in adults may be tried in severe alopecia of acute onset in children, though preliminary results in children do not seem to be as sustained as in the adult patient group.

Case 9.24 A 65-year-old female presented with a 3-month history of scalp hair loss in tufts. She also complained of swelling and bluish red discoloration of the right lower limb and of fatigue. Laboratory evaluation revealed elevated thyroid peroxidase (TPO) and thyroglobulin antibodies (>600 resp. 464 IU/ml; normal: <34 resp. 115 IU/ml), elevated thyreotropin (TSH) levels (15.29 mIU/l; normal: 0.27–4.20 mIU/l), and vitamin D deficiency (42.9 nmol/l). *Borrelia* serology (Western blot) tested positive for VLsE IgMG (different genospecies), p41 IgG (*B. burgdorferi sensu stricto*), and p41 IgM (*B. burgdorferi sensu stricto*). A diagnosis of acute diffuse and total alopecia of the female scalp associated with *Borrelia* infection (acrodermatitis chronica atrophicans), autoimmune thyroid disease, and vitamin D deficiency was made. The patient was successfully prescribed intravenous ceftriaxone 2 g daily during 21 days, topical clobetasol propionate 0.05 % foam twice daily on 5 consecutive days per week for 6 months, thyroid supplementation therapy, and oral vitamin D3 1,500 IU per day: (**a**) before, (**b**) after 3 months, (**c**) after 6 months, and (**d**) after 10 months of treatment

Comment Acute diffuse and total alopecia of the female scalp of Sato-Kuwamora et al., alopecia areata incognita of Rebora, and diffuse alopecia areata all represent the same alopecia areata variant that is characterized by diffuse hair shedding in the absence of the patches otherwise typical for the disease. The condition usually affects women over 40 years of age, who complain of diffuse alopecia and may be misdiagnosed as having telogen effluvium. Since alopecia areata is considered to be an organ-specific autoimmune disease, further laboratory investigation would seem unnecessary. Nevertheless, an increased incidence of other autoimmune diseases, such as autoimmune thyroid disease, is seen among alopecia areata patients, while low vitamin D levels and infections may have an influence on the disease course. Although the reported associations of alopecia areata with various infectious agents have remained controversial and need to be confirmed by epidemiologic studies, it remains conceivable that the antigenic stimulus provided by the infection may entertain the autoimmune reaction underlying the hair loss. Therefore, detection and treatment of possible infection associated with alopecia should be taken into consideration. Vice versa, alopecia

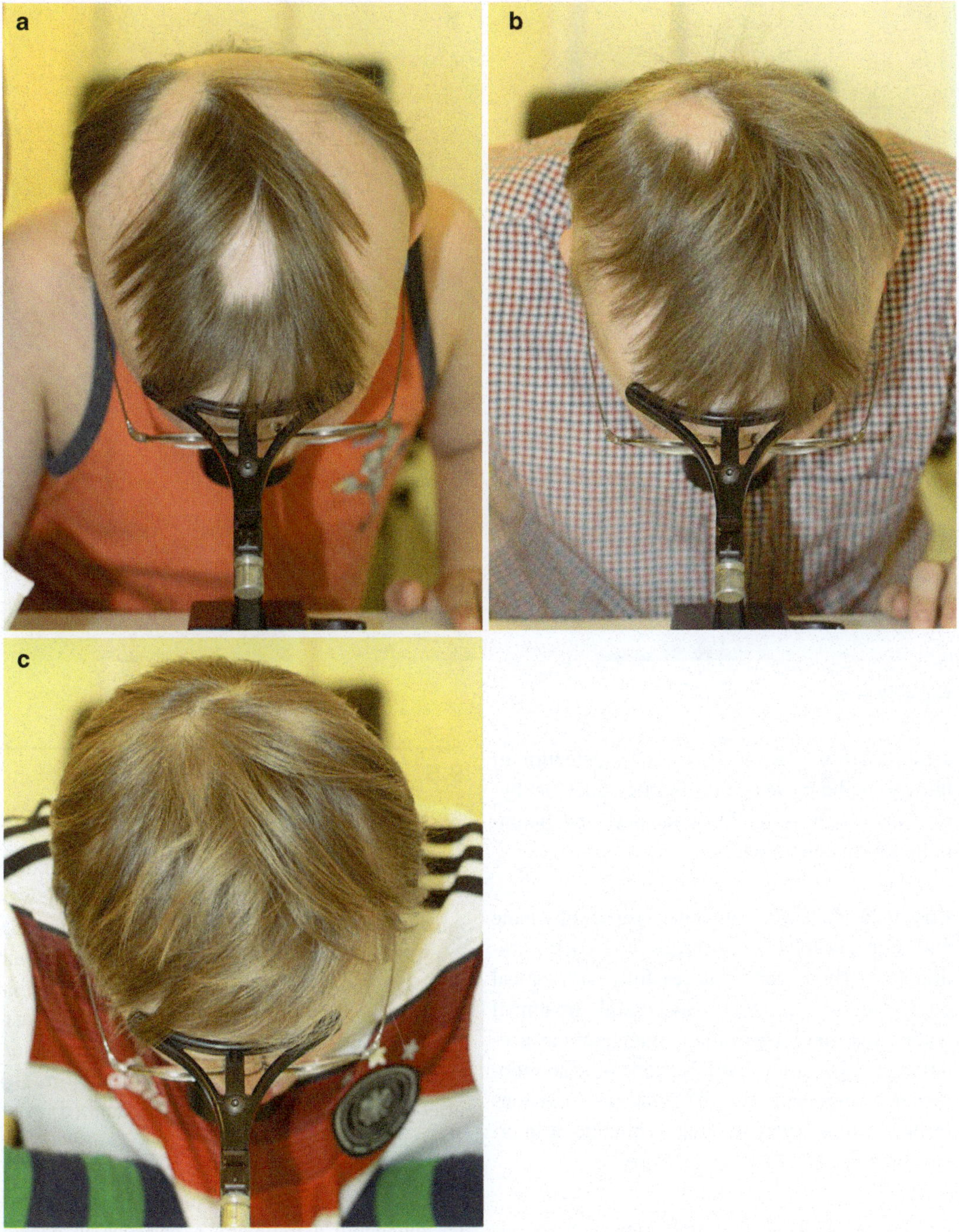

Fig. 9.22 (a–c)

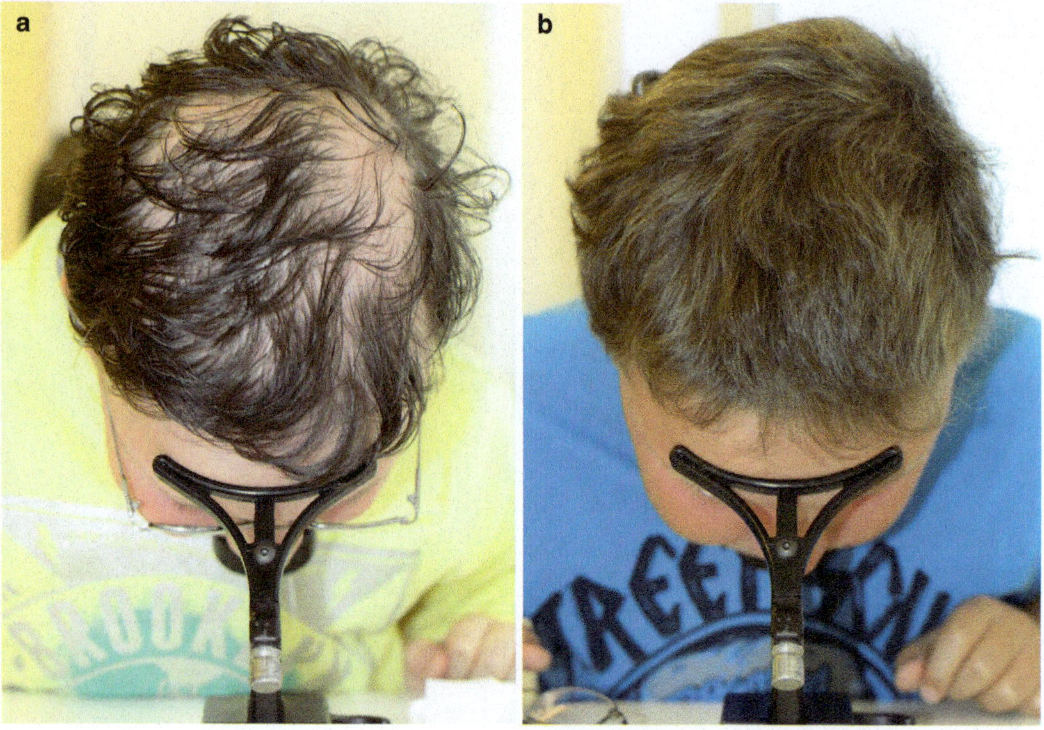

Fig. 9.23 (a, b)

areata itself may act as a marker for detection of hitherto undiagnosed comorbidities, such as thyroid disease, vitamin D deficiency, and potentially serious infections.

Case 9.25 A 32-year-old otherwise healthy male with alopecia areata of the beard of 2 years' duration, formerly treated unsuccessfully with topical corticosteroid ointment. Successful treatment with 5 mg/mL intralesional triamcinolone acetonide: (**a**) just after first injections of triamcinolone acetonide and after (**b**) 2 and (**c**) 4 sessions of intralesional triamcinolone acetonide at intervals of 4 weeks (complete recovery)

Comment Alopecia areata in special locations (face), specifically of the eyebrow and beard, can be successfully treated with intralesional triamcinolone acetonide at lower concentrations than on the scalp (eyebrow: 2.5–5 mg/mL, beard: 5 mg/mL). These regions are particularly sensitive to adverse reactions and unresponsive to topical corticosteroids or calcineurin inhibitors.

9.5 Chemotherapy-Induced Alopecia

Case 9.26 A 50-year-old female who had undergone chemotherapy for breast cancer and was currently taking the aromatase inhibitor letrozole complained of persistent and progressive hair loss. Successful treatment with 5 % topical minoxidil solution b.i.d., L-cystine, medicinal yeast, pantothenic acid-based oral supplementation therapy, and witch hazel shampoo (**a**) before, (**b**) after 3 months, (**c**) after 6 months, and (**d**) after 12 months of treatment

Comment Chemotherapy-induced hair loss is considered a traumatic experience in cancer patient care, since hair loss negatively affects a patient's perception of appearance, body image, and self-esteem. The incidence and severity of the hair loss are variable and related to the particular chemotherapeutic agent and protocol. Moreover, while chemotherapy-induced hair loss has traditionally been categorized as acute diffuse

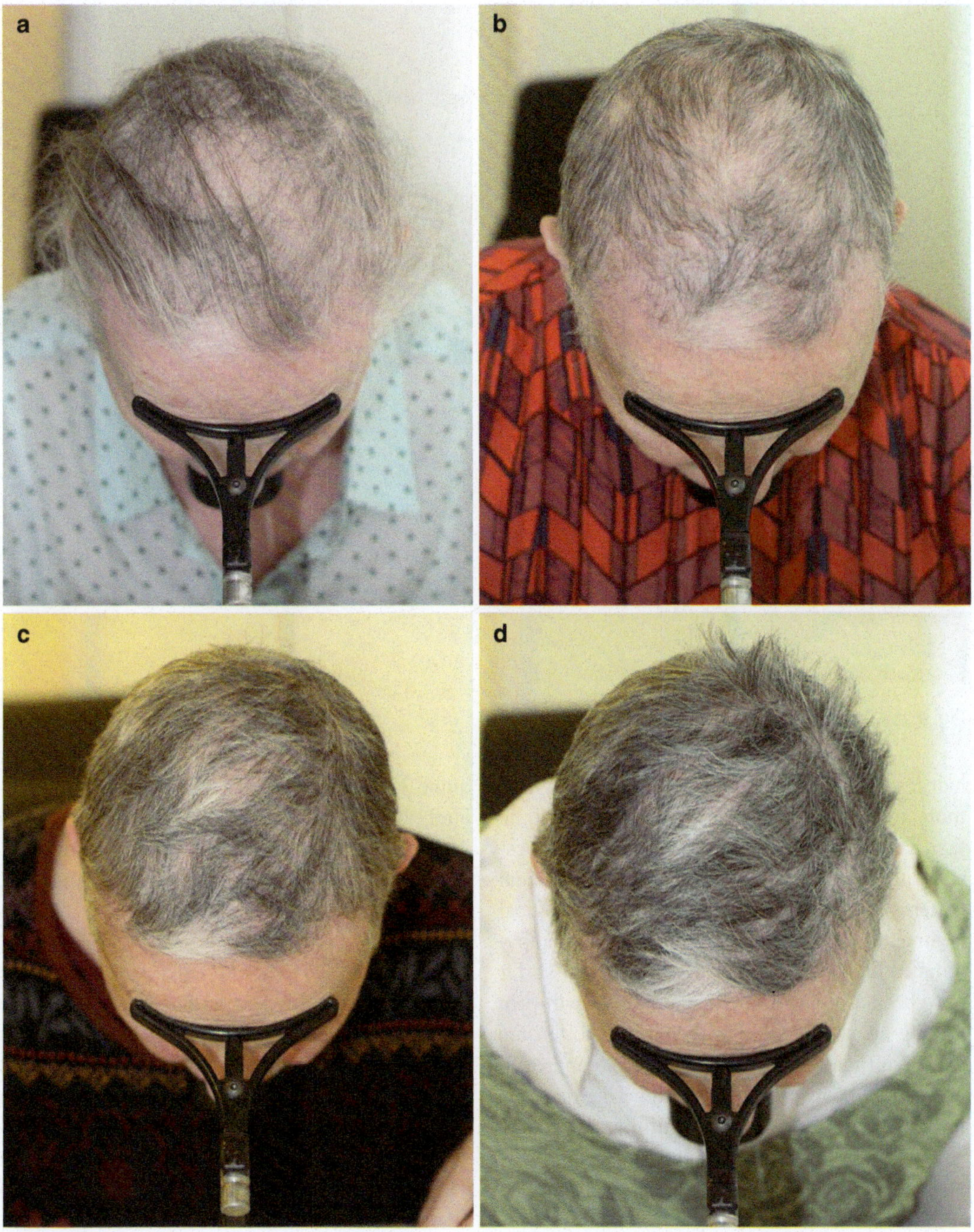

Fig. 9.24 (a–d)

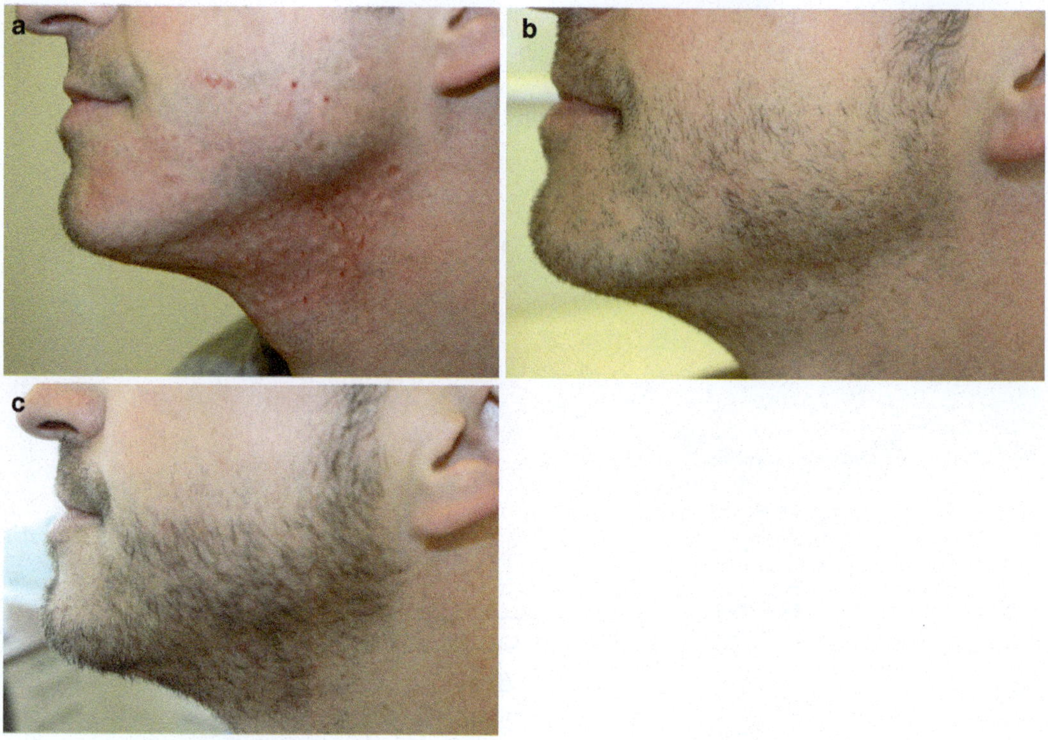

Fig. 9.25 (a–c)

hair loss caused by dystrophic anagen effluvium, more recently it has been pointed out that, in fact, chemotherapy-induced hair loss may present with different pathomechanisms and clinical patterns. So far, no approved pharmacological treatment exists for prevention of chemotherapy-induced hair loss. Among the agents that so far have been evaluated, the topical hair growth-promoting agent minoxidil was able to shorten the duration. Finally, since the estrogen to androgen ratio might be responsible for triggering hair loss in women with genetic susceptibility for androgenetic alopecia, patients following chemotherapy for breast cancer who are under anti-estrogen treatment with aromatase inhibitors may recover some considerable hair with appropriate topical minoxidil therapy.

9.6 Scarring Alopecias

Case 9.27 A 40-year-old female with chronic cutaneous lupus erythematosus of the scalp. Successful treatment with oral hydroxychloroquine 200 mg b.i.d. during the first 4 weeks, thereafter 200 mg once daily, in combination with intralesional triamcinolone acetonide 10 mg/mL: (**a**) before, (**b**) after 3 months, (**c**) after 6 months, and (**d**) after 12 months of treatment

Case 9.28 A 47-year-old female with systemic lupus erythematosus and an inflammatory diffuse effluvium. Successful treatment with intravenous belimumab, oral prednisone 5 mg daily, oral hydroxychloroquine 200 mg b.i.d., 1,200 IU vitamin E daily, 500 mg vitamin C daily, and 0.05 % clobetasol propionate foam twice daily on 5 consecutive days per week: (**a**) before, (**b**) after 3 months, and (**c**) after 6 months of successful treatment

Case 9.29 A 64-year-old female presented with a frontal fibrosing type of alopecia with the clinical and histopathologic findings of cutaneous lupus erythematosus. Successful treatment with 1,200 IU vitamin E and 500 mg vitamin C daily and intralesional triamcinolone acetonide 10 mg/ml: (**a**) before, (**b**) after 3 months, (**c**) after 6 months, and (**d**) after 12 months of treatment

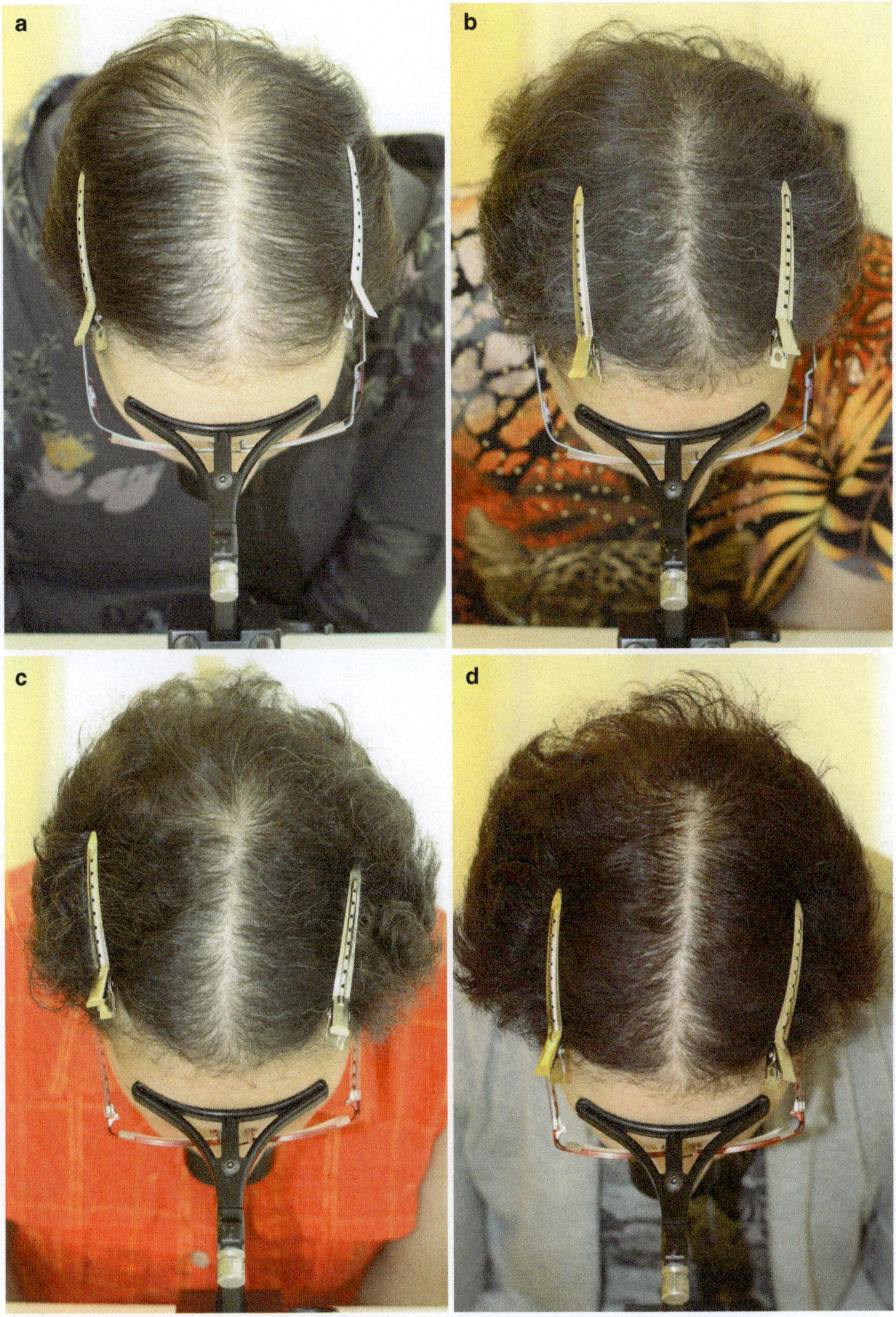

Fig. 9.26 (a–d)

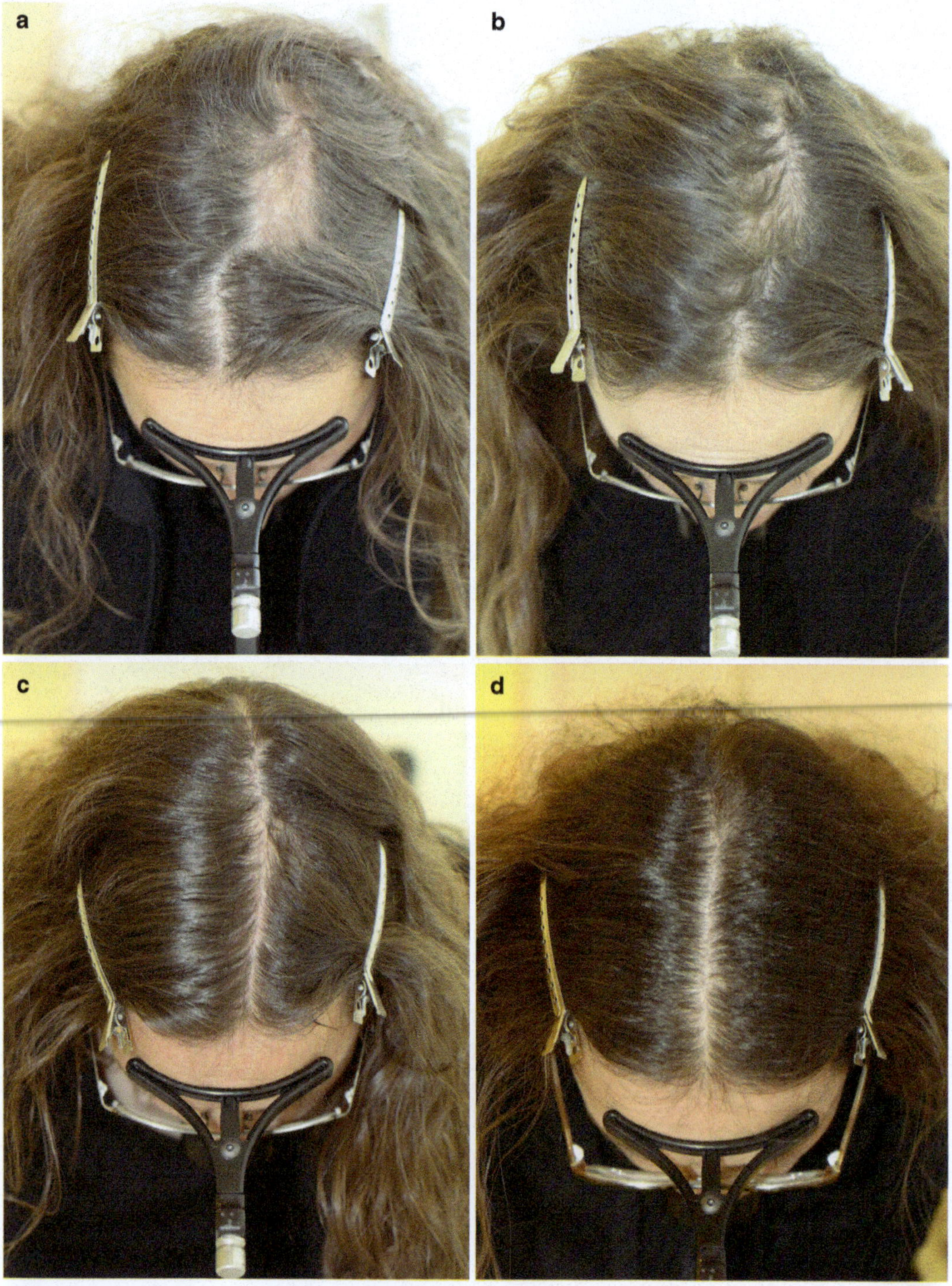

Fig. 9.27 (a–d)

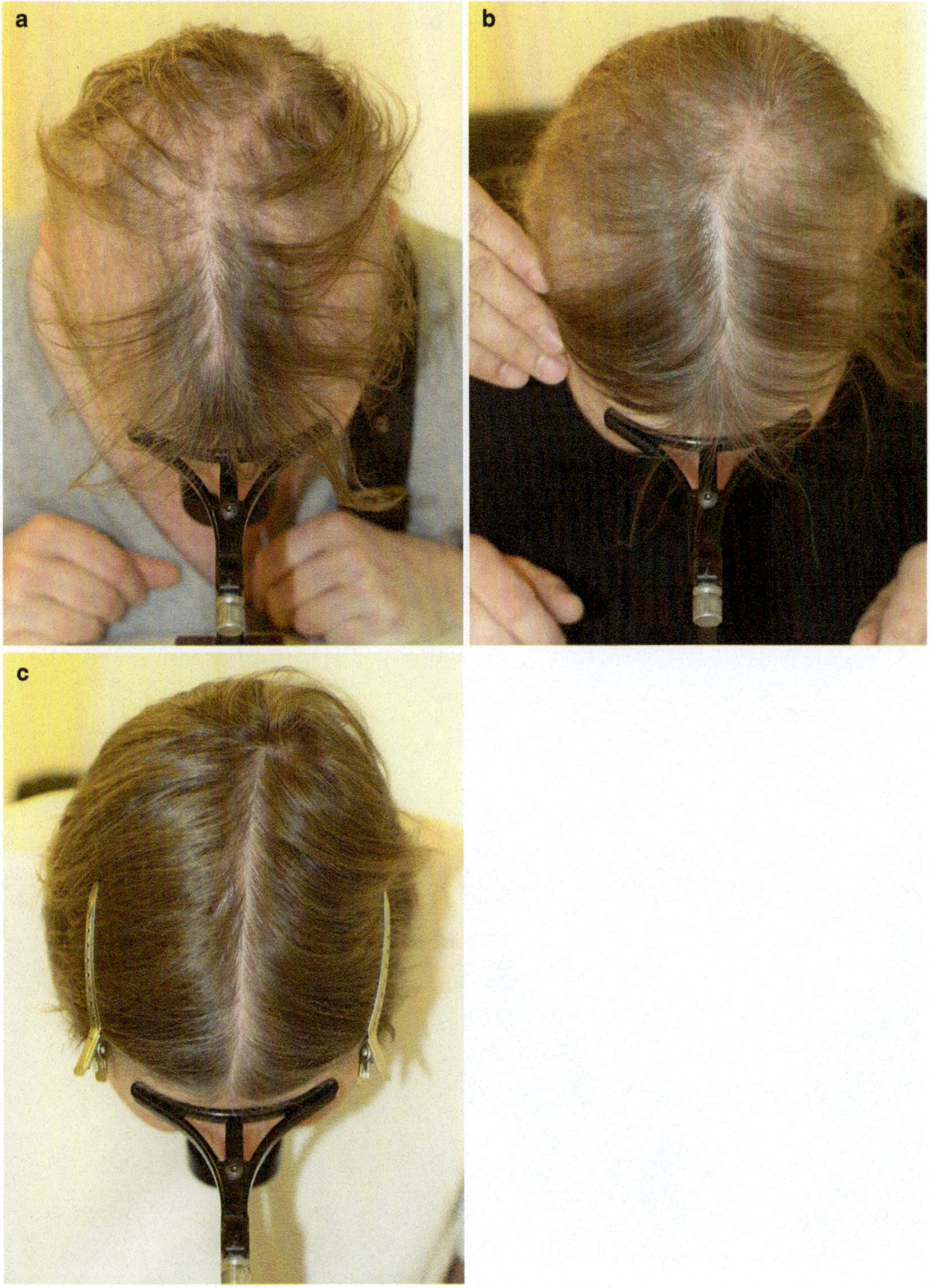

Fig. 9.28 (a–c)

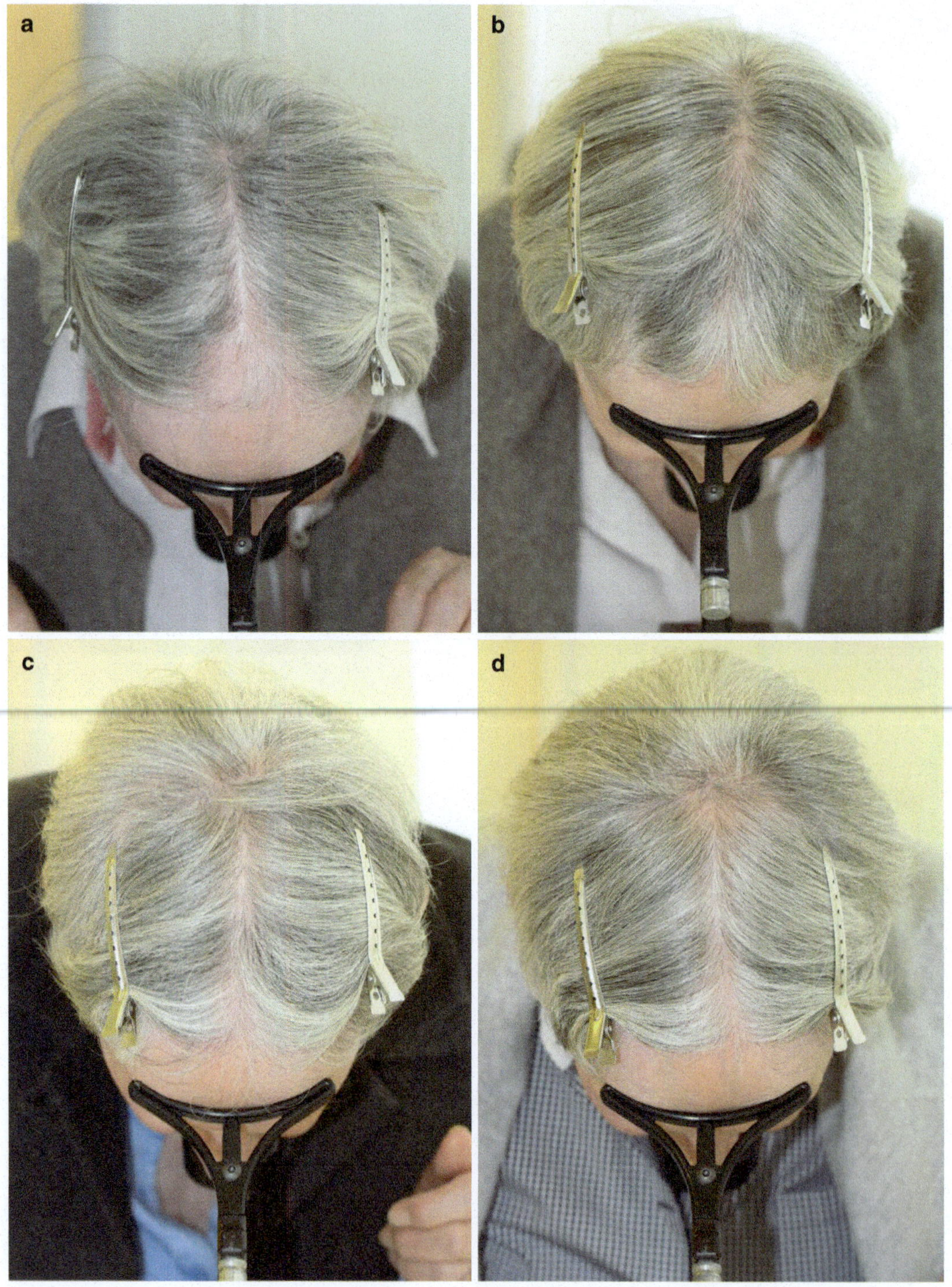

Fig. 9.29 (a–d)

Comment Among the primary cicatricial alopecias, lupus erythematosus is the only one that may be associated with systemic disease. Patients with only discoid lesions of the scalp uncommonly progress to systemic disease. Nevertheless, patients with systemic disease may also have discoid lesions. Because of their high specificity, they have been included in the ACR criteria for the classification as systemic disease. In addition to the focal scarring form of alopecia associated with discoid lupus erythematosus, systemic lupus erythematosus patients experience a diffuse, nonscarring hair loss associated with exacerbations of their lupus disease process. More recently, discoid lupus erythematosus has been observed to also present as a frontal fibrosing type of alopecia, and it has been discussed to what extent a background of androgenetic alopecia may contribute to this particular clinical presentation of the disease.

Case 9.30 A 33-year-old female with folliculitis decalvans. Successful treatment with surgical reduction of scarring alopecia with the use of expander: (**a**) before, (**b**) with expander and areas with active folliculitis to be excised marked in blue, (**c**) 3 months, and (**d**) 6 months after surgery

Case 9.31 A 34-year-old female with folliculitis decalvans. Successful treatment with surgical reduction of scarring alopecia with the use of expander: (**a**) before, (**b**) with expander, and (**c**) 5 months after surgery

Comment Folliculitis decalvans represents a chronic pustulofollicular scalp inflammation resulting in scarring alopecia with hair tufting and centrifugal progression. Invariably pathogenic strains of *S. aureus* can be detected. A recent study provided evidence of the presence of bacterial biofilms at the interface of the hair shaft, which provides an explanation for the chronicity and high relapse rate of the condition even after prolonged systemic antibiotic treatments. Pericin et al. originally proposed that punch excision or excision surgery of hair tufts may provide more sustained results. Since structural changes in the course of scarring alopecia are irreversible, and early interventions usually fail, surgical treatments, such as reduction plasty, in combination with scalp expander technology, should be taken into consideration for best results.

Case 9.32 3 cases of dissecting cellulitis of the scalp successfully treated with subcutaneous adalimumab 40 mg every other week: (**a–c**) before and (**d–f**) after treatment (From: Navarini AA, Trüeb RM (2010) 3 cases of dissecting cellulitis of the scalp treated with adalimumab: control of inflammation within residual structural disease. *Arch Dermatol* 146(5):517–520)

Comment Dissecting cellulitis of the scalp represents yet another chronic inflammatory disease of scalp hair follicles that runs a progressive course eventually resulting in scarring alopecia. The condition is thought to represent a follicular occlusion disorder. Sebaceous and keratinous material within dilated pilosebaceous units accumulates until follicles burst, with subsequent neutrophilic inflammatory reaction and abscess formation. Traditional treatments remain unsatisfactory. In this case series, the inflammation responsible for scarifying tissue destruction was directly targeted by means of the tumor necrosis factor antagonist adalimumab. Histopathologic characteristics demonstrated marked improvement of inflammation, despite persistence of underlying structural disease. Relapse on discontinuation of therapy can be expected depending on persisting structural disease. Therefore, continuous treatment or combined surgical resection of involved areas could be necessary for definitive resolution of disease.

Case 9.33 A 49-year-old black female with central centrifugal cicatricial alopecia. Partially successful treatment with 100 mg oral doxycycline and a compound of topical 5 % minoxidil and 0.2 % triamcinolone acetonide b.i.d., avoidance of traction, chemical hair treatments, and heat: (**a**) before and (**b**) after 2 months of treatment

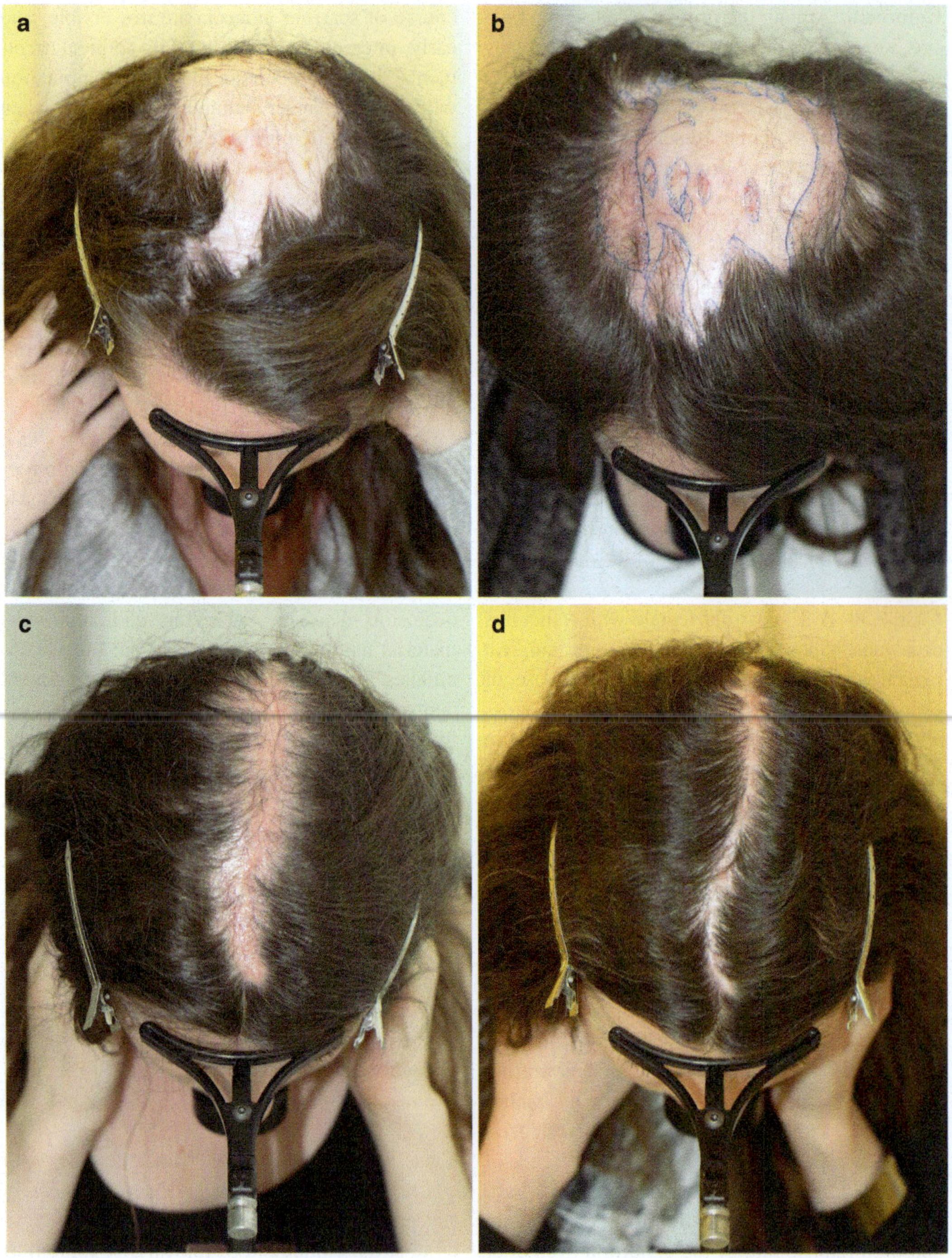

Fig. 9.30 (a–d)

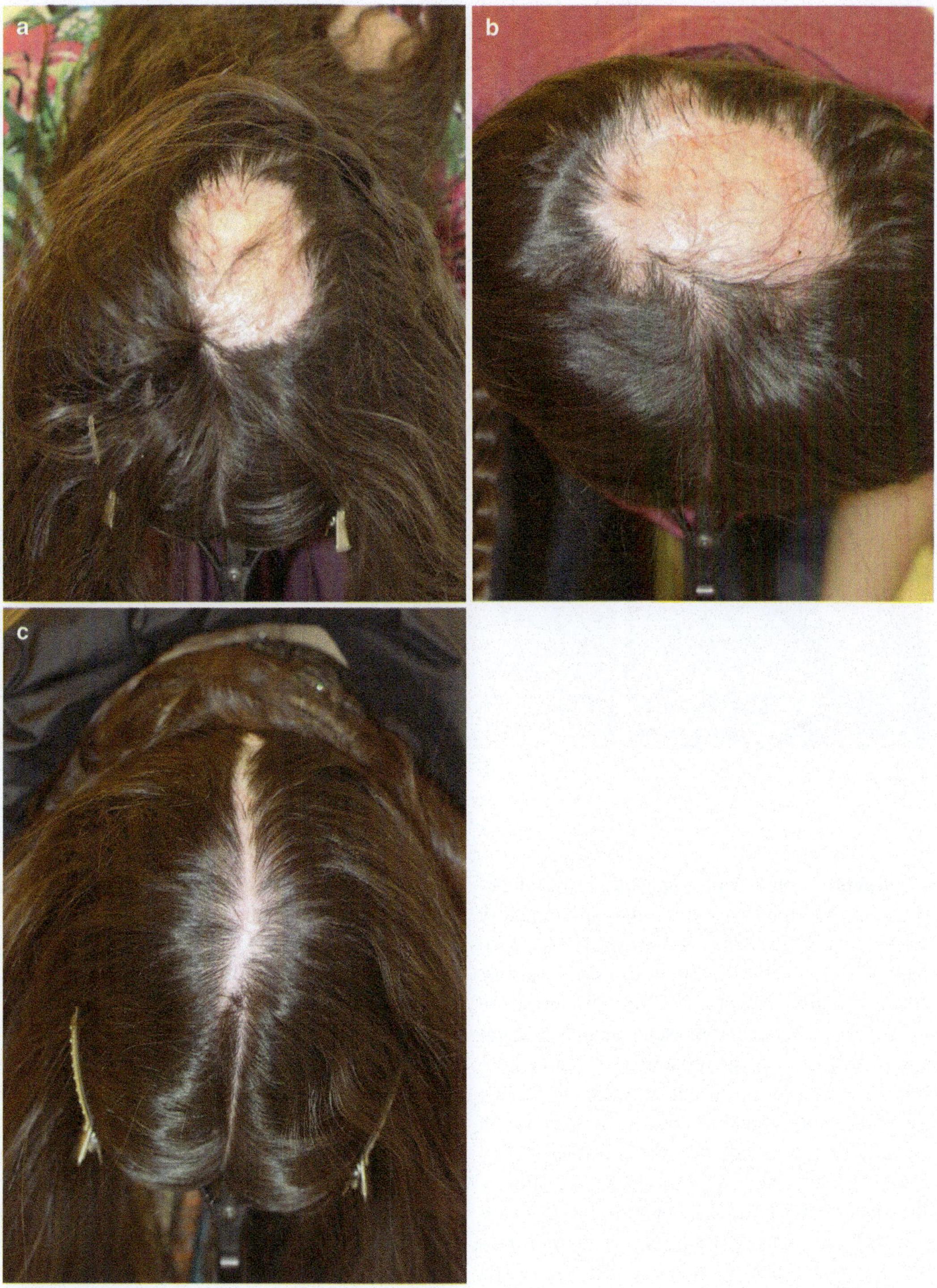

Fig. 9.31 (a–c)

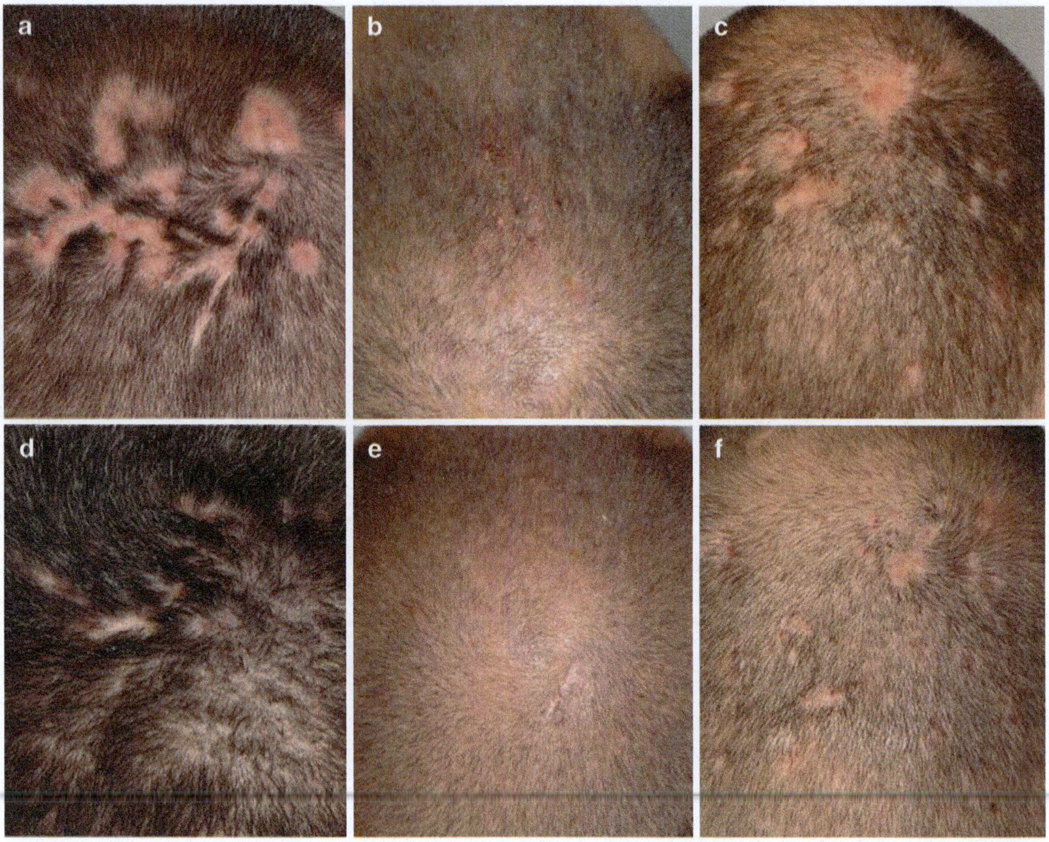

Fig. 9.32 (a–f)

Comment Central centrifugal cicatricial alopecia (CCCA) represents a peculiar inflammatory scarring disease of the African scalp. Its etiopathogenesis has so far remained elusive. However, one hypothesis involves pressure exerted on the internal root sheath leading to damage, which leads to the recruitment of inflammatory cells and the end result of scarring. African Americans are found to be at increased risk because of the curled hair shaft, distinct styling practices, and chemical processing techniques. Risk factors so far identified include diabetes mellitus type 2, bacterial scalp infections, and hairstyles associated with traction. The condition tends to present itself in the 20s and progresses over the following 20–30 years. Prevalence has been found to be highest in women over 50 years (6.7 %). For early detection, one should consider the possibility of CCCA in African Americans with what appears to be female pattern hair loss.

9.7 Red Scalp

Case 9.34 A 24-year-old otherwise healthy female complained of scalp dysesthesia. Clinical inspection revealed telangiectatic erythema of the scalp. Successful treatment with North American Virginian witch hazel (*Hamamelis virginiana*)-based shampoo: (**a**) before and (**b**) after 3 months of treatment. (**c**) Dermoscopic finding before and (**d**) after treatment

Comment Red scalp is a common complaint and may represent a therapeutic challenge in daily clinical practice. The condition was origi-

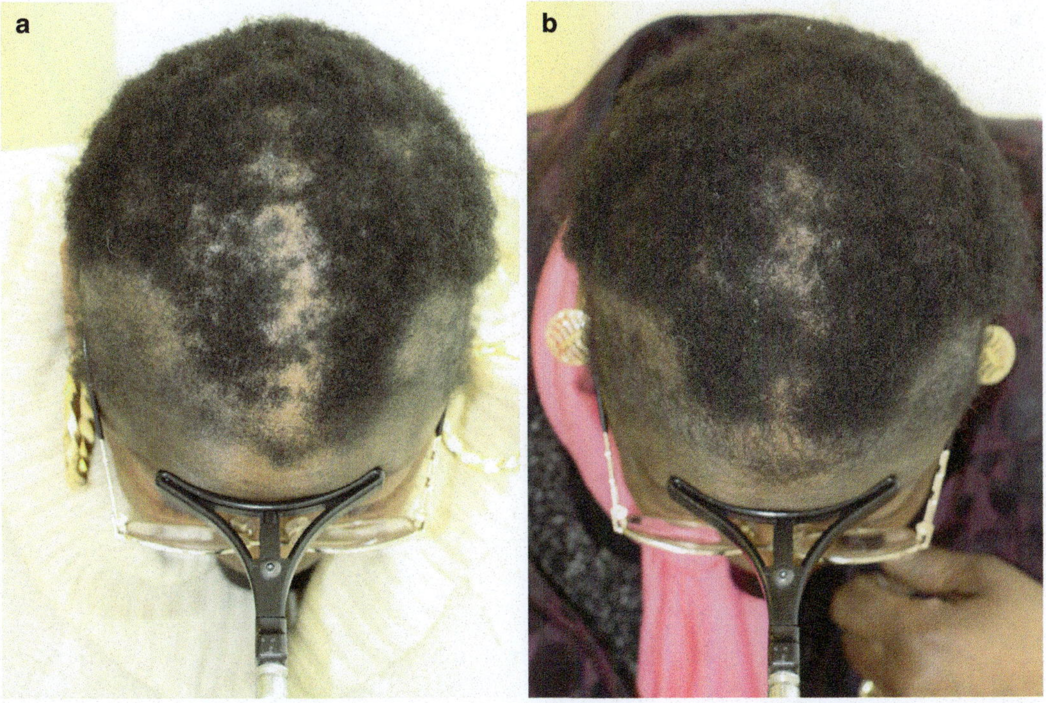

Fig. 9.33 (a, b)

nally described by Thestrup-Pedersen and Hjorth but has largely been ignored. By definition, red scalp is a condition of persistent redness of the scalp, not explained by a specific dermatologic disease of the scalp, with or without sensation of itching or burning, refractory to topical corticosteroids and antiseborrheic agents, and with aggravation in the sun. The most prevalent speculations with respect to its pathogenesis are perifollicular inflammation and/or increased expression of neuropeptide substance P in the vicinity of affected hair follicles. In some cases, there exists some relationship to atopy and atopic disease, in others to rosacea and rosacea-like dermatosis of the scalp. Management begins with protection of the scalp from further noxious environmental, medical, or cosmetic exposures and acting toward appeasement and restoration of the skin. The first step consists in adapting the frequency of hair washing to the condition of the hair and scalp. A mild shampoo must be selected, avoiding ingredients with irritation potential or containing frequent contact allergens. Of particular interest are herbal special care ingredients with anti-irritant activity from traditional phytomedicine, such as North American Virginian witch hazel (*Hamamelis virginiana*).

Case 9.35 A 57-year-old female with burning sensations of the scalp, treated before with antiseborrheic shampoos without success. Clinical examination revealed a red scalp with follicular erythematous and telangiectatic papules strictly within the limits of the scalp hair. On the basis of clinical and histopathologic features of rosacea, treatment was successfully performed with oral tetracyclines (300 mg/day lymecycline): (**a–c**) before and (**d–f**) after treatment. Erythema and follicular papules and pustules disappeared. There remained residual telangiectasia. The patient was recommended to omit topical corticosteroids and to protect scalp from UV exposure (From: Oberholzer PA, Nobbe S, Kolm I et al. (2009) Red scalp disease—a rosacea-like dermatosis of the scalp? Successful therapy with oral tetracycline. *Dermatology* 219:179–181)

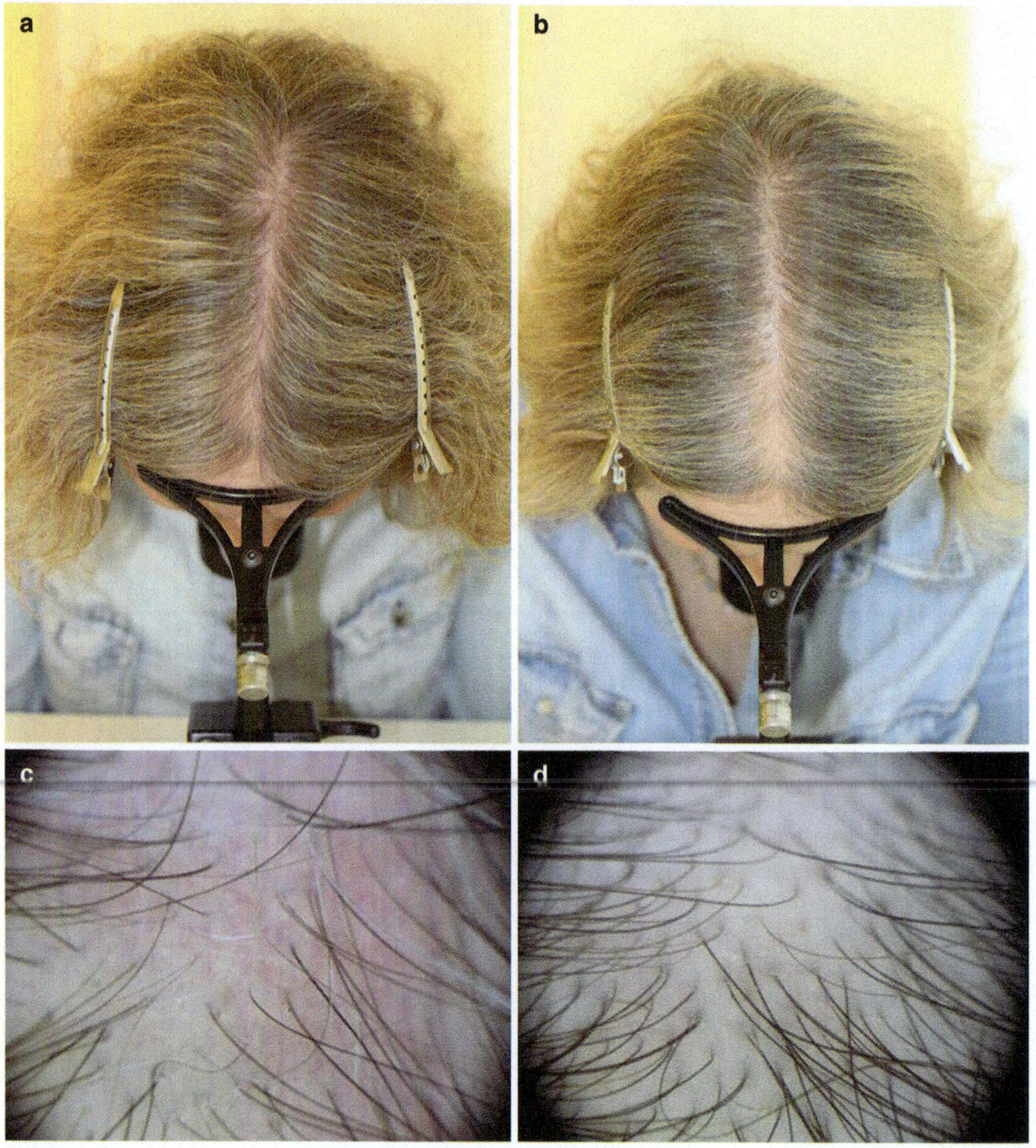

Fig. 9.34 (a–d)

Comment On the basis of clinical, dermoscopic, and histopathologic findings, a subset of patients with red scalp show features of rosacea. Remarkably patients with the telangiectatic variant of rosacea report stinging sensation to the topical application of 5 % lactic acid on the cheeks more frequently than patients with the papulopustular type of rosacea or normal controls. Extrafacial locations of rosacea may be involved more frequently than appreciated because of failure to search, in particular, rosacea affecting the upper forehead and scalp. Accordingly, treatment consists of oral tetracyclines and avoidance of topical corticosteroids and UVR exposure.

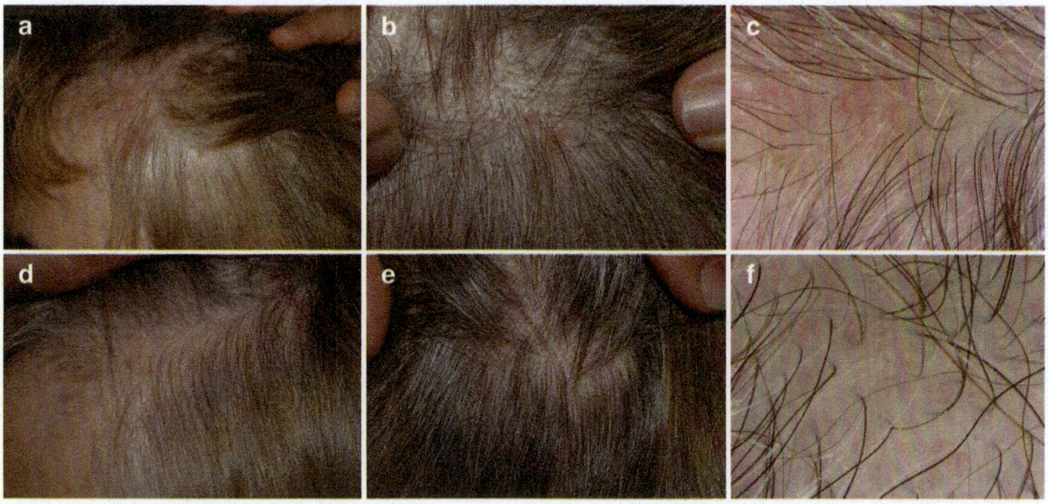

Fig. 9.35 (a–f)

Case 9.36 A 63-year-old male with pruritic, inflammatory lesions of the scalp. (**a**) *Demodex* was extracted from a papulopustular follicular lesion. The patient was successfully treated with oral metronidazole 250 mg bid and 5 % topical permethrin cream, (**b**) before and (**c**) after 30 days' treatment

Case 9.37 A 46-year-old female with female pattern hair loss, Ludwig II, a frontal telogen rate of 23 %, and (**a**) high *Demodex* load on light microscopic examination of hair plucks was started on 5 % topical minoxidil solution b.i.d. and 1 % permethrin lotion 10 min once weekly for 8 weeks. (**b**) Before treatment and after (**c**) 3, (**d**) 6, and (**e**) 12 months of successful treatment, she showed significant regrowth of hair and normalization of frontal telogen rates, despite persistent high load of *Demodex*

Comment Depending upon their genus, parasitic mites embed themselves either in skin or hair follicles in the animal and cause mange in furry mammals. *Sarcoptes spp.* burrow into skin causing sarcoptic mange, while *Demodex spp.* live in follicles causing demodectic mange. In humans, these two types of mite infections are instead known as scabies and demodicosis, respectively. In humans, there is no consensus to what degree *Demodex* mites contribute to disease in humans, since *Demodex* is a common commensal of the pilosebaceous unit. Nevertheless, in humans, *Demodex spp.* have been identified and implied to play a role in papulopustular scalp eruptions, pustular folliculitis of the face, and blepharitis.

9.8 Multitargeted Treatments

Case 9.38 A 45-year-old otherwise healthy Asian male with advanced androgenetic alopecia. Successful treatment with combination therapy with 1 mg oral finasteride and 5 % topical minoxidil solution b.i.d.: (**a**) before, (**b**) after 3 months, (**c**) after 6 months, (**d**) after 12 months, and (**e**) after 24 months of treatment

Case 9.39 A 31-year-old otherwise healthy male with androgenetic alopecia. Successful switch from 1 mg oral finasteride treatment to combination treatment with 0.5 mg dutasteride and 5 % topical minoxidil solution b.i.d.: (**a**) before, (**b**)

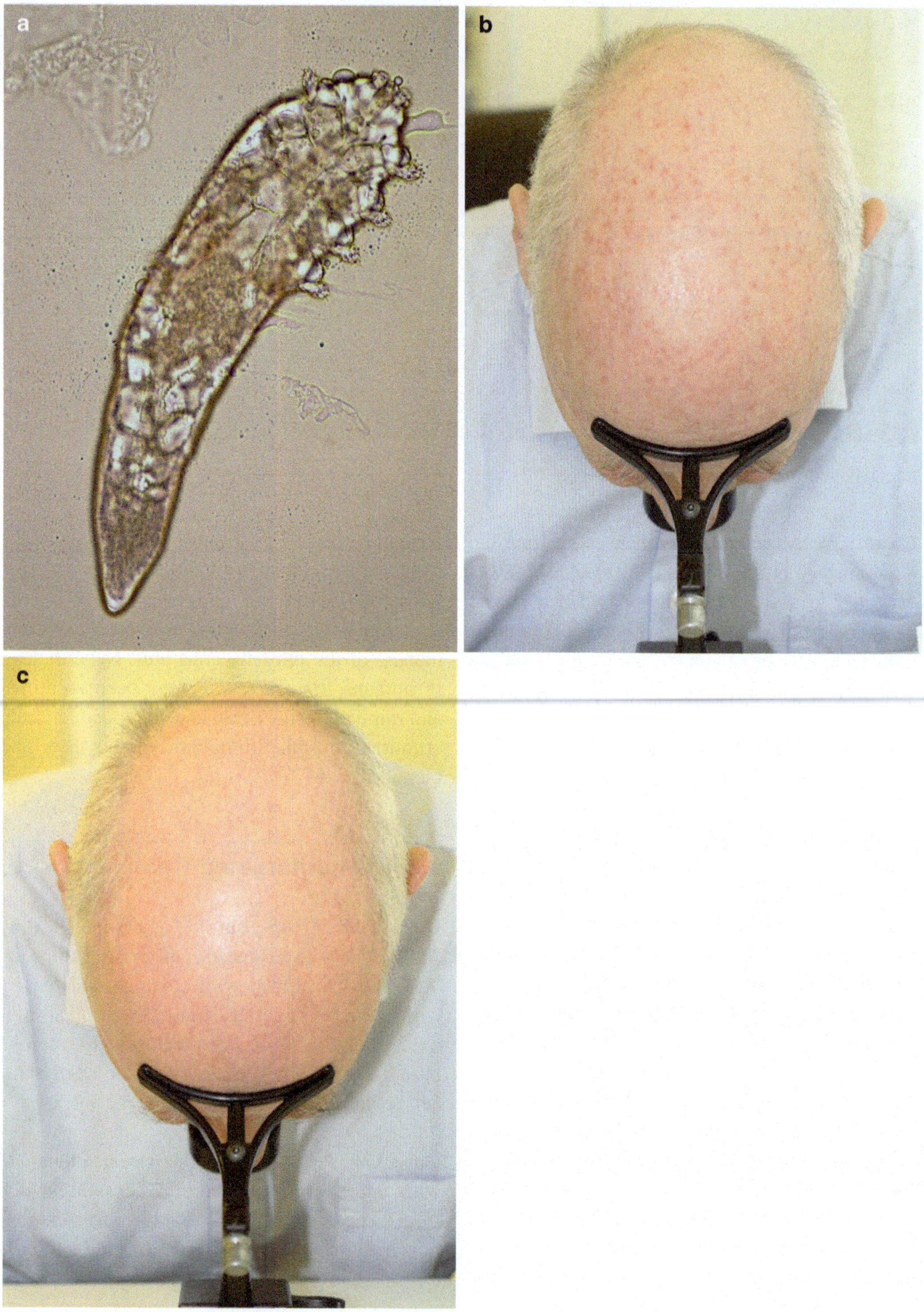

Fig. 9.36 (a–c)

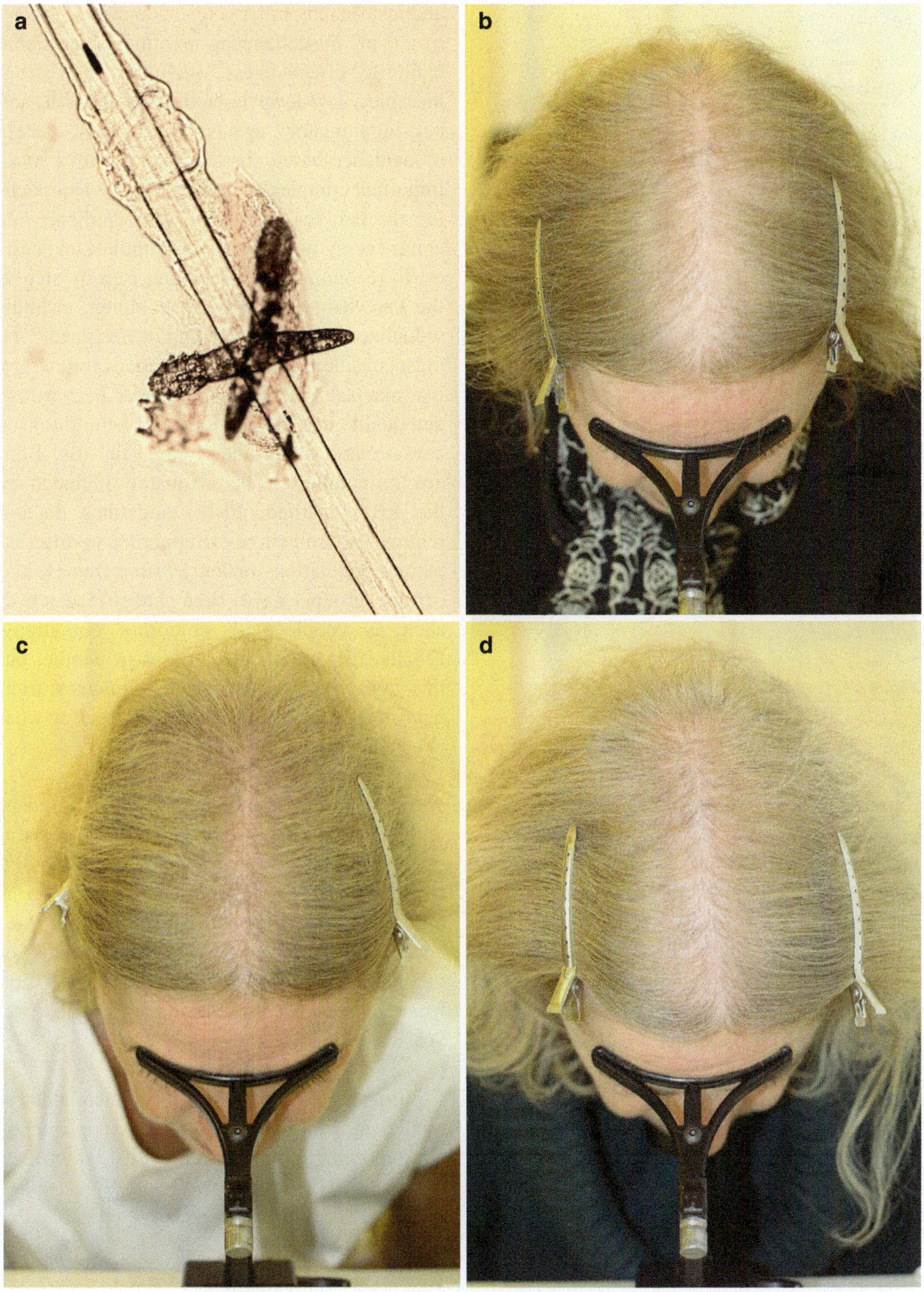

Fig. 9.37 (a–e)

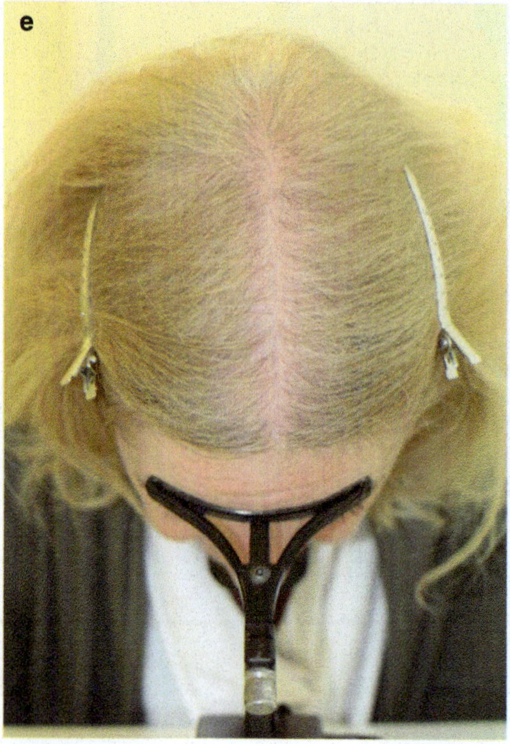

Fig. 9.37 (continued)

after 12 months of treatment with 1 mg oral finasteride, and (**c**) 3 months after switching to 0.5 mg dutasteride and 5 % topical minoxidil solution b.i.d.. After switching from finasteride to dutasteride, the serum dihydrotestosterone dropped from 0.73 nmol/L (normal: 1.05–2.98 nmol/L) to 0.12 nmol/L

Comment Evidence-based medicine (EBM) aims for the ideal that healthcare professionals should make conscientious, explicit, and judicious use of the best available evidence gained from the scientific method to clinical decision making. A European consensus group recently revealed excellent evidence levels for the therapeutic use of topical minoxidil or of oral finasteride for the treatment of androgenetic alopecia and insufficient, or lacking, evidence for a broad panel of miscellaneous treatments available claiming effectiveness, including nutritional therapies, low-level laser therapy (LLLT), and anti-inflammatory agents. The limited success of evidence-based therapies points to a more important complexity of hair loss. By approaching the hair loss patient in a methodical way, commencing with objects the simplest and easiest to recognize, and ascending step by step to the knowledge of the more complex, an individualized treatment plan can be designed. One must consider combination regimens for therapy that may act synergistic to enhance hair growth and quality and the possibility of a multitude of cause-relationships underlying hair loss. Both are too complex to be adequately included by the EBM method. EBM guidelines do not remove the problem of extrapolation to different patient populations or longer time frames, and certain groups have been under-researched, such as people with comorbid conditions. Finally, EBM applies to groups of people, but this does not preclude astute clinicians from using their personal experience in deciding what is best for the individual at hand.

Case 9.40 A 61-year-old male heavy smoker with advanced androgenetic alopecia. Successful treatment with combination therapy of 1 mg oral finasteride and cystine, medicinal yeast, and pantothenic acid-based oral supplementation therapy: (**a**) before and (**b**) after 3 months of treatment. Treatment result exceeds expectation from 5-alpha reductase inhibition in the male >60 years

Comment Since an important commercial interest lies in the value of nutritional supplements, an important question that arises is whether increasing the content of an already adequate diet with specific amino acids, vitamins, and/or

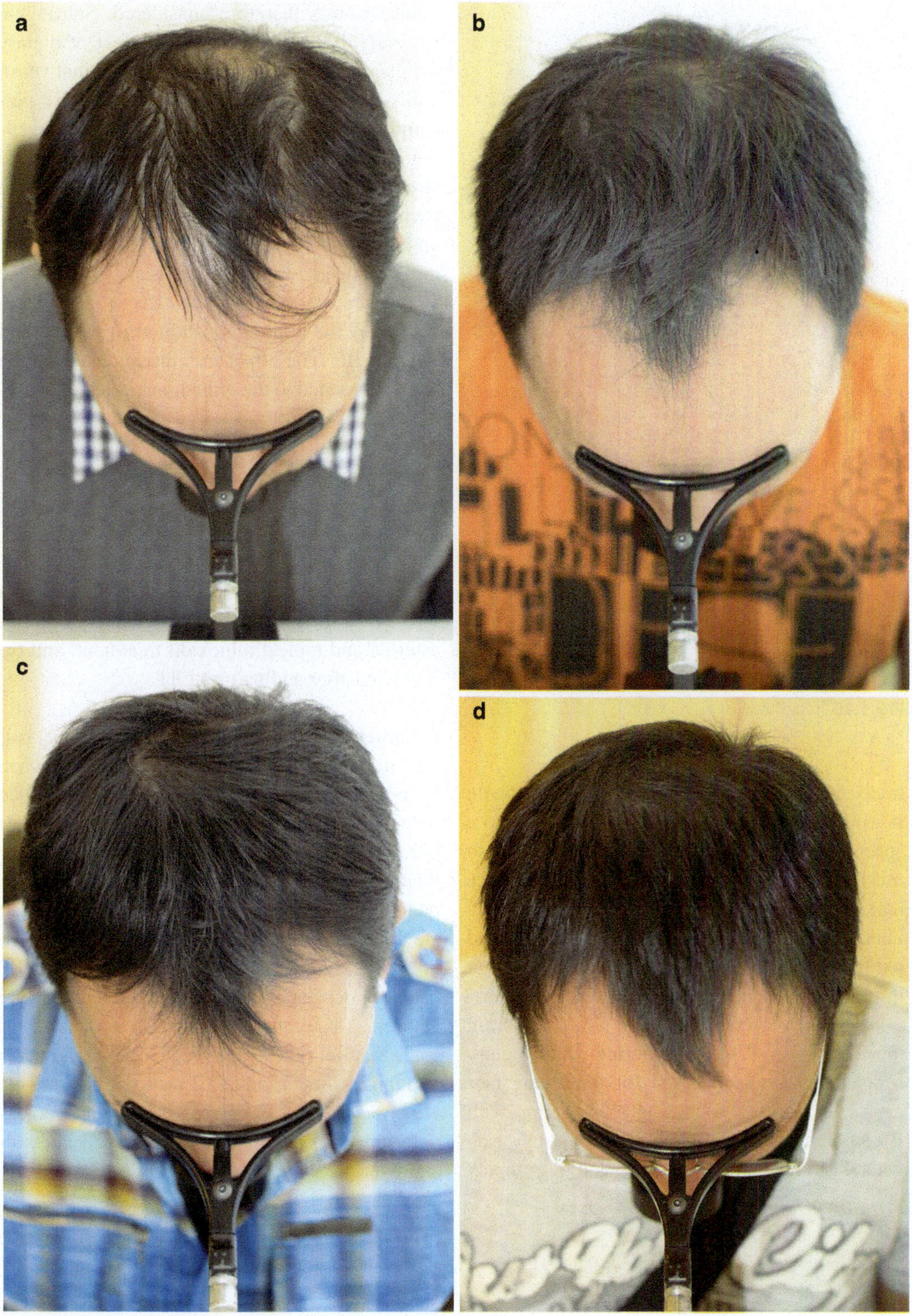

Fig. 9.38 (a–e)

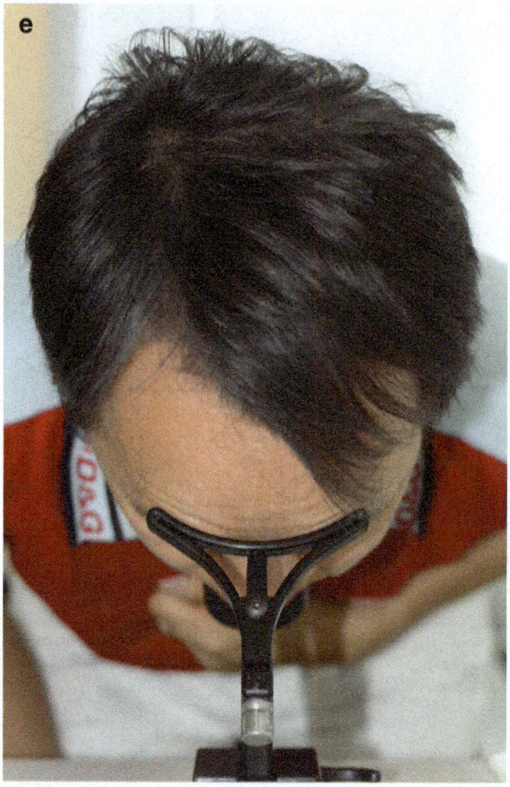

Fig. 9.38 (continued)

trace elements may further promote hair growth. It would appear that unless hair loss is due to a specific nutritional deficiency, there's only so much that nutritional therapies can do to enhance hair growth and quality. However, there are internal and external factors, such as aging and oxidative stress, e.g., from cigarette smoke, that influence hair health to such a degree that nutritional therapy can boost hair that's suffering from these problems. When considering which dietary supplements could be used for improving hair growth in humans, cystine in combination with B-complex vitamins or medicinal yeast, a rich natural source of amino acids and B-complex vitamins, was therefore considered. Starting in the early 1990s, studies on the effect of dietary supplements containing cystine, medicinal yeast, and pantothenic acid (CYP-complex) were performed, showing improvements in hair swelling as a criterion for hair quality, in the tensile strength of the hair fiber, and in anagen rates in the trichogram and phototrichogram. Interestingly, an experiment performed on C57BL/6 mice that developed hair loss when exposed to cigarette smoke demonstrated that this effect could be prevented by the oral administration of cystine and vitamin B6. The effect was interpreted as to be possibly related to the glutathione-related detoxification system.

Case 9.41 A 36-year-old otherwise healthy male with advanced androgenetic alopecia. Successful combination therapy with 1 mg oral finasteride, 5 % topical minoxidil solution b.i.d., and LLLT with the Hairmax LaserComb® three times weekly: (**a**) before, (**b**) after 9 months of oral finasteride and topical minoxidil treatment, and (**c**) 3 months after adding on LLLT

Comment The ability of lasers to induce hair growth was incidentally noted in 1967 when Mester et al. used LLLT to treat cancer in mice with shaved backs. Since then, hypertrichosis has been recognized to be a possible side effect of laser treatment for epilation. Today, the phenomenon is understood to result from suboptimal fluences that are too low to induce thermolysis but high enough to stimulate follicular growth. Eventually, LLLT has been developed for treatment of androgenetic alopecia. The technology appears to work better for some than for others, and predictive factors which will most benefit from LLLT are to be determined. Nevertheless, LLLT represents a safe and potentially effective treatment option for patients with androgenetic alopecia who do not respond or are

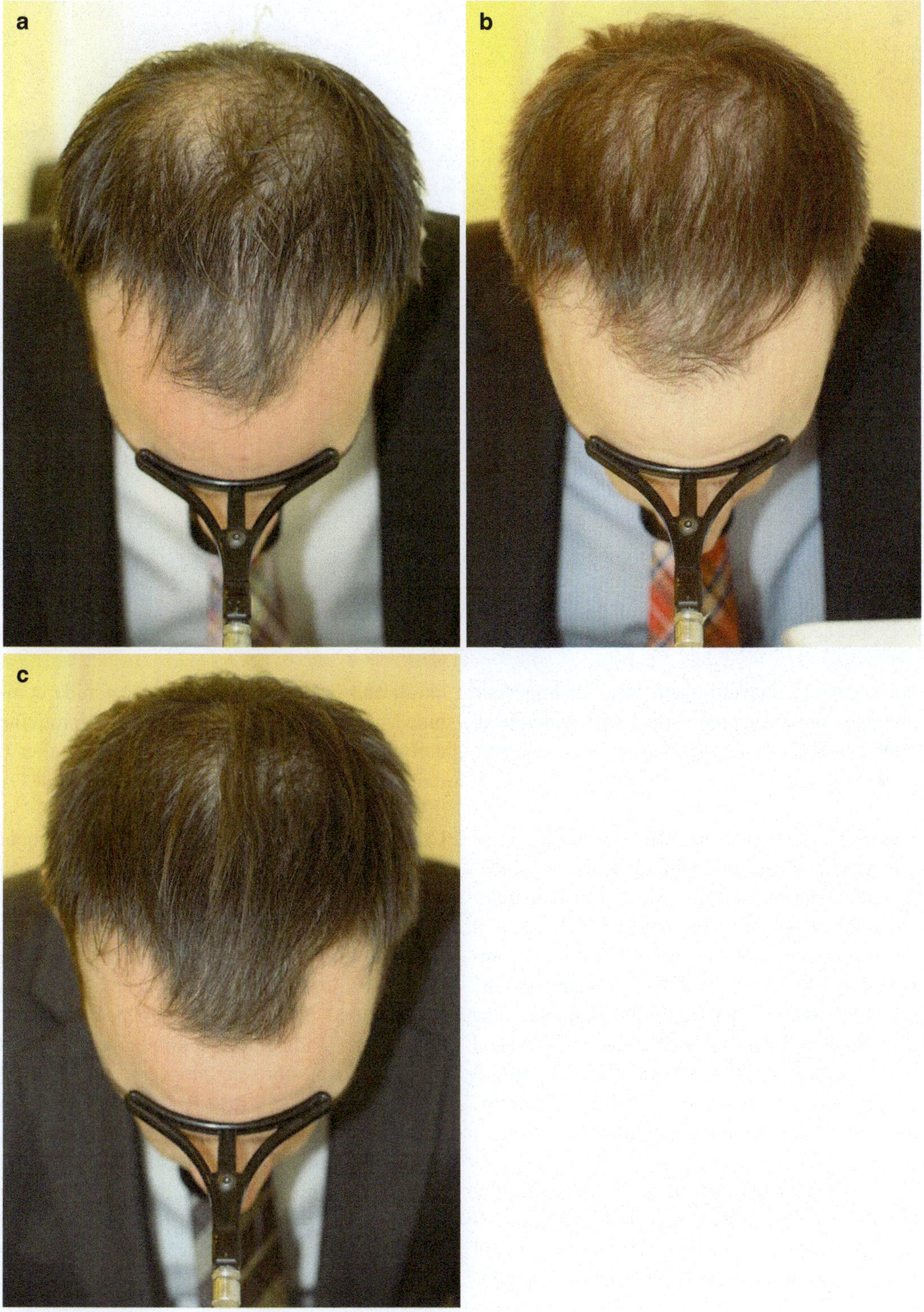

Fig. 9.39 (a–c)

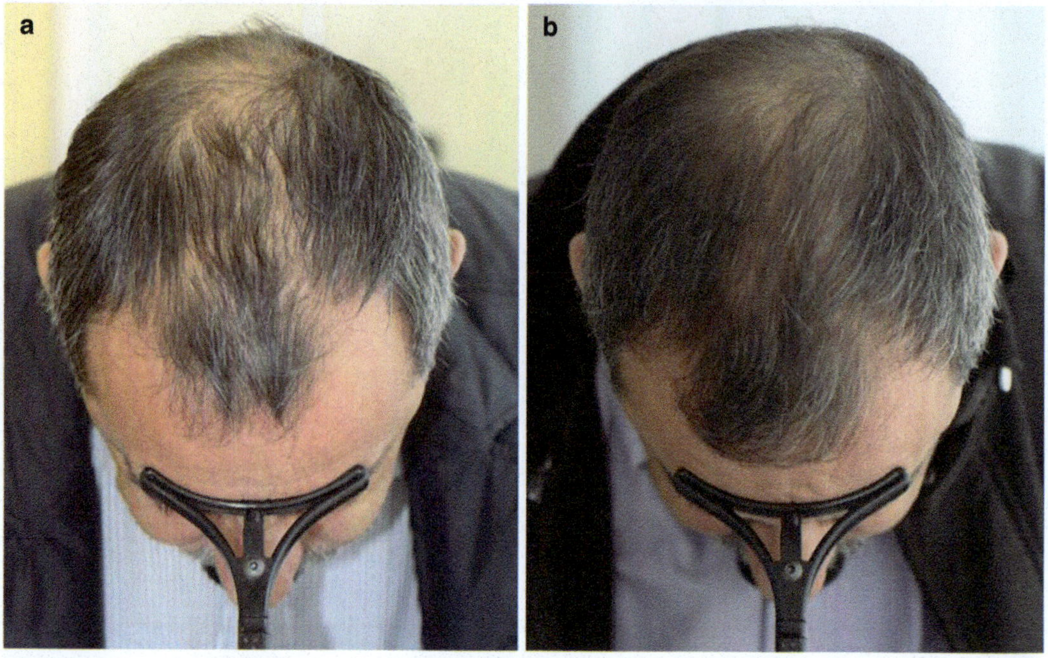

Fig. 9.40 (a, b)

not tolerant to standard treatment of androgenetic alopecia. Moreover, combining LLLT with topical minoxidil and oral finasteride may act synergistic to enhance hair growth.

Case 9.42 A 30-year-old otherwise healthy male with patterned hair loss with evidence of follicular inflammation and fibrosis. Successful treatment with 1 mg oral finasteride and 100 mg oral doxycycline in combination with a topical compound of 3 % minoxidil and 0.2 % triamcinolone acetonide and witch hazel-based shampoo. The last 3 months 1 mg oral finasteride was switched to 0.5 mg oral dutasteride: (**a**) before, (**b**) after 3 months, (**c**) after 6 months, (**d**) after 9 months, and (**e**) after 12 months of treatment

Case 9.43 A 68-year-old otherwise healthy female with fibrosing alopecia in a pattern distribution (cicatricial pattern hair loss). Successful treatment with a topical compound of 5 % minoxidil and 0.2 % triamcinolone acetonide combined with 200 mg oral hydroxychloroquine daily: (**a**) before, (**b**) after 3 months, (**c**) after 6 months, and (**d**) after 12 months of treatment

Comment The limited success rate of treatment of androgenetic alopecia with topical minoxidil or oral finasteride means that further pathogenic pathways must be taken into account. The implication of microscopic follicular inflammation in the pathogenesis of androgenetic alopecia has emerged from several independent studies. Ultimately, follicular microinflammation and fibrosis, frontal fibrosing alopecia, and fibrosing alopecia in a pattern distribution seem to represent a continuum from microscopic inflammation and fibrosis to localized and more generalized forms of clinically perceptible inflammatory scarring alopecia in a patterned distribution (cicatricial pattern hair loss). Surprisingly, the use or addition of topical corticosteroids or of systemic

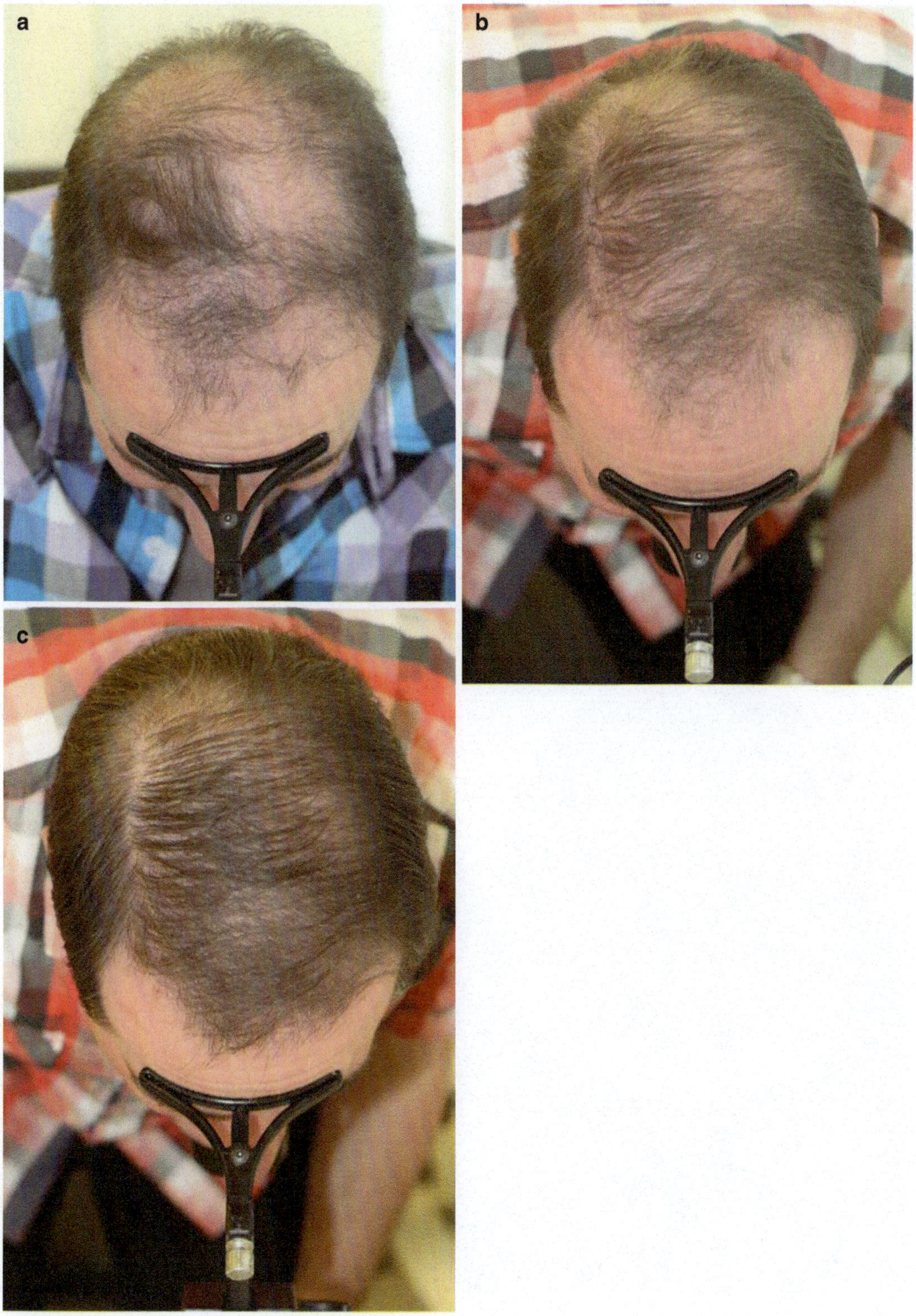

Fig. 9.41 (a–c)

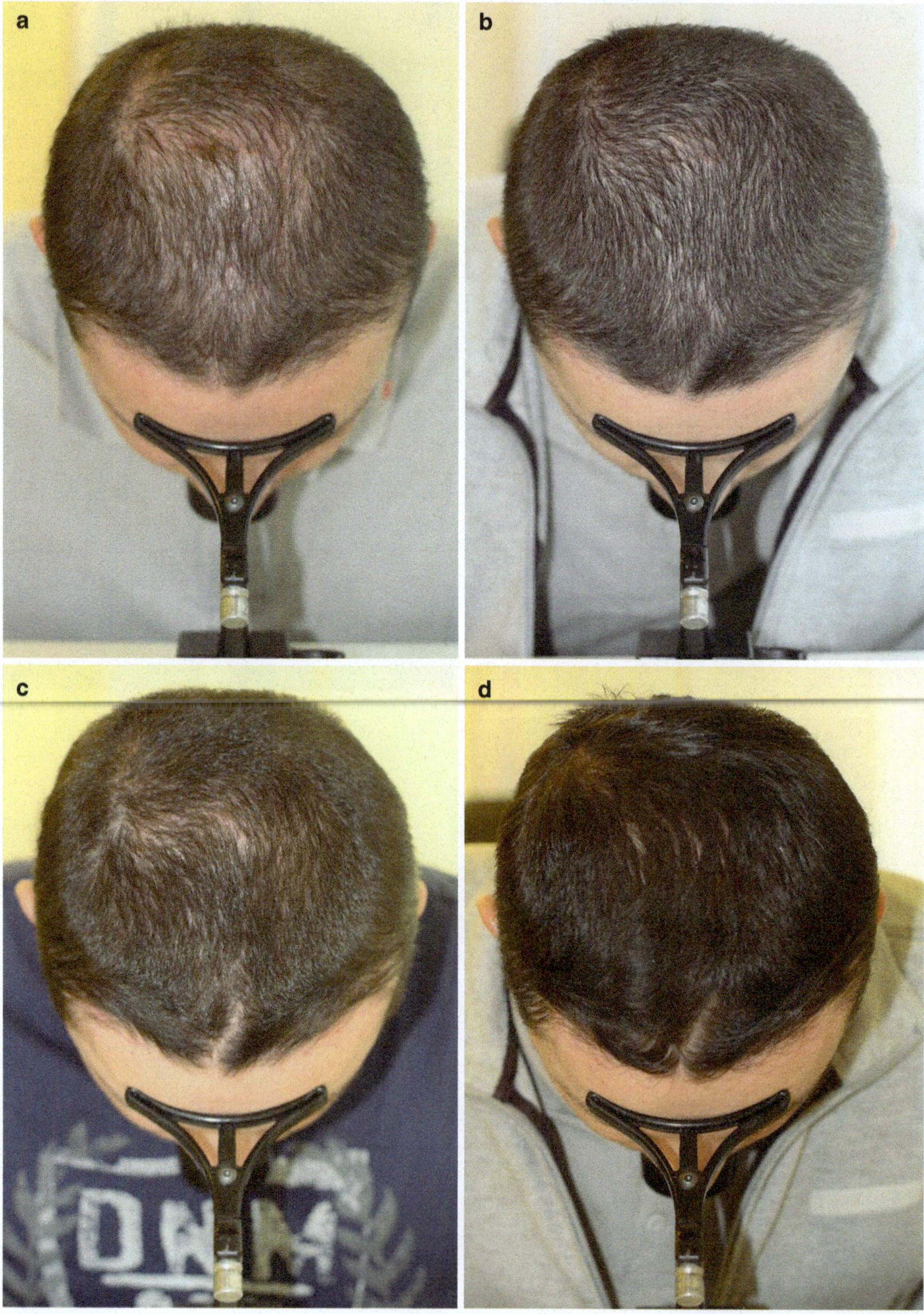

Fig. 9.42 (a–e)

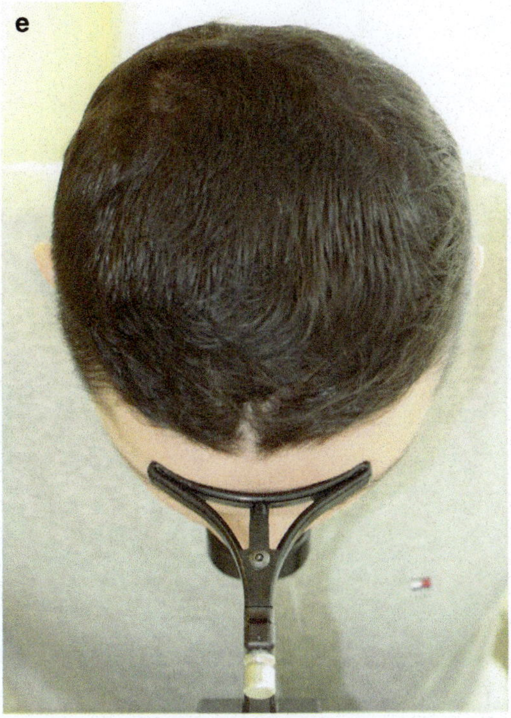

Fig. 9.42 (continued)

anti-inflammatory agents such as oral hydroxychloroquine or oral doxycycline in the treatment plan of androgenetic alopecia with evidence of inflammation and fibrosis has so far not been systematically studied. For now, we can only deduce a putative added benefit by analogy from their preliminary successful use in cicatricial pattern hair loss or in central centrifugal cicatricial alopecia. Oral hydroxychloroquine may also be replaced with oral doxycycline (200 mg daily).

9.9 Hair Transplantation

Case 9.44 A 40-year-old female with frontal fibrosing alopecia. Successful treatment with autologous hair transplantation: (**a**) before and (**b**) 12 months after hair transplantation

Case 9.45 A 45-year-old male with frontal fibrosing alopecia and loss of eyebrows. Successful treatment with autologous hair transplantation: (**a**) before and (**b**) 6 months after eyebrow transplantation

Case 9.46 A 63-year-old female with fibrosing alopecia in a pattern distribution (cicatricial pattern hair loss). Successful treatment with 0.5 mg dutasteride, a compound of 3 % topical minoxidil and 0.2 % triamcinolone acetonide solution b.i.d., and autologous hair transplantation: (**a**) before, (**b**) 1 month after, (**c**) 4 months after, and (**d**) 9 months after autologous hair transplantation. (**e**) Sustained result 2 ½ year after transplantation

Comment Autologous hair transplantation remains the only treatment option for advanced patterned baldness both in males and in females and may be performed in selected cases of cicatricial alopecia including the eyebrows. Modern techniques based on micrografting use the visual qualities of hair and varying design patterns to create the optical illusion of more hair than is actually present. Since hair loss in the course of scarring alopecia is irreversible and early interventions often fail to halt progression

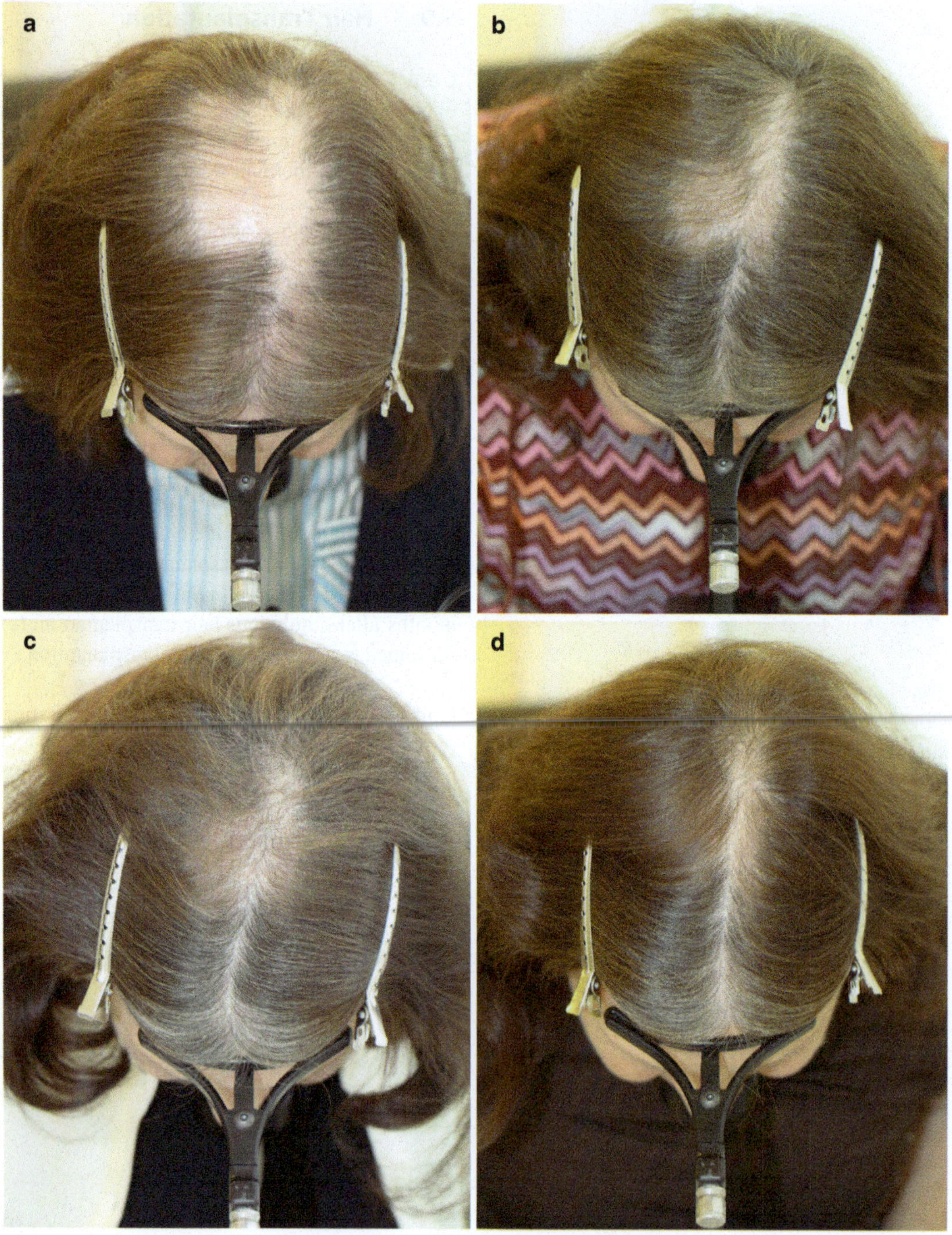

Fig. 9.43 (a–d)

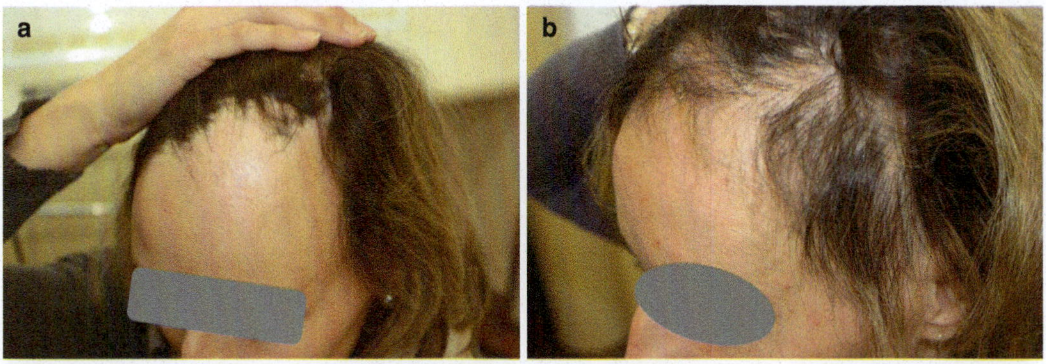

Fig. 9.44 (a, b)

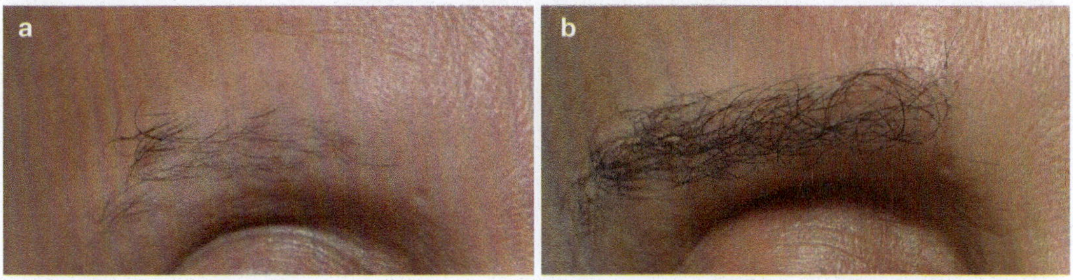

Fig. 9.45 (a, b)

of disease, particularly in frontal fibrosing alopecia, or patients come late, surgical treatments, including autologous hair transplantation, may be taken into consideration. Specifically in diseases such as lichen planopilaris, where surgical trauma may trigger Köbner's isomorphic phenomenon, hair transplantation is usually recommended only if the disease has been in clinical remission for 2 years or may be considered earlier under perioperative immunosuppression (6 weeks pre- to 6 weeks postoperative) with oral cyclosporine A (2.5–5 mg/kg patient body weight). The hair transplantations in Cases 9.44, 9.45, and 9.46 have been performed by Beatrice Banholzer, MD, Formaxis, Zurich, Switzerland, in cooperation with the Center for Dermatology and Hair Disease Professor Trüeb.

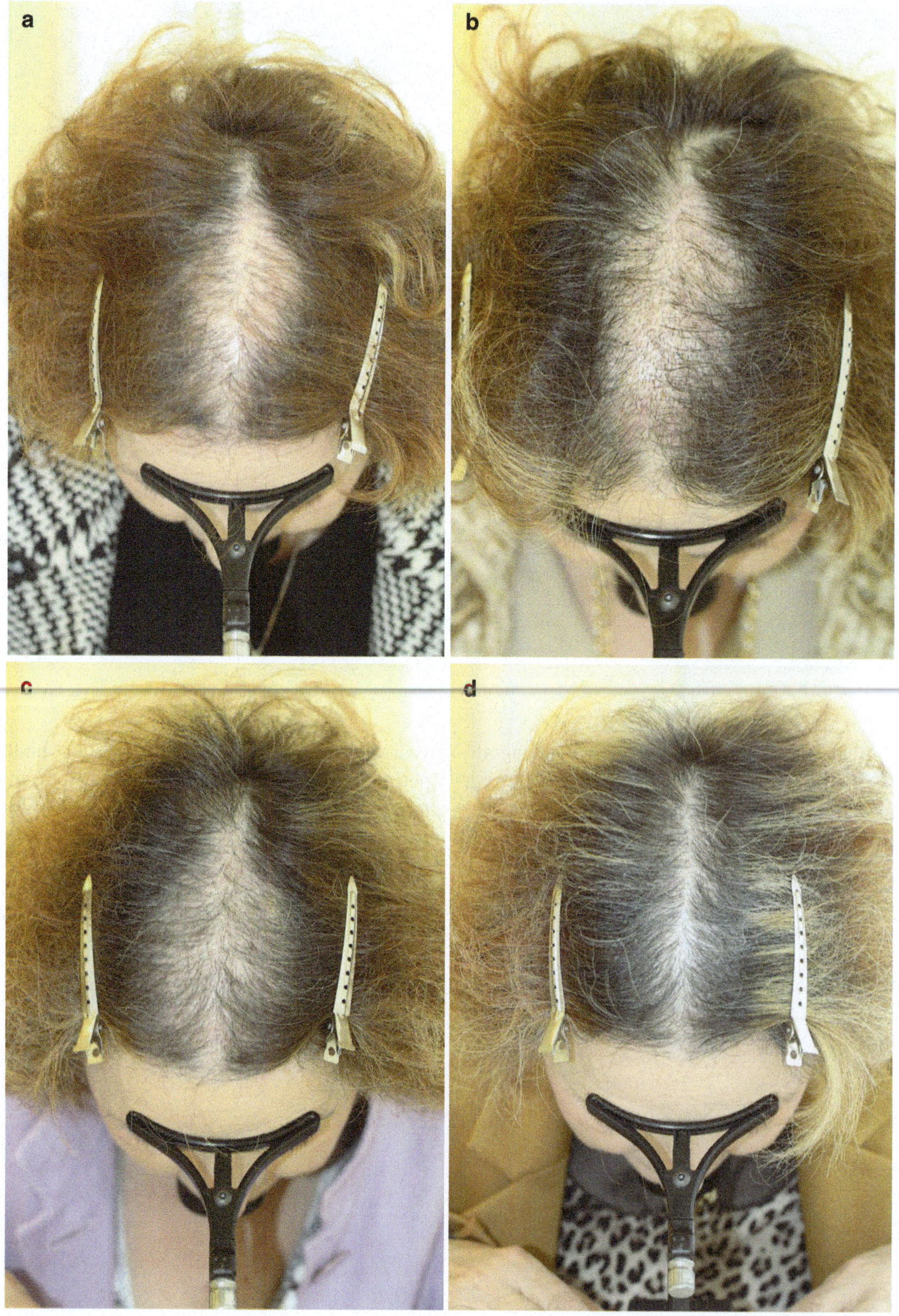

Fig. 9.46 (a–e)

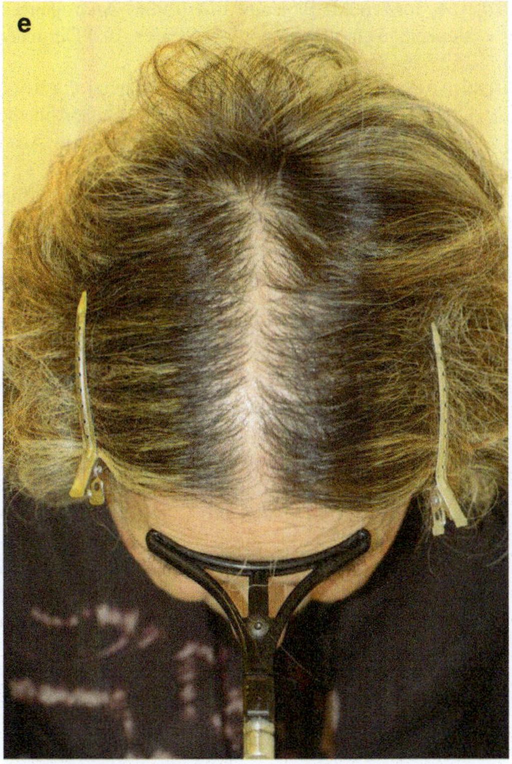

Fig. 9.46 (continued)

Further Reading

Acquiring the Basic Skills to Effective Treatment of Alopecia and Related Conditions

Carnagie D (1977) The quick & easy way to effective speaking. Modern techniques for dynamic communication. Pocket Books, a division of Simon & Schuster, Inc, New York

Trüeb RM (2013a) The difficult hair loss patient: a particular challenge. Int J Trichol 5(3):110–114

Trüeb RM (2013b) Female alopecia. Guide to successful management. Springer, Berlin/Heidelberg

Trüeb RM, Lee WS (2014) Male alopecia. Guide to successful management. Springer International Publishing, Cham

Case Studies

Blumeyer A, Tosti A, Messenger A et al (2011) Evidence-based (S3) guideline for the treatment of androgenetic alopecia in women and in men. J Dtsch Dermatol Ges 9(Suppl 6):S1–S57

D'Agostini F, Fiallo P, Pennisi TM, De Flora S (2007) Chemoprevention of smoke-induced alopecia in mice by oral administration of L-cystine and vitamin B6. J Dermatol Sci 46:189–198

Delamere FM, Sladden MM, Dobbins HM, Leonardi-Bee J (2008) Interventions for alopecia areata. Cochrane Database Syst Rev(2):CD004413

Friedli A, Labarthe MP, Engelhardt E, Feldmann R, Salomon D, Saurat JH (1998) Pulse methylprednisolone therapy for severe alopecia areata: an open prospective study of 45 patients. J Am Acad Dermatol 39:597–602

Gaffney DC, Sinclair RD, Yong-Gee S (2013) Discoid lupus alopecia complicated by frontal fibrosing alopecia on a background of androgenetic alopecia. Br J Dermatol 169(1):217–218

Gubelin Harcha W, Barboza Martínez J, Tsai TF et al (2014) A randomized, active- and placebo-controlled study of the efficacy and safety of different doses of dutasteride versus placebo and finasteride in the treatment of male subjects with androgenetic alopecia. J Am Acad Dermatol 70(3):489–498

Im M, Lee SS, Lee Y et al (2011) Prognostic factors in methylprednisolone pulse therapy for alopecia areata. J Dermatol 38(8):767–772

Iorizzo M, Vincenzi C, Voudouris S et al (2006) Finasteride treatment of female pattern hair loss. Arch Dermatol 142(3):298–302

Joly P (2006) The use of methotrexate alone or in combination with low doses of oral corticosteroids in the treatment of alopecia totalis or universalis. J Am Acad Dermatol 55:632–636

Kyei A, Bergfeld WF, Piliang M, Summers P (2011) Medical and environmental risk factors for the development of central centrifugal cicatricial alopecia: a population study. Arch Dermatol 147(8):909–914

Lonne-Rahm SB, Fischer T, Berg M (1999) Stinging and rosacea. Acta Derm Venereol 79(6):460–461

Mahé YF, Michelet JF, Billoni N et al (2000) Androgenetic alopecia and microinflammation. Int J Dermatol 39:576–584

Matard B, Meylheuc T, Briandet R et al (2012) First evidence of bacterial biofilms in the anaerobe part of scalp hair follicles: a pilot comparative study in folliculitis decalvans. J Eur Acad Dermatol Venereol 27:853–860

Munck A, Gavazzoni MF, Trüeb RM (2014) Use of low-level laser therapy as monotherapy or concomitant therapy for male and female androgenetic alopecia. Int J Trichol 6(2):45–49

Nakajima T, Inui S, Itami S (2007) Pulse corticosteroid therapy for alopecia areata: study of 139 patients. Dermatology 215:320–324

Navarini AA, Nobbe S, Trüeb RM (2009) Marie Antoinette syndrome. Arch Dermatol 145(6):656

Navarini AA, Trüeb RM (2010) 3 cases of dissecting cellulitis of the scalp treated with adalimumab: control of inflammation within residual structural disease. Arch Dermatol 146(5):517–520

Oberholzer PA, Nobbe S, Kolm I et al (2009) Red scalp disease–a rosacea-like dermatosis of the scalp? Successful therapy with oral tetracycline. Dermatology 219:179–181

Pericin M, Trüeb RM (1998) Topical immunotherapy of severe alopecia areata with diphenylcyclopropenone: evaluation of 68 cases. Dermatology 196:418–421

Rebora A (1987) Alopecia areata incognita: a hypothesis. Dermatologica 174:214–218

Sato-Kawamura M, Aiba S, Tagami H (2002) Acute diffuse and total alopecia of the female scalp. A new subtype of diffuse alopecia areata that has a favorable prognosis. Dermatology 205:367–373

Smith A, Trüeb RM, Theiler M et al (2015) Methylprednisolone pulse therapy for severe childhood alopecia areata. Ped Dermatol Apr 15 (Epub ahead of print)

Thai KE, Sinclair RD (2002) Finasteride for female androgenetic alopecia. Br J Dermatol 147:812–813

Thestrup-Pedersen K, Hjorth N (1987) Rod skalp. En ikke tidligere beskrevet harbundssygdom? Ugeskr Laeger 149:2141–2142

Tosti A, Iorizzo M, Botta GL, Milani M (2006) Efficacy and safety of a new clobetasol propionate 0.05% foam in alopecia areata: a randomized, double-blind placebo-controlled trial. J Eur Acad Dermatol Venereol 20:1243–1247

Tosti A, Iorizzo M, Piraccini BM (2005) Androgenetic alopecia in children: report of 20 cases. Br J Dermatol 152:556–559

Tosti A, Piraccini BM, Pazzaglia M, Vincenzi C (2003) Clobetasol propionate 0.05% under occlusion in the treatment of alopecia totalis/universalis. J Am Acad Dermatol 49:96–98

Trüeb RM (2007) Chemotherapy-induced anagen effluvium: diffuse or patterned? Dermatology 215:1–2

Trüeb RM (2014) North American Virginian witch hazel (Hamamelis virginiana)-based scalp care and protection for sensitive scalp, red scalp, and scalp burn-out. Int J Trichol 6(3):100–103

Trüeb RM, Navarini AA (2010) Thomas More syndrome. Dermatology 220(1):55–56

Trüeb RM, Pericin M, Hafner J, Burg G (1997) Tufted hair folliculitis. Hautarzt 48(4):266–269

Trüeb RM, Swiss Trichology Study Group (2004) Finasteride treatment of patterned hair loss in normoandrogenic postmenopausal women. Dermatology 209:202–207

Zinkernagel MS, Trüeb RM (2000) Fibrosing alopecia in a pattern distribution. Patterned lichen planopilaris or androgenetic alopecia with a lichenoid tissue reaction pattern? Arch Dermatol 136:205–211

10 Epilogue: Faith Healing

[9]My son, do not neglect yourself in sickness but pray to the Lord and he will heal you.
…
[12]Then give the physician his place for the Lord created him. Let him not depart from you for his works are necessary.
[13]For there is a time when you must fall into the hands of doctors
[14]and they will beseech the Lord that he bless what they prescribe to relieve and cure for your preservation.

Sirach (Ecclesiasticus) 38:9–14

Faith and knowledge lean largely upon each other in the practice of medicine.

Peter Mere Latham (1789–1875)

Faith healing is healing allegedly through spiritual means. Believers claim that the healing of a person can be brought about by religious faith through prayer and/or rituals that stimulate a divine presence and power toward healing disease. In common usage, faith healing refers to ritualistic practices of communal prayer and gestures, such as laying on of hands, which are claimed to mediate divine intervention in initiating spiritual and factual healing.

> Ultimately, belief in divine intervention in illness and healing is related to religious belief.

Claims that prayer, divine intervention, or the ministrations of an individual healer can cure illness have been popular throughout history, and healings have been reported in connection to prayer, a visit to a religious shrine, or simply a strong belief in a supreme being.

> Healing is referred to as miraculous, when a sick or injured person recovers unexpectedly and in ways that can't be explained medically.

By definition, an event is referred to as miraculous when it is not ascribable to human power or the laws of nature and consequently attributed to a supernatural, especially divine, agency. Such an event may be attributed to a miracle worker, Saint, or faith-based leader. Traditionally, theologians contend that, with divine providence, theistic gods work through created nature yet are free to work without, above, or against it as well.

In his *Tractatus Theologico-Politicus* (published in 1670), philosopher Baruch Spinoza

R.M. Trüeb, *The Difficult Hair Loss Patient: Guide to Successful Management of Alopecia and Related Conditions*, DOI 10.1007/978-3-319-19701-2_10

(1632–1677) challenged this view and claimed that miracles are merely lawlike events whose causes we are ignorant of. We should not treat them as having no cause or of having a cause immediately available.

> Rather the miracle is for combating the ignorance it entails, like a political project.

The miraculous healing of Naaman from his leprosy by the Prophet Elisha in the Old Testament, who advised him to go and wash himself seven times in the Jordan River, then his skin would be restored (2 Kings 5:1–19), may well be viewed today as balneophototherapy for a skin condition that might have been psoriasis rather than leprosy. Nonetheless, there remain a vast number of unexplained miraculous healings, referred to both in the Old and in the New Testaments or related to the visits of religious shrines.

Among the religious shrines with miraculous healing powers, the Sanctuary of Lourdes in France is one of the most prominent, with an estimated 200 million people having visited the shrine since 1860. The spring water from the grotto is believed to possess healing properties, and the Roman Catholic Church has officially recognized 69 healings as miraculous. Cures are examined using Church criteria for authenticity and authentic miracle healing with no physical or psychological basis other than the healing power of the site and water. In fact, the Sanctuary houses a Medical Bureau (Bureau des Constatations Médicales) with the function to transfer medical investigation of apparent cures associated with the shrine of Lourdes to the International Medical Committee of Lourdes (Comité Médical International de Lourdes, CMIL), which consists of an international panel of experts in various medical specialities and of different religious beliefs. CMIL meets annually. A full investigation requires that one of its members investigates every detail of a case in question and reviews the literature around the respective condition to warrant that up-to-date academic knowledge is applied to the final decision.

Traditionally, miraculous healings are believed to happen in response to prayer, and faith healing is best known in connection with Christianity. Specifically, some people interpret the Bible, especially the New Testament, as teaching belief in and practice of faith healing.

> According to New Age spirituality, it is also believed that pathways exist through which attitudes and emotions may have effects on physical health.

The New Age movement is a Western spiritual movement that developed in the second half of the twentieth century. Its central precepts have been described as drawing from both Western and Eastern spiritual and metaphysical traditions and combining them with influences from self-help and motivational psychology. The definition of spirituality (versus religion) relates to every person's inherent quest for ultimate meaning and purpose in life. That meaning can be found in religious belief but may also be broader to include a relationship with a divinity or transcendence, relationships with others, as well as spirituality found in nature, art, and rational thought. Accordingly, the concept of spirituality is found in all cultures and societies. In contrast, religion represents a system of beliefs and practices observed in a specific community and supported by particular rituals that acknowledge, worship, and communicate with or approach the Divine (in Western cultures) or the Ultimate (in Eastern cultures). Unlike faith healing, advocates of spiritual healing make no attempt to seek divine intervention, instead believing in divine energy.

> Either way, from the perspective of neuroscience, spiritual practices, even when stripped of religious beliefs, enhance the neural functioning of the brain in a way that may improve emotional and physical health.

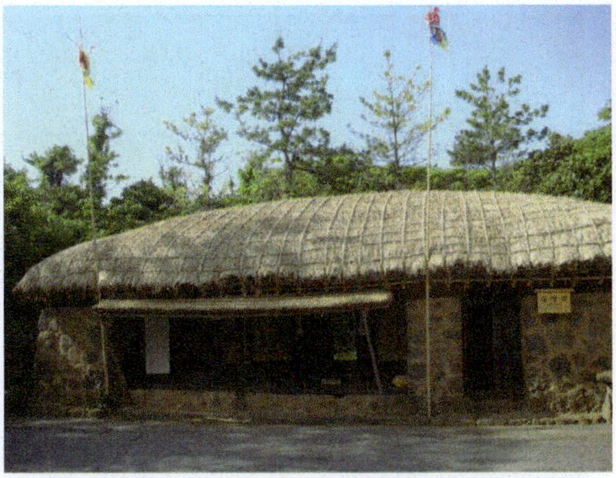

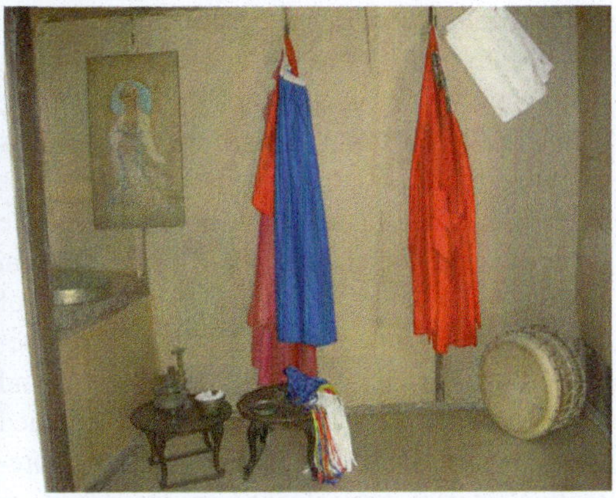

Fig. 10.1 Shaman's house and interior with paraphernalia, Jeju Folk Village, Jeju Island, Korea

10.1 Earliest Cultures

Intimate connection between medicine and religion has existed throughout history, with magic originally playing an important role. Illness was believed to result from malevolent spirits that entered a person, encroaching on vital functions and resulting in the specific features of the disease. Accordingly, treatments were directed at ridding the patient of these spirits in the form of dances, incantations, and sacrifices. These were performed by highly specialized practitioners, called shamans, who engaged in rituals to reach altered states of consciousness in order to encounter and interact with the world of spirits. Although the causes of disease were understood to lie in the spiritual realm, physical methods were also used to heal. Many shamans had expert knowledge of medicinal plants, and herbal treatments were often prescribed to accompany the spiritual incantations. In many places, shamans supposedly learned directly from the plants native to their area, harnessing their effects and healing properties, after obtaining permission from the indwelling spirits. Such practices are apparently very ancient, and Plato (428/427 or 424/423 BC–348/347 BC) wrote in his *Phaedrus* that the "first prophecies were the words of an oak" and that those who lived at that time found it rewarding enough to "listen to an oak or a stone, so long as it was telling the truth."

Today, shamanism survives primarily among some indigenous peoples all over the world (Fig. 10.1). Meanwhile, there is an attempt in some contemporary occult and esoteric circles to reinvent shamanism in a modern form.

The main criticism of modern Western or New Age forms of shamanism involves the notion of cultural appropriation, misrepresentation, and dilution of specific indigenous practices by taking pieces of diverse origins out of their respective cultural contexts and synthesizing them into a set of universal shamanic techniques.

European-based neo-shamanic traditions are focused upon the researched or imagined traditions of ancient Europe, where many mystical practices and belief systems were suppressed by the Christian Church. Some of these practitioners express a desire to practice a system that is based upon their proper ancestral traditions. Some anthropologists and practitioners have discussed the impact of such neo-shamanism as acknowledging indigenous American traditions.

Commonly used in Native American religion and practices, fetishes (derived from the French fétiche, which comes from the Portuguese feitiço, and this in turn from Latin facticius, "artificial" and facere "to make") represent man-made objects believed to have supernatural powers. Specifically, Zuni fetishes are small carvings made from various materials by the Zuni people. Traditionally, the materials used were indigenous to the region. Besides being made from various stones and other materials, each with its unique properties, the contemporary fetish may carry an offering of a smaller animal or a prayer bundle of carved arrowheads with small disk- or tube-shaped beads made of organic shells or ground and polished stones (heishe). It may be adorned with a heishe necklace, feathers, etchings representing ancient petroglyphs, or an etched or inlaid Heart line (Fig. 10.2). These small items are intended to protect and feed the fetish itself.

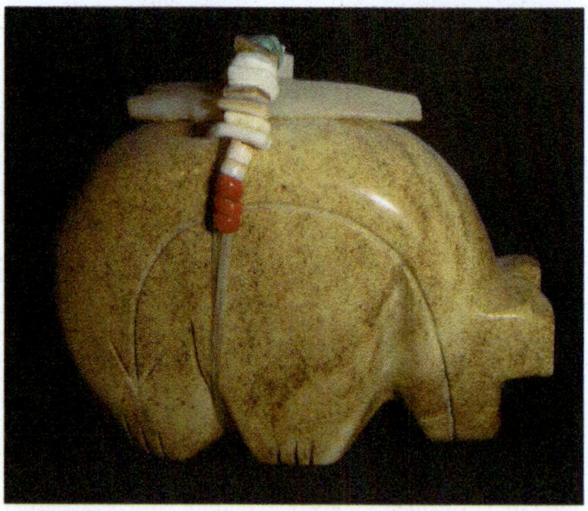

Fig. 10.2 Zuni Bear fetish with heishe necklace and etched Heart line, stone (Artist: Eloise Lee)

Typically, Zuni fetishes depict animals such as the wolf, badger, bear, mountain lion, eagle, mole, frog, deer, ram, and others. These carvings have traditionally served a ceremonial purpose for their creators and depict animals and icons integral to their culture. The bear represented the shaman, the buffalo was the provider, the mountain lion was the warrior, and the wolf was the pathfinder. In tradition, each animal is believed to have inherent powers or qualities that may aid the owner and is therefore also called "power animal."

> Power animals are common to shamanic practice. They are the helping or ministering spirit or familiar which empowers individuals and is essential for the success in any venture undertaken. In the shamanic worldview, most persons have power animals which empower and protect them from harm, like guardian spirits or Angels in the Abrahamic traditions. In these traditions, the power animal may also lend the wisdom or attributes of its kind to those under its protection.

According to Zuni mythology, the Bear fetish has the power to heal and transform human passions into wisdom. They believe that Bear is invaluable whenever one is faced with change or transition and that it can be one's ally when attempting to resolve conflict and forgive oneself or others for errors of the past or when faced with new challenges on the spiritual path. There is a particular kind of depression of the spirit sometimes associated with the deep introspective stage of transition and change. When this occurs, Bear is a reminder that there is a parallel between depression and the natural state known as hibernation, when involvement with the outer world is minimized in order to focus more energy on the inner processes necessary for a successful transition.

> Since the bear is associated with shamans in many traditions, this spirit animal can symbolize healing abilities and stepping into the role of the healer.

Initiates of the "Bear Society" in many Pueblo cultures become members of what might be called the equivalent of the American Medical Association. The "Bear Dance" is an ancient ritual once performed as a healing ceremony, where miraculous healing of mind, body, spirit, and soul has taken place (Fig. 10.3).

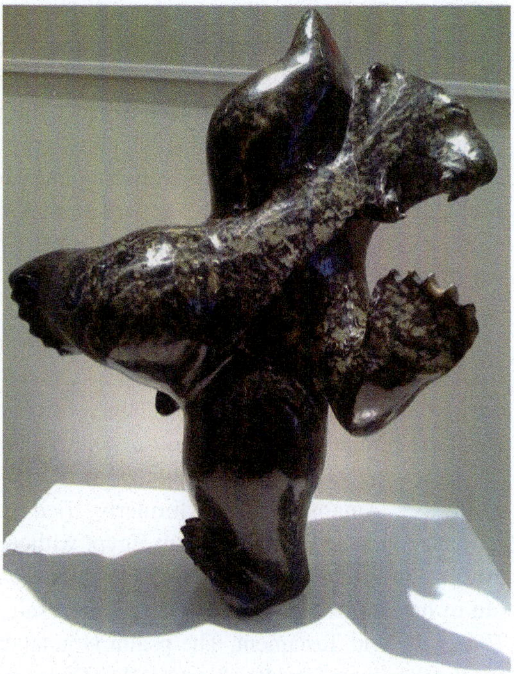

Fig. 10.3 Dancing Bear, serpentine, Inuit (Artist: Kulula Ituluk)

Ultimately, the Kaiser Permanente Center for Health Research in Portland, Oregon, conducted a phase 1 clinical study into the effectiveness of shamanic healing as treatment for chronic face and jaw pain. Twenty-three women diagnosed with temporomandibular joint disorder participated in the study. At the end of treatment only four were clinically diagnosed with the disorder present at the beginning of the study.

The medicine of ancient Egyptian is one of the oldest documented. Until the nineteenth century, the main sources of information about ancient Egyptian medicine were writings from later antiquity, with Greek historian Herodotus (484–425 BC), who visited Egypt 440 BC, being the most prominent to document his observations. Finally, in 1822, the translation of the Rosetta stone by French orientalist Jean-François Champollion (1790–1832) made the translation of the ancient Egyptian papyri possible, including many related to medical matters. A number of medical practices were effective, such as many of the surgical procedures reproduced in the Edwin Smith papyrus and the recommendations in the area of hygiene, such as to wash and shave the body, to look after diet, and circumcision of males. Egyptian medicine was a far-reaching discipline, including many fields, and enjoying an excellent reputation in the ancient world. Doctors in Egypt, like today, were specialists in their particular fields to include pharmacology, dentistry, gynecology, crude surgical procedures, general healing, autopsy, and embalming.

At the same time, the Egyptians held the belief that illness was caused by an angry god or an evil spirit. For this reason, the Egyptian doctor was also part shaman, who performed rituals and incantations for the ill.

There does not appear to have existed a clear distinction between what nowadays one would consider the very distinct callings of priest and physician.

Thus, an Egyptian suffering from an ailment would seek the services of many different types of healers, including priests. The impact of the emphasis on magic is seen in the selection of remedies or ingredients for them. Ingredients were sometimes selected seemingly because they were derived from a substance, plant, or animal that shared characteristics with the symptoms of the patient. For example, an amulet portraying a hedgehog might have been used against baldness. The Ebers papyrus is full of incantations and applications meant to turn away disease-causing demons. Again, religion and magic were an integral part of everyday life in ancient Egypt. Evil gods and demons were thought to be responsible for many ailments, so often the treatments involved a supernatural element, such as beginning treatment with an appeal to a deity. The Egyptian deity Thoth (Greek form of the Egyptian name Djehuty) was of central significance to Egyptian medicine (and magic), because of his

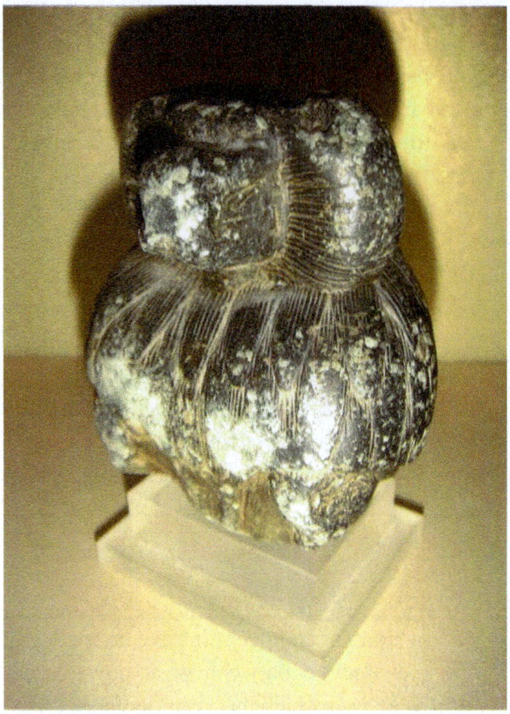

Fig. 10.4 Carved steatite baboon representing Thoth, Egypt, Late Period (712–332 BC)

role as the god of writing, of wisdom, and of balance. No less important to the art of healing was his special capacity to write and to recite what is written. For this reason, Thoth was commonly called upon in healing incantations. In art, he was often depicted as an ibis-headed scribe or as a baboon (Fig. 10.4). Thoth's chief temple was located in the city of Khmun, later called Hermopolis Magna during the Greco-Roman era, in reference to him through the Greeks' interpretation that he was equivalent to their god Hermes.

10.2 Old Testament

The Old Testament is the Christian term for the collection of religious writings by ancient Israelites. For the Israelites, the writings of the Old Testament told of their own unique relationship with God, but the overarching Messianic nature of Christianity has led Christians from the very beginning of faith to acknowledge the Old Testament as a preparation for the New Covenant and New Testament. The books of the Old Testament can be broadly divided into the Pentateuch, which tells how God selected Israel to be his chosen people; the history books telling the history of the Israelites from their conquest of Canaan to their defeat and exile in Babylon; the poetic and wisdom books dealing with questions of good and evil in the world; and the books of the Biblical Prophets, warning of the consequences of turning away from God.

The key feature that distinguished the Israelites from ancient Egypt and other Near Eastern cultures was their monotheism, the belief in only one God, though Egyptian Pharao Amenhotep IV, better known as Akhenaton (reign: 1353–1336 BC, Amarna Period), formerly tried to introduce monotheism in Ancient Egypt without avail, with striking similarities between the wording of his "Great Hymn to the Aten" and Psalm 104 in the Old Testament. The psalm is notable among the others for describing YHWH (Yahweh or Jehovah) explicitly as creator deity. German philosopher and theologian Johann Gottfried Herder (1744–1803) remarked, "It is worth studying the Hebrew language for ten years in order to read Psalm 104 in the original."

> In the Old Testament, Jehovah-Rapha, translated "I am the Lord your Physician" or "I am the Lord who heals you," is one of the seven redemptive names for Jehovah God.

Healing in the Bible is often associated with the ministry of specific individuals, including Abraham (Gen 20:1–18), Moses (Num 12:1–15), Elijah (1 Kings 17:17–24), and Elisha (2 Kings 4:8–17; 2 Kings 4:18–37; 2 Kings 5:1–14; and 2 Kings 13:21). Exodus 15:26 points to God as the source: "[26]If you will listen to the voice of the Lord your God, and obey it, and do what is right, then I will not make you suffer the diseases I sent on the Egyptians, for I am the Lord who heals you." Faith is trusting the God who heals. Another key distinction is the relationship between moral failure and illness. God's response to people for breaking his laws was to punish with sickness, though illness was not the only punishment. God also diminished resources, made the land barren, or sent enemies to attack in order to discipline his chosen people. The book of Deuteronomy consistently states that health and wealth are the rewards of God for obedience, whereas sickness and misfortune are his punishments. The Psalms, Proverbs, and the Prophets continue this theme.

When the Israelites set out from Mount Hor toward the Red Sea, they had to make a detour around the land of Edom (Num 20:21, 25). Frustrated and impatient, they complained against Jehova and Moses (Num 21:4–5), and God sent venomous snakes among them. For the sake of the repentant, Moses was instructed by God to erect a serpent of bronze (the Nehushtan) that was to be used to save those who looked upon it (Num 21:4–9). Eventually, King Hezekiah (reign: 715/716-687 BC) instituted a religious iconoclastic reform and "…broke up the bronze serpent that Moses had made, because the people of Israel had begun to worship it by burning incense to it; even though, as King Hezekiah pointed out to them, it was merely a piece of bronze" (2 Kings 18:4).

Ultimately, the serpent of bronze in Numbers 21 has become a well-known symbol to Christians because of referral to it by Jesus in the Gospel of John (John 3:14–15): "[14]And as Moses in the wilderness lifted up the bronze image of a serpent on a pole, even so I must be lifted up upon a pole, [15]so that anyone who believes in me will have eternal life." In this passage, Jesus obviously foresaw his forthcoming crucifixion and established the significance of the cross as spiritual healing from the curse of sin.

The worship of serpent deities is found in several ancient cultures, particularly in religion and mythology, where snakes were mostly regarded as entities of renewal and strength. Ancient Mesopotamians believed that snakes were immortal because they could shed their skin and appear forever youthful. Ancient Egyptians worshiped snakes, notably the cobra. Serpents could also be evil and harmful, as referenced in the "Book of the Dead," in which spell number 39 was made to call upon the repulsion of an evil snake into the netherworld: "Get back! Crawl away! Get away from me, you snake! Go, be drowned in the Lake of the Abyss, at the place where your father commanded that the slaying of you should be carried out." The patron goddess of Upper Egypt, Wadjet, was represented as a cobra-headed woman. She later became a protective emblem on the pharaoh's crown and was said to "spit fire" at the pharaoh's enemies. Another early depiction of Wadjet is a cobra entwined around a papyrus stem, beginning in the predynastic period (prior to 3100 BC), and thought to be the first image of a snake entwined around a staff symbol. Before the arrival of the Israelites, snake cults were well established in Canaan in the Bronze Age (c. 3300–1200 BC), since archaeologists have uncovered serpent cult objects in Bronze Age strata at several pre-Israelite sites in Canaan.

In Ancient Greece, a particular type of nonvenomous snake was used in healing rituals. In honor of the god of medicine and healing, these snakes were introduced at the founding of each new temple of Asclepius throughout the classical world. These snakes slithered around freely on the floor in dormitories where the sick and injured slept. From about 300 BC onward, the cult of Asclepius grew very popular and pilgrims flocked to these temples of healing (Asclepieia) to be cured of their ailments. To this day a species of nonvenomous pan-Mediterranean serpent, the Aesculapian snake (*Zamenis longissimus*), is named after the god.

The snake-entwined staff of Asclepius (the Asklepian) remains a symbol of medicine until today. The erroneous use—especially in the United States—of the staff with two snakes and wings carried by the Greek god Hermes (the Caduceus: Fig. 10.5), instead of the correct Asklepian with only a single snake, as a symbol of medicine originates from the adoption of the Caduceus as its insignia by the US Army Medical Corps in 1902.

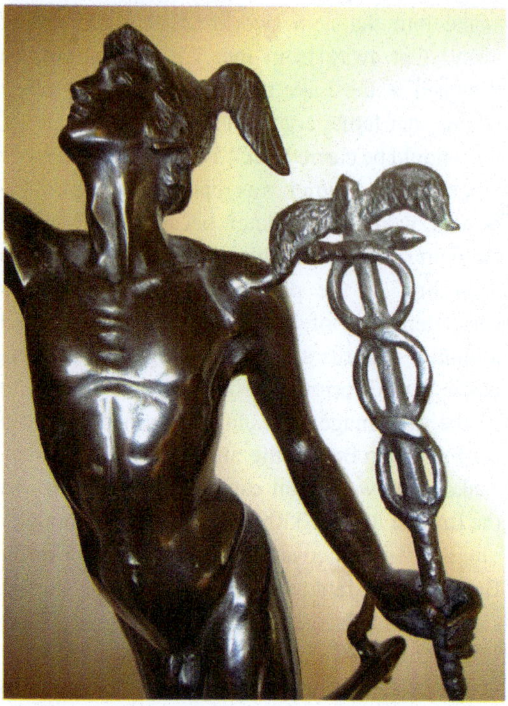

Fig. 10.5 Greek god Hermes holding Caduceus, bronze (From the author's desk)

Finally, taking up serpents or "snake handling" is a religious ritual still practiced in modern times in a small number of Pentecostal churches in rural areas of the United States, particularly the "Church of God with Signs Following." The practice is said to have originated in 1909 with "Church of God" preacher George Went Hensley (1880–1955) who became obsessed with a passage from the New Testament: "[18]They will be able to handle snakes with safety, …; and they will be able to place their hands on the sick and heal them" (Mark 16:18). Eventually, Hensley himself succumbed to a fatal snake bite sustained during a religious service.

10.3 New Testament

The New Testament is the second major part of the Christian biblical canon. Its contents deal explicitly with first-century Christianity. Therefore, the New Testament has frequently accompanied the spread of Christianity around the world and reflects and serves as a source for Christian theology.

> The number of specific healings recorded in the Old Testament bears no comparison with those recorded in the Gospels and Acts. In fact there are only twelve recorded in the four millennia of Old Testament history, far less than Jesus or his disciples sometimes achieved in a single day.

The types of healings seem to have a deeper symbolic meaning, such as cures from blindness (Matthew 9:27–31; Mark 10:46–52), deafness (Matthew 9:32–34), paralysis (Mark 2:1–12), and possession by demons (Mark 4:35; Mark 5:1–20), and a prerequisite for a miraculous healing was faith. The symbolism of symptoms bears remarkable analogies to the symptomatology patients with conversion disorder display, which today's psychoanalysists would attribute to the subconscious as they relate to the failing of the particular organ in question (i.e., hysterical blindness or paralysis).

Nevertheless, the Gospels also testify that Jesus cured physical ailments well outside the capacity of first-century medicine. Most dramatic perhaps is the case of "…a woman who had been sick for twelve years with a haemorrhage. [26]She had suffered much from many doctors through the years and had become poor from paying them, and was no better but, in fact, was worse. [27]She had heard all about the wonderful miracles Jesus did, and that is why she came up behind him through the crowd and touched his clothes" (Mark 5:26–27). Sure enough, as soon as she had touched him, the bleeding stopped and she knew she was well. After healing her, Jesus tells her, "Daughter, your faith has made you well; go in peace, healed of your disease" (Mark 5:34). In at least two more instances, Jesus credited the sufferer's faith as the means of being healed (Mark 10:52; Luke 19:10) but at the same time endorsed the use of medical assistance, when he praised the Good Samaritan for acting as a physician (Luke 10:33).

Jesus called his twelve disciples to him and gave them the authority to heal every kind of sickness and disease (Matthew 10:1). He told his followers to heal the sick and stated that signs such as healing are evidence of faith. Jesus also told his followers to "[8]Heal the sick, raise the dead, cure the lepers, and cast out demons" (Matthew 10:8). The apostle Paul believed healing is one of the special gifts of the Holy Spirit (1 Corinthians 12:9) and that the possibility exists that certain persons may possess this gift to an extraordinarily high degree. God gave Paul the power to do miracles to the extent "[12]so that even when his handkerchiefs or parts of his clothing were placed upon sick people, they were healed" (Acts 19:12), ultimately laying the basis to the cult of Relics in the Catholic and Orthodox Churches.

To the Protestant reformers Luther (1483–1546) and Calvin (1509–1564), the age of faith healing ended with the demise of the Apostles, and that view has prevailed in churches associated with the Reformation. Nevertheless, miraculous healing practices continue to prevail in the Catholic and Orthodox faiths and have been revived among certain Protestants by the Charismatic Movement and particularly the Pentecostals originating in the twentieth-century in the United States.

10.4 In Catholicism

The Roman Catholic Church represents one of the oldest religious institutions and has played a prominent role in modeling Western civilization. It maintains that it is the only true Church founded by Jesus Christ in the first century AD in the province of Judea of the Roman Empire. The New Testament records Jesus' activities and teachings, his appointment of the twelve Apostles, and his instructions to them to carry on his vocation. In an event known as Pentecost, the coming of the Holy Spirit upon the Apostles is understood to signal the beginning of the public ministry of the Catholic Church. Catholic doctrine teaches that the contemporary Catholic Church is the continuation of this early Christian community, that its bishops are the successors of the Christ's Apostles, and that the Pope, the Bishop of Rome, is the only successor to Saint Peter who has Apostolic primacy.

The earliest evidence of the use of the term Catholic Church is found in the "Letter to the Smyrnaeans" that Ignatius of Antioch wrote ca. 107 AD to Christians in Smyrna. Urging Christians to remain closely united with their bishop, he wrote: "Wherever the bishop shall appear, there let the multitude (of the people) also be; even as, wherever Jesus Christ is, there is the Catholic Church." From the second half of the second century AD, the word began to be used to mean non-heretical, "because Catholics claimed to teach the whole truth, and to represent the whole Church, while heresy arose out of the exaggeration of some one truth and was essentially partial and local." In 380, Roman Emperor Theodosius I (347–395 AD, reign from 379 to 395 AD) eventually limited the use of the term "Catholic Christian" exclusively to those who followed the same faith as Pope Damasus I of Rome (305–384 AD, papacy from 366 to 384 AD).

The Catholic Church defines its mission as spreading the Gospel of Jesus Christ, administering the Sacraments (Baptism, Eucharist, Reconciliation, Confirmation, Marriage, Holy Orders, and Anointing of the Sick), and exercising charity. Catholic worship is highly liturgical, focusing on the Mass (or Divine Liturgy) in which the sacrament of the Eucharist (or Holy Communion) is celebrated. The Catholic Church practices closed communion, and only baptized members of the Church in a state of grace are customarily recognized to receive the Eucharist. Catholic social teaching emphasizes support for the sick, the poor, and the afflicted through the corporal works of mercy.

> Suffering is essential to the Christian view of the world, and it leads to spiritual renewal.

This view suggests an unavoidable tension between the fate of the soul and the fate of the body. The former is the realm of theology, and the latter of medicine. Nevertheless, throughout the history of Christianity, care for disease and suffering by a physician has been understood not only as appropriate but as a vocation, since the physician is viewed as an instrument of God. This position is consistent with the practice, beginning in the fourth century, of monastic clergy establishing hospitals and facilities for the needy and the old. This approach promoted practical treatment of disease. At the same time, however, and in contrast to this more pragmatic approach to providing relief for the suffering, accounts of miraculous healings began to emerge, many with the use of relics representing the Saints.

The Catholic Church, in particular, holds the Blessed Virgin Mary, as mother of Jesus Christ, in special regard and reveres in its "Apostles' Creed" the community of Saints.

> Miracle healings have allegedly taken place at the sites of apparitions of the Blessed Virgin Mary, such as Lourdes, or by intercession of the Saints.

A Saint (from Latin *sanctus*) is an individual who has fulfilled the criteria set for sainthood by a religious institution. Though the term is mostly commonly used in Christianity, the concept also may apply to other religions. The Roman Catholic Church has more than 10,000 Saints. While some may assume that honoring Saints is something the Church set up later, in fact, it was part of Christianity from the beginning. The first Christian Saints were martyrs who had sacrificed their lives for their faith during the persecution of Christians. Starting with the first martyrs of the early Christian Church, Saints were chosen by public acclaim. Though this was a more democratic way to recognize saints, some Saints' stories were distorted by legend, and some never existed. Gradually, the bishops and finally the Vatican took over authority for approving Saints. Canonization, the process the Church uses to nominate a Saint, has only been introduced in the tenth century. The process begins after the death of a Catholic whom people regard as holy, often many years after death in order to give perspective on the candidate. The local bishop investigates the candidate's life and writings for heroic virtue or martyrdom and orthodoxy of doctrine. Then a panel of theologians at the Vatican evaluates the candidate. After approval by the panel and cardinals of the Congregation for the Causes of Saints, the Pope proclaims the candidate "venerable." The next step, "beatification," requires evidence of a miracle (except in the case of martyrs). Since miracles are considered proof that the person is in heaven and can intercede for us, the miracle must take place after the candidate's death and as a result of a specific petition to the candidate. Only after one more miracle will the Pope canonize the Saint (this includes martyrs as well). The title of Saint tells us that the person lived a holy life, is in heaven, and is to be honored by the universal Church.

Christian hagiography deals with the account of the Saints' lives and passion, and Christian iconography with the Saints' depiction in religious art. Most Catholic churches are full of images of Saints—in stained glass windows, sculptures, murals, and mosaics. Appreciation of religious art is deepened by knowledge of what is depicted and why, and that includes all the mysterious figures carrying various objects and dressed in different ways. Saints are only sometimes labeled with their names. The clues to their identity are rather given in their appearance or in what they are holding. These objects may be the instruments of martyrdom, representations of events in their lives, or symbols of their teachings and are called the Saint's attributes.

Roman Catholic tradition has made Saints the patrons or protectors of various aspects of human life, and they are invoked for particular reasons. A patron Saint is regarded as an advocate in heaven of a craft, activity, or person.

> Patron Saints, because they have already transcended to the metaphysical, are believed to be able to intercede effectively for the needs of their special charges.

Some consider it a special devotion to God by displaying humility in asking a Saint for intercession rather than expecting to be answered themselves. Intercessory prayer may also be a petition made to God on behalf of others. The doctrine of Saintly intercession goes back to the earliest church. They point to such scriptural passages as Tobit 13:12–15; Revelation 5:8; Revelation 8:3–4, which depicts heavenly beings offering the prayers of mortals before God; and James 5:16, where all those in heaven can be presumed to be living righteously, which states the prayer of the righteous is powerful and effective. The justification for calling upon a Saint in prayer is that the Saints are both close to God, because of their holiness, and accessible to humans. Historically, the belief matched the earthly patterns of patron–client relations that were the normal way of attempting to deal with the bureaucracy of the later Roman Empire and the very personal governmental processes of the Middle Ages. The Saints were seen as God's courtiers in a Heaven that was often imagined as resembling somewhat the courts of earthly rulers.

The number of protector Saints for the medical profession, specifically the "Anargyroi" (Greek for "Unmercenaries," i.e., Saints who received no payment for their medical services), and for dermatologic conditions is large. The affiliation of a protector Saint to specific condition usually relates to actual facts in the lives of the saints and their depiction in Christian iconography, e.g., St. Lawrence is invoked for burns because he was put to death by being roasted on a gridiron, and St. Bartholomew is invoked for skin diseases since images of his martyrdom depict him with his skin draped over his arm. St. Mary Magdalene is patron Saint for hairdressers. Surprisingly, there is no existing protector Saint for hair loss or trichologists, though St. Agnes of Rome would seem a worthy candidate: According to the *Legenda Aurea* (Golden Legend) of Jacobus de Voragine (1230–1298), St. Agnes of Rome was a member of the Roman nobility born 291 and raised in a Christian family. She suffered martyrdom during the reign of the Roman Emperor Diocletian (284–305), on January 21, 304. The Prefect Sempronius wished Agnes to marry his son, and on Agnes' refusal he condemned her to death. As Roman law did not permit the execution of virgins, Sempronius dragged Agnes naked through the streets to a brothel. As she prayed, her hair grew and covered her body. When led out to die she was tied to a stake, but the bundle of wood would not burn, whereupon the officer in charge of the troops drew his sword and beheaded her, or, in some other texts, stabbed her in the throat. In the fourth century, Constantia, the daughter of the Roman Emperor Constantine (reign 312–337), built a basilica on the site of her tomb. Agnes' bones are conserved in the church of Sant' Agnese fuori le mura in Rome, built over the catacomb that housed Agnes' tomb. Her skull is preserved in a side chapel in the church of Sant' Agnese in Agone in Rome's Piazza Navona.

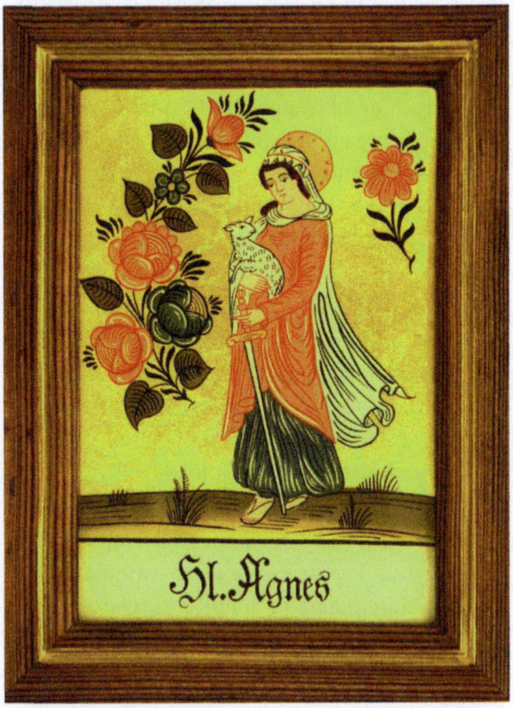

Fig. 10.6 St. Agnes of Rome, reverse glass painting with gold leaf, Tyrolean, contemporary

In Christian iconography, St. Agnes is depicted with long and beautiful hair and a lamb as her attribute (Fig. 10.6), since her name resembles the Latin word "agnus," which means "lamb." The name is actually derived from the Greek word "agnon" meaning "chaste, pure, sacred." In the past, her feast day was the occasion for the blessing of the lambs, whose wool was used by the nuns of Saint Agnes in Rome to weave the palliums of archbishops. Traditionally, St. Agnes of Rome is regarded patron saint of chastity, girls, betrothed women (she chose Christ as her betrothed), rape victims, virgins, and gardeners, since virginity is symbolized as a closed garden.

In fact, St. Agnes of Rome seems most appropriate as protector Saint for women with hair loss and patron Saint for trichologists on the basis of (1) her historic *passio* (miraculous growth of long hair); (2) her attribute in Christian iconography (the lamb, notably the Australian Hair and Wool Research Society is one of the original and major international, nonprofit organization bringing together premier doctors and scientists involved in treatment and research of hair disorders); and (3) her feast day on January 21st, when seasonal hair growth is peaking at its maximum.

Yet another Saint whose legend is relevant to the act of miraculous healing is Veronica. According to Roman Catholic tradition, St. Veronica was a pious woman of Jerusalem in the first century AD. When she saw Jesus carrying his cross to Golgotha, she was moved with pity and gave him her veil that he might wipe his forehead. The event is commemorated by the Sixth Station of the Stations of the Cross. Jesus accepted the offering, held it to his face, and then handed it back to her with the image of his face then miraculously impressed upon it. This piece of cloth became known as the Veil of Veronica. In his "History of the Church," Roman historian and exegete Eusebius (260/265–339/340 AD) gives account how at Caesarea Philippi lived the woman whom Christ healed of an issue of bleeding (Mark 5:26–27). Legend was not long in providing the woman of the Gospel with a name. In the West she was identified with Martha of Bethany, and in the East she was called Berenike, a name meaning "bearer of victory" and appearing in as early a work as the "Acts of Pilate" (from the apocryphical "Gospel of Nicodemus"). The section about Pilate is a purported official document composed of accounts from the praetorium at Jerusalem reporting events in Judea to Emperor Tiberius (reign: 4–37 AD) referring to the crucifixion of Jesus, and his miracles. The name "Veronica" itself is a Latinization of Berenike. Folk etymology has attributed its origin to the words for true (Latin: vera) and image (Greek: eicon).

Little is known about the fate of Pilate, but tradition has filled the gap with a body of legend. Eusebius quotes some early apocryphal accounts, which relate that Pilate fell under misfortunes during the reign of Caligula (37–41), was exiled to Gaul and eventually committed suicide there in Vienne. Other details come from less credible sources. His body, says the Mors Pilati ("Death of Pilate"), was thrown first into the Tiber, but the waters were so "disturbed by evil spirits" that the body was taken to Vienne and sunk in the river Rhône. As the waters of the Rhône likewise rejected Pilate's corpse, the corpse's final disposition was in a deep and lonely mountain tarn, which, according to later tradition, was on a mountain, still called Pilatus (actually pileatus or "cloud capped"), overlooking Lucerne, Switzerland (Fig. 10.7). Every Good Friday, the body is said to re-emerge from the waters and wash its hands.

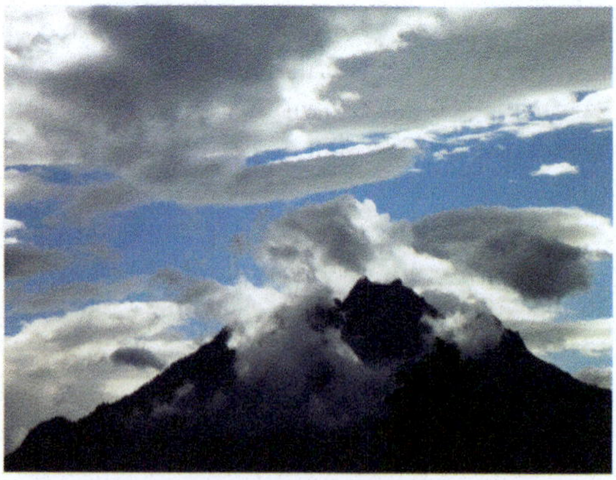

Fig. 10.7 Mount Pilatus, Switzerland (With courtesy of Thomas Trüeb, President of the Synodical Council of the Roman Catholic Church of Lucerne 2014 and 2015)

There is no reference to the story of St. Veronica and her veil in the canonical Gospels. The closest is the miracle of the woman who was healed by touching the hem of Jesus' garment, whose name was later identified as Veronica by the apocryphal "Acts of Pilate." The story was later elaborated in the eleventh century by adding that Christ gave her a portrait of himself on a cloth. According to some versions, St. Veronica later traveled to Rome to present the cloth to the Roman Emperor Tiberius whom she cured from an ailment by virtue of the miraculous properties of the Veil.

Ultimately St. Veronica was mentioned in the reported visions of Jesus by Sister Marie of St. Peter (1816–1848), a Carmelite nun who lived in Tours, France, and started the devotion to the Holy Face of Jesus. In 1844, Sr. Marie reported that in a vision, she saw St. Veronica wiping away with her veil the spit and mud from the face of Jesus on his way to Calvary. She said that sacrilegious and blasphemous acts today are adding to the spit and mud that St. Veronica wiped away that day. According to Sr. Marie of St. Peter, in her visions Jesus told her that he desired devotion to His Holy Face in reparation for sacrilege and blasphemy. The Devotion to the Holy Face of Jesus was eventually approved by Pope Leo XIII in 1885.

Today, there exist at least six images which bear a marked resemblance to each other and which are claimed to be the original Veil, or a direct copy of it. Each is enclosed in an elaborate outer frame with a gilded metal sheet within, in which is cut an aperture where the face appears. At the lower extreme of the face there are three points which correspond to the shape of the hair and beard of the Christ.

To distinguish at Rome the oldest and best known of these images, it has been called the vera icon (true image), which in common tongue soon became "Veronica." Nevertheless, in 1999, German Jesuit Father Heinrich Pfeiffer, Professor of Art History at the Pontifical Gregorian University, challenged the authenticity of the Veil at Rome and announced at a press conference that he had found the true Veil in a church of a Capuchin monastery in the small village of Manoppello, Italy, where it had been since 1660. According to local belief, an anonymous pilgrim arrived in 1508 with the cloth inside a wrapped package. The pilgrim gave it to Doctor Giacomo Antonio Leonelli, a physicist famous in astrology and other liberal arts, who was sitting on a bench in front of the church. Leonelli went into the church and opened the parcel containing the Veil. At once he went out of the church but he did not find the bearer of the packet.

In religion, a relic usually consists of the physical remains or personal effects of a Saint preserved for purposes of veneration as a tangible memorial. The word relic comes from the Latin *reliquiae*, meaning "remains" or "something left behind" (the same root as relinquish). One of the earliest sources that purports to show the efficacy of relics is found in 2 Kings 13:20–21: "So Elisha died and was buried. In those days bandits gangs of Moabites used to invade the land in each spring. Once some men who were burying a friend spied these marauders and so they hastily through his body in the tomb of Elisha. And as soon as the body touched Elisha's bones, the dead man revived and jumped to his feet!"

With regard to relics that are objects, an often cited passage is Acts 19:11–12, which says that Paul's handkerchiefs were imbued by God with healing power.

Many tales of miracles were attributed to relics beginning in the early centuries of the Church. These became popular during the Middle Ages. These miracle tales made relics much sought after during the Middle Ages. By the late Middle Ages the collecting of, and eventually dealing in, relics had reached such proportions that, in the absence of real ways of assessing authenticity, relic-collectors became prey to the unscrupulous, and some extremely high prices were paid for forgeries.

Early on, Augustine (354–430 AD) denounced impostors making a profit from the sale of spurious relics. Later, Charlemagne (742/747/748–814) ordered that "the false names of martyrs and the uncertain memorials of Saints should not be venerated," and in the Fourth Lateran Council in 1215 the Church condemned such abuses such as counterfeit relics and exaggerated claims. Finally, the Council of Trent of 1563 enjoined bishops to instruct their flocks that "the holy bodies of holy

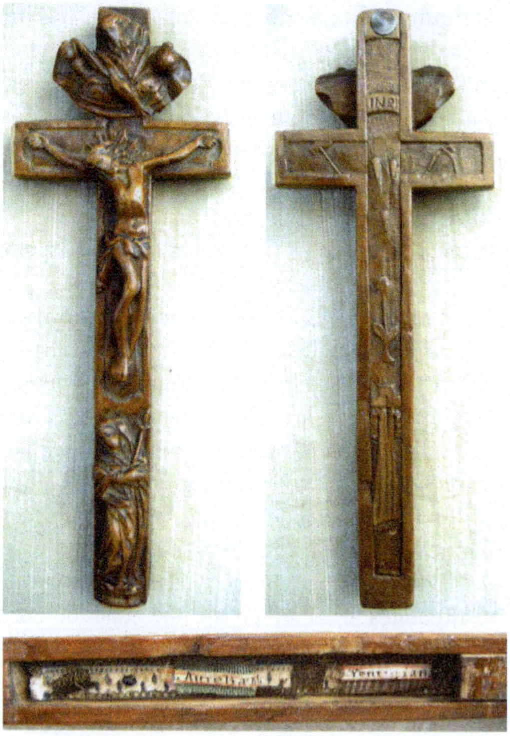

Fig. 10.8 Reliquary, Roman Catholic, Southern Germany, ca. 1800

martyrs … are to be venerated by the faithful, for through these (bodies) many benefits are bestowed by God on men," while "in the invocation of Saints, the veneration of relics and the sacred use of images, every superstition shall be removed and all filthy lucre abolished." Eventually, sixteenth-century reformers such as Martin Luther (1483–1546) opposed the use of relics since many had no proof of historic authenticity, and they eventually objected even to the cult of Saints.

A reliquary is a container for the Holy relics (Fig. 10.8). These may be the physical remains of Saints, such as bones, pieces of clothing, or some object associated with Saints or other religious figures.

> Reliquaries provide a means of protecting and displaying relics, which many believe are endowed by God with the grace of miraculous powers.

The use of reliquaries became an important part of Christian practices from at least the fourth century on and is venerated in the Oriental Orthodox, Eastern Orthodox, Roman Catholic, and some Anglican Churches. They range in size from simple pendants or rings to coffin-like containers, to very elaborate ossuaries. Many were designed with portability in mind, often being exhibited in public or carried in procession on the Saint's feast day or on other holy days. Pilgrimages often centered around the veneration of relics. The faithful often venerate relics by bowing before the reliquary or kissing it. Those churches which observe the veneration of relics make a clear distinction between the honor given to the Saints and the worship that is due to God alone.

10.5 In Other Confessions

The Eastern Orthodox Church also identifies itself as the present-day continuation of the theology and episcopacy established by Jesus Christ through his Apostles, and traces its development back to the earliest church established by St. Paul and the Apostles, through the ancient Roman Empire and its continuation in the Byzantine Empire. Today it represents the second largest Christian church with an estimated 225–300 million adherents, primarily in Eastern Europe, especially Greece and Southeastern Europe, throughout the Middle East and across Russia. The Church's structure is composed of several self-governing ecclesial bodies, each geographically and often nationally distinct but unified in theology and worship.

A form of religious art peculiar to the Orthodox Church, is the icon. The Orthodox believe that the first icons of Christ and the Virgin Mary were painted by Luke the Evangelist. In the icon-painting Christian traditions, the icon is generally a flat panel painting depicting Jesus, Mary, the Saints, Angels, or the Holy Cross. In stark contrast to pagan art, creating free-standing, three-dimensional sculptures of holy figures was resisted by Christian tradition throughout centuries out of the belief that demons inhabited the respective sculptures. In obedience to the commandment to withhold producing graven images, Orthodox icons may never exceed three-quarter bas relief. Icons are filled with symbolism and tend to be formulaic, following a prescribed methodology for how a particular person should be depicted, including hairstyle, body position, clothing, and background details. Therefore, icon painting is not primarily an opportunity for artistic expression.

In the Eastern Orthodox Christian tradition there are reports of particular, wonderworking icons that emanate myrrh (a fragrant oil believed to be Holy), or perform miracles upon petition by believers. They are understood as miracles performed by God through the interception of the respective Saint depicted on the icon, rather than result from magical properties of the painted wood itself.

Therefore, all icons are considered to be sacred from a theological point of view, and are supposed to be miraculous by nature, at the same time representing a means of spiritual communion between the earthly and heavenly realms.

Two Saints with peculiarities relating to the hair, one female and the other male, frequently found on icons of the Eastern Orthodox Church are St. Mary of Egypt and St. Onuphrius. In both, long hair covers their body. In a spiritual context, hair has been recognized to have two perceived symbolic meanings: long, uncut hair is seen as a withdrawal from worldly concern and vanities, while shaven hair is a symbol of celibacy and chastity. The symbolism of hair in Christian iconography has previously been discussed by Navarini and Trüeb in "Beneath the nimbus—the hair of the Saints."

St. Mary of Egypt was born in Egypt and at the early age of twelve left her home for the city of Alexandria where for upward of 17 years she lived an extremely dissolute life. Some authorities refer to her as a public prostitute during this period, but in her *Vita* she states that she often refused the money offered for her sexual favors. She said she was driven by an insatiable desire and an irrepressible passion, and that she mainly lived by begging, supplemented by spinning flax. On the occasion of a pilgrimage to Jerusalem for the Feast of the Exaltation of the Holy Cross, she embarked for Palestine, not however with the intention of making the pilgrimage, but with the prospect that on board the ship she would encounter numerous men to pay for her passage by offering her sexual favors. On the Feast of the Exaltation of the Cross, she joined the crowds toward the church where the sacred relic was venerated, hoping to encounter in the gathering new victims whom she might allure into sin. The turning point in her life came when she tried to enter the Church of the Holy Sepulchre for the celebration and was barred from doing so by an unseen force. Realizing that this was because of her impurity, she was struck with remorse, and on seeing an icon of the Virgin Mary outside the church, she prayed for forgiveness and promised to become an ascetic. Then she attempted again to enter the church, and this time was permitted in. Having adored the Holy Cross and kissed the pavement of the church, she returned to the icon to give thanks, and while praying there for guidance as to her future course, she heard a voice telling her that if she crossed the Jordan, she would find rest. That same evening Mary reached the Jordan and received absolution and afterward Holy Communion in the monastery dedicated to St. John Baptist on the bank of the River Jordan. The following day she crossed the river and wandered eastward into the desert that stretches toward Arabia to live the rest of her life as a hermit in penitence. Here she had lived absolutely alone for 47 years, when the monk and priest St. Zosimas of Palestine, who had come out from his monastery to spend Lent in the desert, unexpectedly encountered her. She was completely naked and almost unrecognizable as human. As soon as they met, she called Zosimas by his name and recognized him as a priest. She asked him for his mantle to cover herself with, and then she narrated the strange and romantic story of her life to him manifesting marvelous clairvoyance. On returning to the monastery, Zosimas related her life story to the brethren, and it was preserved among them as oral tradition until it was written down by St. Sophronius (560–638).

St. Onuphrius was one of the Desert Fathers who made such a deep impression on Eastern spirituality, around the time that Christianity was emerging as the dominant faith in the Roman Empire of the third and fourth centuries. At the time, Christians felt compelled to go out into the bearness of the desert to live in prayer in a harsh environment of extreme heat and cold, with little to eat or drink, and surrounded by dangerous animals and robbers. It is uncertain when Onuphrius exactly lived. The account of Paphnutius the Ascetic, who encountered him in the Egyptian desert, forms the sole source for our knowledge of the life of St. Onuphrius. According to this account, Paphnutius undertook a pilgrimage to study the hermits' way of life. Wandering through the desert, on the 17th day, Paphnutius came across a wild figure covered in hair and only with a loincloth of leaves. Frightened, Paphnutius fled, but the figure called him back, crying: "Come down to me, man of God, for I am a man also, dwelling in the desert for the love of God." Paphnutius turned back to the wild figure, who introduced himself as Onuphrius and explained that he once had been a monk at a large monastery in the Thebaid, but now had lived the life of a hermit for 70 years, enduring extreme thirst, hunger, and all the discomforts of the desert. He further explained that it was his guardian Angel who had brought him to this desolate place. Paphnutius accompanied Onuphrius to his hermit's cell, and they conversed until sunset, when bread and water miraculously was found on the outside of the cell. They spent the night together in prayer, and in the morning Paphnutius discovered that Onuphrius was near death. Paphnutius asked the hermit if he should occupy his cell after his death, but Onuphrius told him "that may not be, thy work is in Egypt with thy brethren." Onuphrius though asked Paphnutius for a memorial with incense in Egypt in remembrance of him, then blessed the traveler, and finally passed away. Due to the rocky ground, Paphnutius could not dig a grave, and therefore covered Onuphrius' body in a cloak, leaving the hermit's body in a cleft among the rock. At that moment, Onuphrius' cell crumbled, which Paphnutius understood to be a sign that he should not remain. Images of St. Onuphrius were conflated with those of the medieval "wild man." In art, he is depicted as a wild man covered with hair or a long beard and wearing a girdle of leaves (Fig. 10.9).

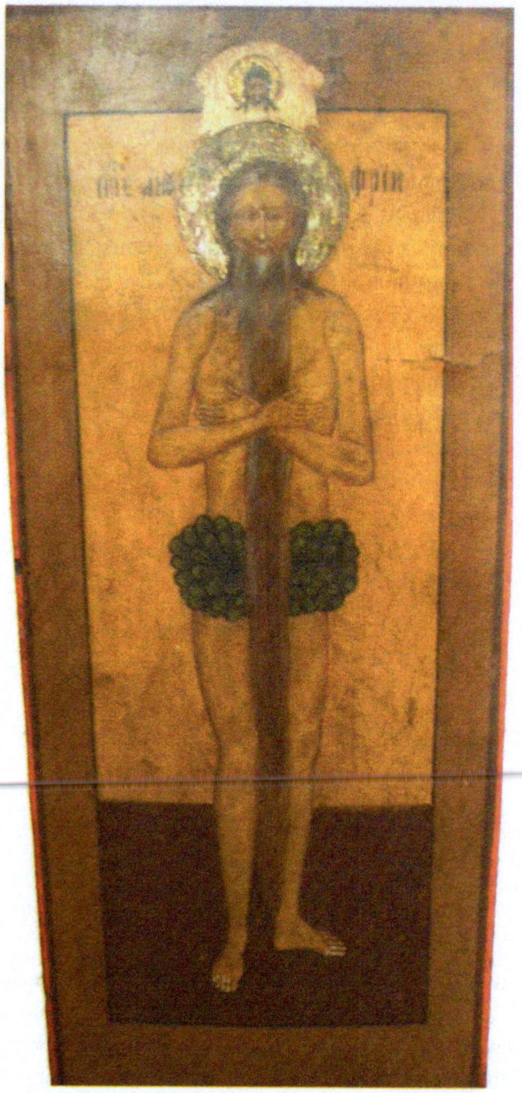

Fig. 10.9 Icon of Saint Onuphrius, Russian Orthodox, Russia, eighteenth century

Christianity in Ethiopia dates back to the first century AD, and this long tradition makes Ethiopia unique among the sub-Saharan African countries. The earliest and best known reference to the introduction of Christianity in Ethiopia is in the New Testament (Acts 8:26–38), when Philip the Evangelist converted an Ethiopian court official in the first century AD. After being shipwrecked and captured at early age, Frumentius (died ca. 383, Ethiopia) was carried to Axum where he was treated well. At the time, there was a small population of Christians living there who sought refuge from Roman persecution. Once of age, Frumentius was allowed to return to his homelands; however, he chose to stay at the request of the queen. In doing so, he began to promote Christianity through the lands. During a trip to meet with church elders, Frumentius met with Athanasius, Archbishop of Alexandria (296/298–373) who was second in line to the Pope. After recommending that a bishop be sent to proselytize, a council decided that Frumentius be appointed as bishop to Ethiopia. By 331 AD, Frumentius returned to Ethiopia, where he was welcomed with open arms by the rulers who were at the time not yet Christian. Ten years later, through the support of the kings, the majority of the kingdom was converted and Christianity was declared the official state religion. Finally, with the emergence of Islam in the seventh century, Ethiopia's Christians became isolated from the rest of the Christian world, being the only region of Africa to survive the expansion of Islam as a Christian state.

While the West understands medicine and art to represent separate realms, Ethiopians consider them to be closely connected. Challenging our narrow view on art, Ethiopians deem artworks to be active forces that ensure health. The power of Ethiopian artworks to heal believers reveals an interrelationship between art and religious faith, and their effect on physical and mental health. In Ethiopia, customized protective scrolls that entwine sacred imagery with textual prayers have been prescribed by traditional healers for over 2000 years. These were carried by the individual to whom they were specifically given to shield them from harm. The iconography of the scrolls includes representations of Saints and of talismanic seals that were modeled on the seal of God revealed to King Solomon. The respective seals feature geometric patterns and stylized representations of multiple faces or eyes that indicate prayers for divine intervention. Healing scrolls usually have the form of long, narrow, and often segmented, vertical strips of parchment covered with handwritten texts (protective prayers, and spell-casting formulas) combined with the aforementioned images. The parchment used for healing scrolls was made from the skin of a sheep that was sacrificed for the benefit of the patient. The scroll had to match the patient's height to protect him from head to toe. Its contents are prayers against demons or possessing spirits, lines from Gospels, petitions to the Saints for protection, and recitations of the various names of God. The texts alternate with visual images, such as Angels, demonic faces with large staring eyes, a grid with a central face, and the net of Solomon, with which the Biblical king caught demons (Fig. 10.10). What is apparent in every detail of the object is a believed-in vivacity that was created to generate live spiritual power in the material world. Out of this reason, devotees would carry healing scrolls everywhere during the day and at night would hang them spread out on the walls of their homes.

> In all religious traditions, written or graphic inscriptions are endowed with sacred attributes, for they are considered both the embodiment of the Divine and a powerful means for transmitting religious teachings. The capacity of the written word to bring about change in people's lives lends itself to contexts of divination, healing, and other forms of spiritual mediation, in addition to prayer, devotion, and states of heightened awareness.

To understand healing from the perspective of the Eastern Religions, a useful starting point is to consider the Eastern concept of mind. The mind is nonphysical, and its nature is pure, limitless, and all-encompassing, like the sun shining without obstruction in a clear sky. The problems or sickness we experience are like clouds in the sky obscuring the sun. Just as the clouds temporarily block the sun but are not of the same nature as the sun, our problems and sickness are temporary and the causes of them can be removed from the mind.

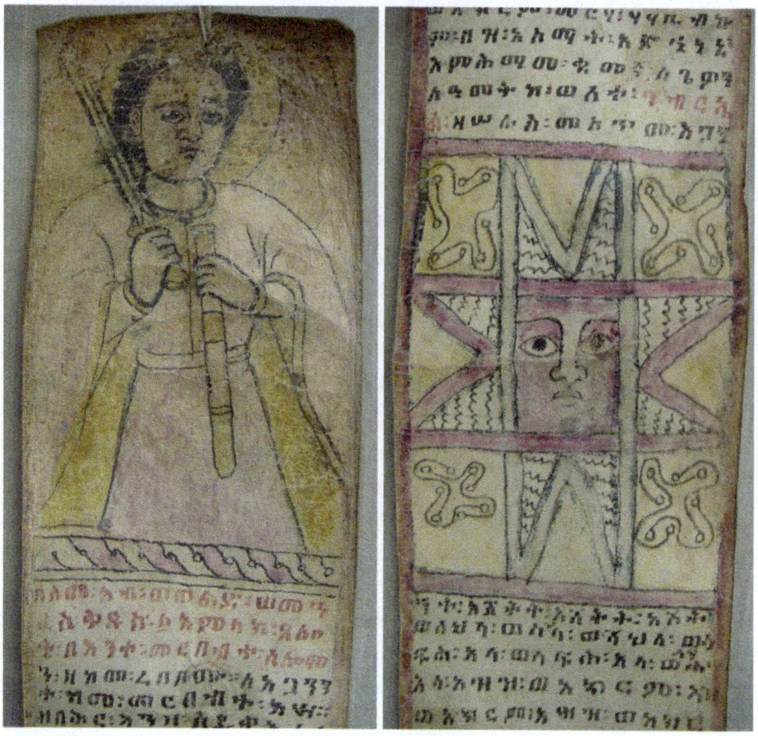

Fig. 10.10 Healing scroll with depiction of Archangel Michael and Seal of Solomon, Ethiopian Orthodox, Ethiopia

From the Buddhist perspective, the mind is the creator of sickness and health. In fact, the mind is believed to be the creator of all problems. Therefore, the methods employed by faith healers are to condition the minds of patients into having a certain mental attitude with the result that certain favorable psychological and physiological changes invariably take place. In this context, there are a number of discourses in the Teaching of the Buddha that indicate that various forms of illness were eradicated through the conditioning of the mind.

In India, especially people who suffer from mental illness frequently employ faith healing as an alternative to psychiatric treatment. Faith healing often takes place in the temple of a Hindu deity. In Indian philosophy, each deity represents Universal Consciousness, Soul, or one Self—the unchanging reality that is veiled by the world and from which the world itself is derived. As such, in worship, one indirectly worships the singularity hidden behind the mask of the deity's personality, which is grounded in the world.

> The person who calls on faith healing moves beyond his or her own personality, or worldly self, to surrender to and discover his or her true Self in the deity.

In Hinduism, the conch or shankha is a sacred emblem of the Hindu preserver god Vishnu. It is at the same time acknowledged to represent the most ancient blown instrument. According to Indian mythology, the demon Shankhasura defeated the Gods, and the Vedas were lost to the bottom of the ocean. The devas appealed to Lord Vishnu for help. In his fish incarnation Matsya Avatara, the Lord defeated Shankhasura and shaped from the demon's head and ear the conch. When Lord Vishnu blew the conch, the "Om" sound emanated from it, and from this the Vedas re-emerged. Therefore, all knowledge enshrined in the Vedas is understood to be an elaboration of "Om." The conch is thus named after Shankhasura. It is still used as a trumpet in Hindu ritual.

The sonorous sound of the conch, its spiral form, and the sound of the ocean represent the beginning of existence: The blowing of the conch salutes and honors the Lord of Creation. It was the divine sound "Om" and primordial sound of creation. Therefore, devotees blow the Shankh before the supreme God with sentiments of welcoming Him in their hearts at the beginning of worship. The blowing of the conch is said to purify the environment from evil, and the sound from the conch is acknowledged to awaken one from ignorance and increase positive attributes in the atmosphere, such as courage, hope, determination, willpower, and optimism, ultimately bringing good luck, and prosperity. The spiral form of the conch represents the infinite space that gradually expands in a clockwise direction and is symbolic of the human journey through birth, life, and reincarnation. Ultimately, the shell's hard casing is understood to protect life.

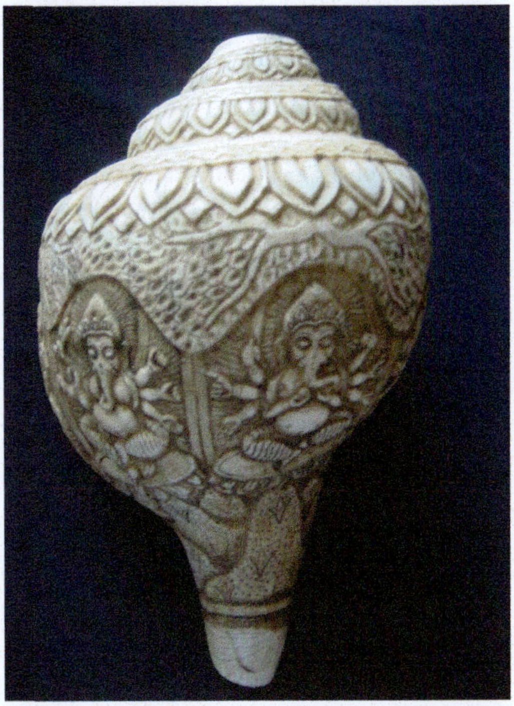

Fig. 10.11 Tibetan carved 5 Ganesha Naga Conch Shell Shankha

"Shankham" also derives etymologically from Sanskrit "Shum" which means something good, and "Kham" meaning water. Therefore, Shankham is the conch holding the sacred water. The water from the Shankha is said to purify the sinner and is believed to cure ailments which cannot be cured by other medicines. Therefore, Shankha powder is also used in several Ayurvedic medicines.

The example of a Conch Shell Shankha depicted in Fig. 10.11 is adorned with the elephant-headed deity Ganesha in five varied postures. Unlike other deities, the depiction of Ganesha shows wide variations and specific patterns changing over the ages. Ganesha is a popular deity of the Hindu pantheon that is widely worshiped. His image is found throughout India and Nepal, and devotion to Ganesha is widely diffused, extending beyond India and to Buddhists. Although he is known by many attributes, Ganesha's elephant head makes him easy to identify. One of his popular forms, Heramba-Ganapati, has five elephant heads. Ganesha is revered as the remover of obstacles and the patron of arts and the sciences.

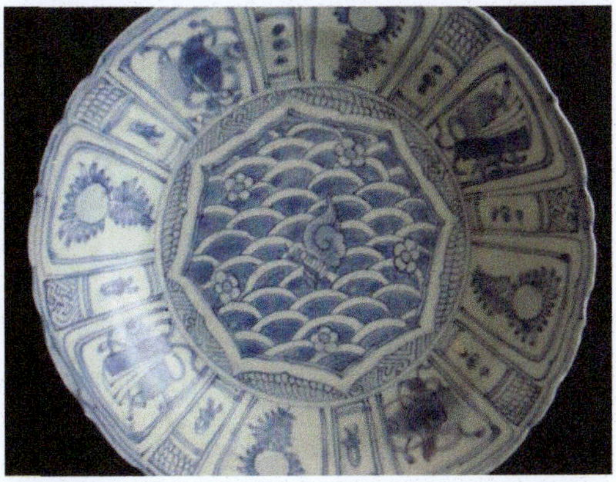

Fig. 10.12 Chinese Kraak *blue* and *white* porcelain charger, Wanli Period (late Ming dynasty), from Captain M. Hatcher Collection

In Chinese Buddhism, the conch shell signifies a prosperous journey. The piece of Chinese Kraak porcelain in Fig. 10.12 depicts a conch rising out of the waves of the sea. It originates from the Captain M. Hatcher Collection of sunken cargo. In 1999, Hatcher succeeded to make one of the biggest shipwreck finds of the twentieth century, the cargoes of which have provided valuable scholarly information. The immense treasure of Chinese Porcelain dating from the fifteenth through nineteenth century salvaged from the South China Sea was recovered from the Chinese Junk Tek Sing ("True Star") that sank in 1822. The Tek Sing was one of the last of the great Chinese ocean-going junks, part of a tradition stretching back to the days of early Ming Dynasty fleet admiral Zheng He (1371–1433) and the legendary Treasure Ships. The Tek Sing was a maritime disaster of epic proportions with nearly 2000 people on board when it sank and has come to be labeled the "Titanic of the East."

Finally, to turn back to Christianity, the scallop shell is the emblem of St. James, the patron Saint of pilgrims. So the shell came to symbolize a pilgrimage.

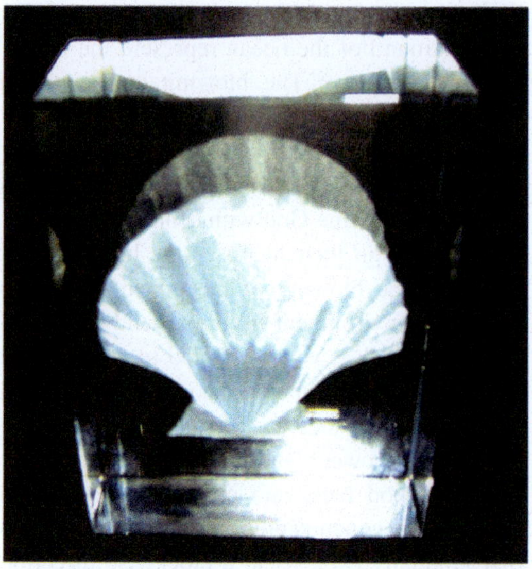

Fig. 10.13 Scallop shell, laser etched in crystal glass, from Santiago de Compostela, Spain, contemporary (Gift from a patient)

A pilgrimage is a journey or search of moral or spiritual significance. Typically, it is a journey to a location of importance to an individual's creed and faith. Such locations may be commemorated with shrines or temples that devotees are encouraged to visit for their own spiritual benefit: to be healed or have questions answered or to achieve some other spiritual benefit.

Originally, Christian pilgrimage was made to sites related to the birth, life, crucifixion, and resurrection of the Christ. Later, pilgrimages began to be made also to places associated with the Apostles, Saints, and Christian martyrs, as well as with apparitions of the Holy Mary. A popular pilgrimage site of the past and present is Santiago de Compostela, in Galicia, Spain, in reference to the Apostle St. James the Greater. Recently, it has gained much popularity through contemporary film and literature, such as literature Nobel Prize laureate Paul Coelho's *O Diario De Um Mago* (1987), American Actress Shirley Maclaine's *The Camino: A Journey of the Spirit* (2000), German entertainer Hape Kerkeling's *Ich bin dann mal weg: Meine Reise auf dem Jakobsweg* (2006), and American drama film "The Way" (2010), directed, produced, and written by Emilio Estevez, starring his father Martin Sheen. The example of a laser-etched glass (by SEYART, Spain) depicted in Fig. 10.13, representing the scallop shell, is a souvenir from Santiago de Compostela, presented by a patient as a token of gratitude to the Center for Dermatology and Hair Diseases Professor Trüeb.

10.6 The Scientific Basis

[18]Anyone presenting his own ideas is looking for praise for himself, but anyone seeking to honour the one who sent him is a good and true person.
John 7,18

Observation as a means of acquiring knowledge played a central role in the development of modern science, including medicine. The emphasis on observation and experimentation diminished the influence of religious authority. Early on, St. Thomas of Aquinas (1225–1274) took a conciliating position in making the statement "that for the knowledge of any truth whatsoever man needs divine help, that the intellect may be moved by God to its act." However, he believed that human beings have the natural capacity to know many things without special divine revelation, even though such revelation occurs from time to time, "especially in regard to such (truths) as pertain to faith."

In our times, a number of ardent antireligious stances have emerged, resulting in best-selling publications, such as Sam Harris' *The End of Faith* (2004), Richard Dawkins' *The God Delusion* (2006), and Christopher Hitchens' *God Is Not Great: How Religion Poisons Everything* (2007).

The Bible took its point with respect to "false teachers" in an explicit and timeless manner: "[10]But these men mock and curse at anything they do not understand, and, like animals, they do whatever they feel like, thereby ruining their souls. [11]Woe upon them! For they follow the example of Cain who killed his brother; and, like Balaam, they will do anything for money; and like Korah, they have disobeyed God and will die under his curse" (Jude 10–11). "[13]… They wander around looking as bright as stars, but ahead of them is the everlasting gloom and darkness that God has prepared for them" (Jude 13). "[16]These men are constant gripers, never satisfied, doing whatever evil they feel like, they are loudmouthed 'show-offs,' and when they show respect for others, it is only to get something from them in return" (Jude 16).

Sam Harris is a contemporary critic of religion and advocate of scientific skepticism. In 2009, he received a Ph.D. degree in cognitive neuroscience at the University of California, Los Angeles, using functional magnetic resonance imaging to carry out research into the neural basis of belief. Harris' basic message is that the time has come to freely cast doubt on the traditional concept of religious faith. He criticizes Judaism, Christianity, and Islam which he declares to be monolithic and prepared to do harm to others only for the sake of religion and apprehends that the survival of civilization is at risk because of the taboo against questioning religious conviction. According to Harris, this taboo hampers progress toward more enlightened approaches to spirituality and ethics. Ultimately, Harris argues that religion is particularly rampant with bad ideas, he calls "one of the most perverse misuses of intelligence ever devised." He compares modern religious beliefs to the myths of the Ancient Greeks, which were once accepted as fact but are considered obsolete today. In *The End of Faith*, Harris proposes that religious dogma is flawed in that such beliefs are based on faith rather than on evidence and experience. Harris' view is that religion is essentially a failed science and states that "religion was the discourse we had when all causes in the universe were opaque" such that religion developed as a consequence of humans' "cognitive imperative" to seek explanations coupled with an earlier ignorance of the natural order of the world. Harris is convinced that religion is "losing the argument" with science, given the escalating popularity of science on almost all fronts within the past 100 years. As an example, he states that, given today's knowledge of epilepsy, most parents would not send their epileptic children to exorcists. Harris also predicts that science holds the potential to one day fathom the basis of spirituality and feelings of otherworldliness connected with religion and religiousness.

Richard Dawkins is an evolutionary biologist and atheist who made the gene-centered view of evolution popular. He is a prominent critic of creationism, i.e., the religious belief that humanity, life, and the universe were created by a deity, without recourse to evolution. Dawkins has passionately opposed the inclusion of intelligent design, i.e., the view that certain features of the universe and of living things are best explained by an intelligent cause, not an undirected process such as natural selection, in science education, challenging it to be "not a scientific argument at all, but a religious one." Dawkins became an eminent critic of religion and has made the statement that religion is both a source of conflict and a justification for belief without evidence. He deems faith as belief that is not based on evidence and "one of the world's great evils." Dawkins rose to celebrity in public appearances debating on science and religion since the publication of *The God Delusion* in 2006, which became an international best seller. Its success has been acknowledged by some as indicative of a change in the contemporary cultural *Zeitgeist* and has been identified with the rise of "New Atheism." Dawkins suggests that atheists should be proud, not apologetic, stressing that atheism is evidence of a healthy mind.

Finally, Christopher Hitchens is a noted critic of religion and "antitheist," who stated that an individual "could be an atheist and wish that belief in God were correct" but that "an antitheist is someone who is relieved that there's no evidence for such an assertion." Hitchens spoke out against the Abrahamic religions (Judaism, Christianity, and Islam) or what he called "the three great monotheisms." When questioned what he considered to be the "axis of evil," Hitchens replied "Christianity, Judaism, Islam—the three leading monotheisms." In his book *God Is Not Great: How Religion Poisons Everything*, Hitchens expanded his criticism to include all religions. According to Hitchens, the idea of a god or a supreme being is a totalitarian belief that obliterates individual freedom and that free expression and scientific discovery should replace religion as a means of teaching ethics and defining human civilization. Hitchens died 2011 from esophageal cancer, a disease that he acknowledged was most likely the consequence of his lifelong heavy smoking and drinking. Prior to his death, *Asteroid 57901 Hitchens* was named after him.

Nonetheless, the recent past has witnessed a scientific interest in examining the relationship between religion and medicine in a genuinely embracing way.

Over one thousand research studies have quantitatively examined the relationships between religious involvement, Christian or non-Christian, health, and longevity. These have been summarized by Harold Koenig from Duke University Medical Center, Durham, North Carolina, USA, in his book *Medicine, Religion, and Health: Where Science and Spirituality Meet* (2008). Koenig is co-director of Duke's Center for Spirituality, Theology, and Health. According to Koenig the newer research is of much higher quality than earlier. Ultimately, this research activity has prompted consensus conferences, partially supported by the National Institutes of Health (NIH), and come up with recommendations for methodological advances and future studies. Most studies have addressed the effect of religious behavior or spiritual practices on mental health and the immune, endocrine, and cardiovascular systems, resulting in many positive results.

The studies and conclusions have also prompted criticism, pointing out flaws in study design, methodology, and interpretation of collected data. These have been summarized by Richard Sloan in his book *Blind Faith: The Unholy Alliance of Religion and Medicine* (2006). Sloan is professor of behavioral medicine at Columbia University Medical Center, New York City, New York, USA. Sloan also makes the point clear that "Much of the support for pursuing connections between religion and health is based on favouring subjectivity over rationality, faith over reason. Because religion relies heavily on faith, it needs not depend upon the objectivity that science demands. Religious truths do not require scientific verification. To suggest otherwise is to completely misunderstand the nature of faith" (*sic*). Because almost all studies examining relationships between religion and health are observational in nature, confounding factors represent one of the most important flaws. In many studies, religious activities are more likely to be markers than mechanisms of good health. Finally, if enough comparisons are conducted in a study, one will almost certainly come up with some finding that achieves apparent significance, but the validity of that conclusion is questionable. Therefore, more research is needed to identify how these relationships operate and whether they are causal.

There is no doubt though that religious beliefs and spiritual practices have positive effects on (1) personal coping with illness and (2) behavioral self-control.

Religious involvement can help a person cope with the psychological stress caused by a particular disease and its sequelae. By improving coping, religious beliefs may also have the potential to impact on physical health and disease outcome, given the effect of stress and negative emotions on physiological systems, such as the immune, endocrine, and cardiovascular systems. Moreover, an individual's ability to cope may affect motivation toward self-care, willingness to cooperate with planned treatment, and ability to comply with medical treatments. Ultimately, religious or spiritual involvement is more prone to protect from negative health behaviors, such as heavy smoking and drinking, gluttony, promiscuity, and anger binges. 1 Corinthian 3:16,17 ("[16]Don't you realize that all of you together are the house of God, and that the spirit of God lives among you in his house? [17]If anyone defies and spoils God's home, God will destroy him. For God's home is holy and clean, and you are that home") may have caused some confusion when trying to determine if St. Paul meant the physical bodies of individual Christians or the church community when he referred to the "temple."

For many with faith, 1 Corinthian 3:16,17 has been an effective call to take self-responsibility for one's own health.

Eventually, modern neuroscience has drawn its attention to the association between religious or spiritual experience, brain function, and health. Andrew Newberg is an American neuroscientist who is Director of Research at the Myrna Brind Center for Integrative Medicine at Thomas Jefferson University Hospital, Adjunct Professor of Religious Studies, and Associate Professor of Radiology at the University of Pennsylvania School of Medicine, USA. He has been a prominent researcher in the field of nuclear medical brain imaging. In particular, his research has focused on the development of neurotransmitter tracers for the evaluation of religiosity. In the early 1990s, he began to research the connection between brain function and religious and spiritual experiences. In this work, also referred to as "neurotheology," Newberg described the possible neurophysiological mechanisms associated with religious and spiritual experiences. His initial investigations included the use of functional brain imaging to study Buddhists in meditation and Franciscan nuns in prayer. In one of his recent publications *How God Changes Your Brain: Breakthrough Findings from a Leading Neuroscientist* (2010), he looks from both scientific and practical angles at how faith and meditation can enhance our brain function and health.

The aim of science is to understand how the natural world operates. The sciences all follow certain basic principles. They depend upon systematic observation and employ methods that attempt to identify the connections between events and phenomena in an unbiased way. Ultimately, they state their hypotheses in ways that allow for testing and, importantly, for disconfirmation.

Hypotheses based on supernatural explanations cannot be scientific, because they can never be disconfirmed. Science operates in a reductionist way, and if one tries to understand a spiritual experience from a scientific perspective, ultimately one is going to reduce it.

Moreover, from a scientific point of view, anecdotes are not evidence, no matter how gripping, dramatic, and heartfelt they may be. Anecdotal evidence is unsystematic and may be highly misleading. Scientific conclusions require systematic data collection. The body has the capacity to heal naturally. While this natural healing process may be assisted, the body's own self-healing mechanisms often will counter effectively. It has been estimated that up to 75 % of patients would get better even if no medicine was given. A typical example is the spontaneous remission rate in alopecia areata that has been estimated to be 30 % within 6 months, 50 % within 1 year, and 80 % within 3 years. If a remission occurs any time following the ritualistic ministration of a faith healer, it may be erroneously attributed to the respective intervention.

Psychosomatic illnesses are the most amenable to "miraculous" healings.

There exist a great variety of often impressive ailments, ranging from functional back pains or headaches to hysterical blindness and paralysis, that have been recognized to be highly responsive to the power of suggestion.

On the other hand, even illnesses that have definite somatic causes may also be partially responsive to the so-called mental medicine. For example, techniques of "visualization" in which the patient is instructed to focus mentally on his or her condition and envision its cure have been successfully used in conjunction with traditional medicine (Fig. 10.14a, b). Just as physical illness can be exacerbated by stressful life events, positive attitudes may enhance the body's self-healing capacities.

Finally, some of the most dramatic evidence staged by supposed faith healers is actually the result of trickery, and fraud performed in the guise of holiness is more common than many are ready to acknowledge. Prominent examples are the ministries of Rev. Peter Popoff, an American televangelist of German origin and self-proclaimed prophet and faith healer, and Dallas-based American televangelist Walter V. Grant Jr., both exposed by retired stage magician and paranormal investigator James Randi in his book *The Faith Healers* (1987).

Popoff is an exponent of the Charismatic Movement adopting beliefs and practices similar to Pentecostals. Fundamental to the movement is the use of spiritual gifts. These are the supernatural graces (charismata) which individual Christians

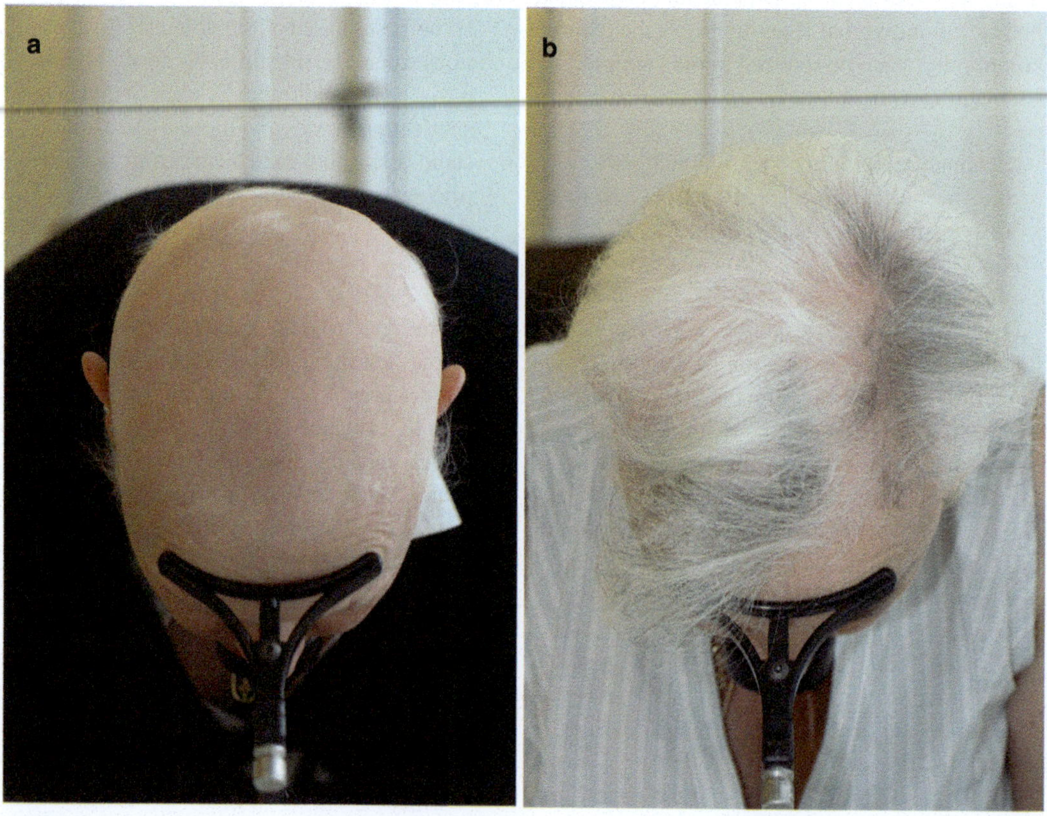

Fig. 10.14 (**a**, **b**). Successful treatment of alopecia areata totalis in a 47-year-old woman with symptom-oriented autosuggestion therapy: (**a**) before and (**b**) after 12 months

need to fulfill the mission of the church. They are described in the New Testament, with the gift of healing specifically declared in 1 Corinthians 12:9 and 28. Popoff initially gained popularity in the 1980s, until in 1986 his method of receiving information about revival attendees from his wife via an in-ear receiver was exposed to the public.

Grant adorns himself in tailored suits with monogrammed shirts and luxurious jewelry. Although he suffers himself of a stammer, he declares to give the blind sight and make the lame walk. As exposed by Randi, one of Grant's tricks was similar to Popoff's, except that instead of using an in-ear receiver, members of his staff conversed with attendees before the healing service took place in order to gather pertinent information.

According to Randi in 1987, Popoff took in almost $4 million per year. Financial data is not available for Popoff's ministry following 2005 because they changed from a for-profit business to a religious organization, making it tax-exempt. Popoff purchased a home in Bradbury, California, for $4.5 million in 2007 and drives a Porsche and a Mercedes-Benz. In 1996, an Internal Revenue Service investigation into Grant's ministry resulted in Grant's imprisonment for tax evasion. He was found guilty of failing to report taxable income in the purchase of two homes, including his $1 million residence. An undercover videotape was alleged to show Grant admitting the use of money from church members as a down payment on a $1.2 million home overlooking a Desoto, Texas, country club and not reporting it as income.

Inappropriate financial conduct in association with religion should always prompt suspicion, in view of the fact that in the Bible, both in the Old and in the New Testaments, the Prophet Elisha refused to accept the gifts offered for the healing of Naaman (2 Kings 5:16), and the Apostle Peter rebuked the sorcerer Simon for wanting to acquire God's gift of healing with money (Acts 8:9–23), respectively. Finally, with respect to the staging of "miraculous" healings on public television, the Christ himself directed those who received healing from him, not to tell anyone, and did not approve of anyone asking for a sign just for the spectacle of it, describing such as coming from an "evil, faithless nation" (Matthew 12:39,40).

Originally, Pentecostals thought it was sinful to take medicine or receive care from doctors. Over time, Pentecostals moderated these views; nonetheless, a minority continues to rely exclusively on prayer and divine healing. For example, doctors in the United Kingdom reported that a minority of Pentecostal HIV patients was encouraged to stop taking their medications and parents were told to stop giving medicine to their children, trends that placed lives at risk. This is evident both in reduced life expectancy for adults and higher mortality rates for children. Critics have also made note of serious damage resulting from misleadingly labeled "healings," where patients falsely consider themselves cured and withdraw from medical treatment. Therefore, reliance on faith healing to the exclusion of other forms of treatment can have a negative impact on public health when it reduces or eliminates access to modern medical practice.

In conclusion, religious or spiritual involvement and medical care can work wonderfully together, while the neglect of the one or the other may influence patient outcomes negatively.

Spiritual objects depicted in Figs. 10.2, 10.3, 10.4, 10.5, and 10.6 and 10.8, 10.9, 10.10, 10.11, 10.12, and 10.13 may be viewed on request and by special appointment at the Center for Dermatology and Hair Diseases Professor Trüeb

Further Reading

http://en.wikipedia.org/wiki/Faith_healing
http://en.wikipedia.org/wiki/Lourdes_Medical_Bureau
http://en.wikipedia.org/wiki/New_Age
The Catholic Living Bible (1971) Tyndale House Publishers Inc, Wheaton

Earliest Cultures

http://en.wikipedia.org/wiki/Fetish
http://en.wikipedia.org/wiki/Shamanism
Lurker M (2002) An illustrated dictionary of the gods and symbols of Ancient Egypt. Thames & Hudson, London
McManis K (1995) A guide to Zuni Fetishes & Carvings. Treasure Chest Books, Tucson
Meadow K (2003) Shamanic experience. A guide to psychic powers. Bear & Company, Rochester
Nunn JF (1996) Ancient Egyptian medicine. The British Museum Press, London

Old Testament

http://en.wikipedia.org/wiki/Aesculapian_snake#History
http://en.wikipedia.org/wiki/Caduceus
http://en.wikipedia.org/wiki/Nehushtan
http://en.wikipedia.org/wiki/Old_Testament
http://en.wikipedia.org/wiki/Snake_handling
http://en.wikipedia.org/wiki/Wadjet

New Testament

Hinsen P (2008) Die heilende Kraft der Bibel. Verlag Katholigsches Bibelwerk, Stuttgart
http://en.wikipedia.org/wiki/New_Testament
Moser RW (2012) Jesus Christus, der Arzt. Krankheit und Heilung in der Bibel. Paulusverlag, Freiburg

In Catholicism

de Voragine, Jacobus, translation from Latin by Benz, Richard (2004) Die Legenda Aurea: Das Leben der Heiligen, 14th edn. Gutersloher Verlagshaus, Gütersloh, pp 103–106.
Fenzl F (2003) Wunderheilungen. Aufzeichnungen beglaubigter Geschehnisse. Nympenburger, München
Gory E (2005) Lexikon der Heiligen, vol 6. Deutscher Taschenbuch Verlag/Auflage, München
http://en.wikipedia.org/wiki/Catholicism
http://en.wikipedia.org/wiki/Relic
http://en.wikipedia.org/wiki/Saint_Veronica
Martin J (2006) My life with the saints. Loyola Press, Chicago
Tanner L (2010) Willst Du gesund werden? Gottes Wege zum Heil. Mit Unterscheidungshilfen zu alternativen Heilpraktiken. Weg Verlag, Koblenz
Trüeb RM (2009) St. Agnes of Rome: patron saint for women with hair loss? Dermatology 219:97–98
Woodward K (1996) Making saints: how the Catholic Church determines who becomes a saint, who doesn't and why. Touchstone/Simon and Shuster, New York

In Other Confessions

http://en.wikipedia.org/wiki/Christianity_in_Ethiopia
http://en.wikipedia.org/wiki/Icon
http://en.wikipedia.org/wiki/Pilgrimage
http://en.wikipedia.org/wiki/Shankha
Pattanaik D (2006) Myth = Mithya. A handbook of Hindu mythology. Penguin Books, London
Trüeb RM, Navarini AA (2010) Beneath the nimbus–the hair of the saints. Arch Dermatol 146:764

The Scientific Basis

Hines T (1988) Pseudoscience and the paranormal. Prometheus Books, Buffalo
Koenig HG (2008) Medicine, religion, and health. Where science and spirituality meet. Templeton Science and Religion Series, West Conshohocken
Newber A, Waldman MR (2009) How god changes your brain. Breakthrough findings from a leading neuroscientist. Ballantine Books Trade Paperbacks, New York
Nickel J (1993) Looking for a miracle. Weeping icons, relics, stigmata, visions & healing cures. Prometheus Books, New York
Randi J (1987) The faith healers. Prometheus Books, New York
Sloan RP (2006) Blind faith. The unholy alliance of religion and medicine. St. Martin's Griffin, New York
The Catholic Living Bible (1971) Tyndale House Publishers Inc, Wheaton
Vuckovic NH, Gullion CM, Williams LA, Ramirez M, Schneider J (2007) Feasibility and short-term outcomes of a shamanic treatment for temporomandibular joint disorders. Altern Ther Health Med 13: 18–29

Name Index

R.M. Trüeb, *The Difficult Hair Loss Patient: Guide to Successful Management of Alopecia and Related Conditions*, DOI 10.1007/978-3-319-19701-2

Subject Index

R.M. Trüeb, *The Difficult Hair Loss Patient: Guide to Successful Management of Alopecia and Related Conditions*, DOI 10.1007/978-3-319-19701-2

B

C

D

E

I

K

L

O

P

The manufacturer's authorised representative in the EU is Springer Nature Customer Service Centre GmbH, Europaplatz 3, 69115 Heidelberg, Germany. If you have any concerns regarding our products, please contact ProductSafety@springernature.com

Printed and bound by CPI Group (UK) Ltd, Croydon, CR0 4YY
22/09/2026
02221056-0009